a textbook of motor development

second edition

a textbook of motor development

charles b. corbin, editor, contributing author
Arizona State University

contributing authors

Karen DeOreo
Kent State University
Kent, Ohio

Jacqueline Herkowitz
Ohio State University
Columbus, Ohio

William Hottinger
Wake Forest University
Winston-Salem, North Carolina

Jack Keogh
University of California
Los Angeles, California

Aileene Lockhart
Texas Woman's University
Denton, Texas

Robert M. Malina
University of Texas
Austin, Texas

Joel Rosentswieg
Texas Woman's University
Denton, Texas

Michael J. Stewart
Kansas State University
Manhattan, Kansas

Harriet Williams
University of Toledo
Toledo, Ohio

wcb
Wm. C. Brown Company Publishers
Dubuque, Iowa

Contents

Preface

This book was written as a text for students of motor development whether they be educators, psychologists, physicians, parents, or interested students of other vocations. For years motor development, an integral part of total human development, has been given only minimal attention with the bulk of the focus in human growth and development being given to intellectual, social, and emotional development. The attention which was given to the motor domain was limited to a study of a restricted few motor behaviors and such factors as height, weight, and body proportions.

The first edition of this *Textbook of Motor Development* was a pioneer effort in that it went beyond the study of human physical growth to present a total picture of motor development. The text was one of the first and most widely adopted of its kind. This second edition provides the reader with a source book-text which summarizes the most recent literature to provide a total picture of the motor development process. Normative information is presented to help the reader understand how the hypothetical "typical" child develops in the motor domain, but beyond that theoretical and practical information is presented to aid the reader in understanding and helping *all* people, typical or atypical, achieve their own potential for motor development.

A close look at the table of contents reveals that the reader will study physical growth as a factor accompanying motor development, fundamental motor skill learning and refinement, physical fitness development, perceptual-motor development, and factors influencing motor development including biologically related factors as well as socially and environmentally related factors. This broad coverage of motor development provides the basis for understanding the motor characteristics of people all ages and the potential of these people for attaining optimal motor performances whether in work or in play.

Regardless of the orientation of the reader, the book should provide a vast source of useful information. The chapters are numbered sequentially and are divided into 12 distinct sections. This makes it easy for users to pick and choose sections which are most relevant to their own interests should they decide not to use the entire text. Chapters are brief by design. Each contains much factual information which is more palatable in short concise chapters than in fewer, but longer chapters. A multiple authorship was decided upon in an attempt to draw more fully from the combined knowledge, experience, and critical thinking capacity of the top people in the area of motor development. No single author could have provided the total expertise of the many authors who contributed to the writing of this book.

After a brief introduction, which establishes the place of motor development in the total developmental process, a new but brief section discussing the physical growth factors underlying motor development is presented. Chapters 3 through 9 focus on motor development from prior to birth through the school years. Special features in these chapters include descriptions and complete illustrations of basic fundamental skills. Checklists which are useful in observing and evaluating these skills are also provided. This information concerning fundamental skills is new to the second edition. The need to use a supplemental text to cover this information is no longer necessary. In the chapters which describe motor performances of children, summary tables and figures are used extensively. This is done to present normative data in the most concise and simple method possible. A special section which includes practical guidelines for facilitating motor development and for implementing youth sports programs is provided.

Because motor development is a continuous process which extends from conception to death, a new section on motor development in adolescence and adulthood has been included in this edition. While the growing years are still the focus, the new section makes the coverage of the motor development process more complete. As with the first edition, a separate section on motor behavior evaluation, a synthesis chapter, and a complete index are included.

In addition to the new sections on growth, fundamental skills, practical applications, adolescence and adulthood, all of the text information has been updated based on the most recent research findings available. The reader will recognize duplication of concepts and material throughout the text—this is to be expected. Authors of the caliber of those contributing to this volume are anxious that their words not be taken out of context. They desire that their readers realize that when they are considering specific areas of specialization, they do so with full regard for the wider integrated picture of motor development. It is imperative that the reader understand the commitment of the authors to the concept of the totality of man. This commitment allows *each* author to discuss his or her specialized material as a separate entity. Where there is repetition, the repetition serves to add strength and appropriate emphasis.

Charles B. Corbin
Editor-Contributing Author

Section 1   Introduction

Introduction

1

Charles B. Corbin
Kansas State University

When should children be able to throw a ball? Do children learn to play automatically? How important is movement behavior to the teenager? Can an adult learn new motor skills? How much activity can older adults tolerate? These and many other questions often go unanswered when studying human growth and development. But humans are active, moving animals and motor or movement development is an essential part of total development. The purpose of this book is to acquaint the reader more fully with the motor aspects of the total human growth and development process.

SOME GENERAL DEVELOPMENT CONCEPTS

Prior to discussing the specific aspects of motor development it is necessary to clarify several general concepts of human development which have specific implications to a study of motor development.

The Continuity of Human Development

Perhaps one of the most important principles of human and motor development is the Principle of Continuity. Because much of growth takes place early in life, we have a tendency to consider the study of motor development as the study of children only. While the focus on children is appropriate, motor development does not stop at any particular age. It is important to consider motor development as a continuing process which starts before birth and continues until death. Just as we have much to learn about the motor development of infants and children, we have much to learn about motor development of adolescents and adults of all ages.

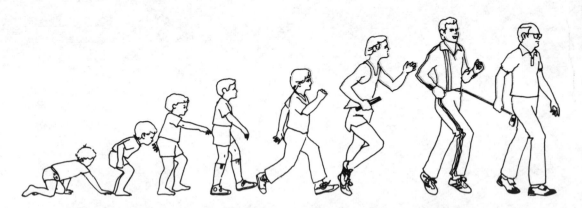

Figure 1.1. Motor development is a continuous process.

Totality of Human Development

Even though much credence has been given the idea that a person is one integrated organism rather than a disintegrated sum of unrelated parts, the study of human development frequently proceeds with little reference to the totality of the person. For example, a simple schematic model for describing the development of humans (see fig. 1.2.) has been widely used to relate the nature of the human development process. If the general categories presented in figure 1.2 are to be used, it would seem more logical to depict (see fig. 1.3) the developmental process as one in which each aspect of development is a small thread intertwined with all others in comprising the total individual. Each small circle reflects a specific developmental factor which relates and overlaps with all others. The overlap is so frequent and so great that individual threads are often indistinguishable. While the chapters that follow are related to the study of factors specifically related to motor performance, it should be recognized that

P = Physical   I = Intellectual
S = Social   E = Emotional
M = Motor   O = Other

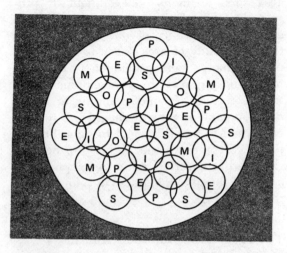

Figure 1.3. An integrated concept of human development.

the comments are put forth in an effort to help the reader better understand a few more of the threads of total human development.

The Specificity of Motor Behavior

While it may seem inconsistent with the concept of the Totality of Development, human performance itself is specific. Each individual possesses specific abilities but those who excel in one area do not necessarily excel in others. The idea, for example, that an individual is either bright or dull, physically fit or unfit, has given way to the notion that each individual has specific capabilities within each performance area. It is necessary to study each specific factor of human performance. As our understanding of individual differences in each specific developmental factor improves, so will our

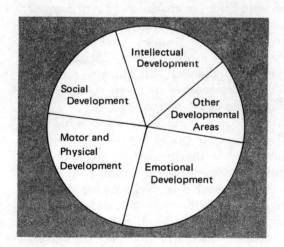

Figure 1.2. A disintegrated concept of human development.

understanding of the total human developmental process. Thus, the study of a specific area such as motor development as presented in this text, contributes to our knowledge of the totality of development. Further, the study of areas such as motor task performance, perceptual-motor development, and physical fitness development contribute to a better understanding of motor development. In no way should this text be construed to be an attempt to describe motor development alone; rather the book is intended to describe motor development as a part of the total integrated development of the individual.

The Progressive Nature of Human Development

A person is not skinny one day and fat the next. Neither is a child a child one day and an adult the next. Many factors contribute to changes in behavior as the child grows older and, of course, no single factor is responsible for any single behavioral change. However, it can be said that humans are more alike than they are different. Regardless of the reason, whether heredity, maturation, or environment, most children grow taller and heavier, learn to walk and run, and learn to perform the tasks of our society. As adults they take on a unique personal movement style appropriate for their own work and leisure demands. In studying motor development it is convenient to study the norm. "Normal" people display subtle changes in motor behavior from day to day, month to month and year to year. This text attempts to describe some of the *progressive* behavioral changes which are characteristic of most children and adults. At the same time attempts are made to describe the unique nature of the motor development

process. All people follow a progressive developmental pattern although the rate of progress through each stage of development varies with each individual.

The Individuality of Development

People develop in similar ways but no two people are alike. Each person has his or her own unique abilities and capabilities. Of course the unique nature of each person is a result of the combination of all the unique but specific factors which comprise the total being. The concept of individuality is especially important since an understanding of each person's unique nature is necessary if we are to help each person grow toward the ultimate goal — becoming a fully functioning healthy individual.

SUMMARY

As outlined in the preface, the purpose of this text is threefold: (1) to describe characteristic motor development patterns with an emphasis on children; (2) to suggest reasons, whether familial or environmental, regarding why people develop as they do; and (3) to project ideas regarding the possible "potential" of humans for motor performance when given optimal conditions for development.

With these three purposes in mind the five basic concepts of human development presented in the proceeding pages of this chapter take on special meaning. The discussion presented in the following chapters is intended to describe *specific* aspects of *progressive* motor development which will contribute to a better concept of the *totality* of *continuous* development but with special reference to the unique nature of every *individual*.

Section 2   Growth

Physical Growth 2

Jacqueline Herkowitz
Ohio State University

Basic to the study of motor development is the study of physical growth. Growth is an increase in the size of a living thing or any of its parts. Today, the terms growth, development, maturation, heredity, and environment are frequently used together: with *growth* implying anatomical changes and differentiation within structures; *development* implying the emergence and expanding of capabilities of the individual to provide progressively greater facility in functioning; *maturation* implying change in the complexity of structure which makes it possible for a structure to begin functioning or to function at higher levels; *heredity* implying the genetic inheritance of an individual; and *environment* implying habits and circumstances of living. Though the discussion of childhood and adolescence is separated for other sections of this book, this chapter will include a discussion of physical growth from early childhood through adolescence to set the stage for the study of all aspects of motor development throughout life.

In the past, researchers have employed two major methods of studying growth; the *cross-sectional* and the *longitudinal*. The cross-sectional method involves the measuring or testing of different groups of children at different ages. In such studies large groups are often tested and the results expressed as averages for those groups. Many of the norms now used, such as those for height and weight, were collected this way. By using the cross-sectional method it becomes possible to determine what is generally expected of most children at a given age and how deviance from these expectations are normally found in the population.

The longitudinal method, on the other hand, involves measuring the same children over a number of years. Collecting data in this way requires more time but is a more reliable method of determining growth trends. The longitudinal method can also be used to study individual patterns of growth and speed of growth. The cross-sectional method cannot.

Growth is often graphically represented in two ways; by distance curves and velocity curves. Measurements taken on a single individual at intervals can be plotted against time to produce a graph of progress (e.g., Figure 2.3). A graph of this sort is called a distance curve, since any point on it indicates the distance the body has traveled along the road to maturity.

Another way of presenting the same data is shown in Figure 2.1, in which increments in growth, within specified time intervals, are plotted against time. Such a curve shows the variation in the rate of growth with time, and is therefore known as a velocity curve.

This chapter shall be divided into three sections. The first section describes age, sex, and individual differences in growth in height and weight, the second section concerns itself with the growth rate of various body tissues. The third section deals with changes in body proportions.

HEIGHT AND WEIGHT

Significant age, sex, and individual differences in growth in height and weight exist and carry with them a number of implications for the study of motor development.

Velocity Curves

The growth patterns for height and weight are characterized by alternating periods of faster and slower growth (Figures 2.1 and 2.2). The first period of fast growth occurs in infancy; the second period, known as the adolescent spurt, occurs in early adolescence. Following this second spurt, growth slows down and, especially in height, ceases at maturity. By the elementary school years the child is already in the middle period of slower growth. The early elementary school years are characterized by decelerating growth in height (Figure 2.1). At approximately 9 years, girls begin their adolescent growth spurt which reaches a peak

in the 12th or 13th year. Boys begin their growth spurt around 11 years and reach their maximum gains, which are greater than those of girls, in the 14th or 15th year. The exact age of the adolescent spurt will vary somewhat from group to group.

In weight (Figure 2.2), the school-age child increases in momentum slowly each year until girls reach a peak at about 12 and boys at about 14 years. The peak in weight tends to lag behind that of height by 6 months or more. Thus, many children have a brief filling out period after their rapid growth in height. Growth in height generally ceases somewhere between 16 years and the early twenties. Growth in weight for the average adolescent probably stops in the early twenties.

Distance Curves

From birth to 12 years of age, boys tend to be slightly taller than girls. Between 12 and 14 years, girls tend to be taller than boys. Between 14 and 18 years, boys become increasingly taller than girls. Eventually boys assume their adult height advantage. This is examined graphically in Figure 2.3. Between 2 and 4 years of age, boys tend to be slightly heavier than girls.

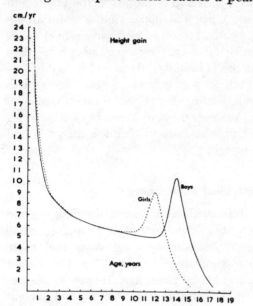

Figure 2.1. Typical individual velocity curves for height. (Tanner, J. M. et al. *Archives of Diseases in Childhood*. Vol. 41, 454-471, 1966.)

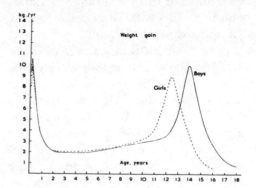

Figure 2.2. Typical individual velocity curves for weight. (Tanner, J. M. et al. *Archives of Diseases in Childhood*. Vol. 41, 454-471 1966.)

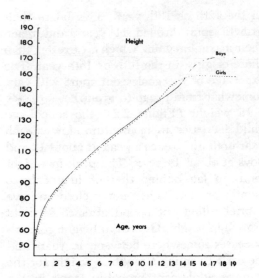

Figure 2.3. Typical individual distance curves for height. (Tanner, J. M. et al. *Archives of Diseases in Childhood.* Vol. 41, 454-471, 1966.)

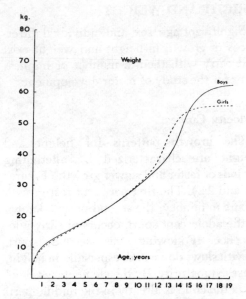

Figure 2.4. Typical individual distance curves for weight. (Tanner, J. M. et al. *Archives of Diseases in Childhood.* Vol. 41, 454-471, 1966.)

Between 4 and 11 years, there is no discernable difference in weight between the sexes. Between 11 and 15 years, girls are frequently heavier than boys. Between 15 and 18 years, this relationship reverses itself to reflect progress toward the characteristic greater weight of most boys (Figure 2.4).

Boys grow in height from a range of about 18½ to 21 inches at birth to a range of 66 to 74 inches at 18 years; in weight from a range of 6½ to 9½ pounds at birth to a range of 120 to 169 pounds at 18 years. Girls grow from a range of approximately 18½ to 21 inches and 6½ to 9 pounds at birth to a range of 62 to 67 inches and 104 to 160 pounds at 18 years. These approximate figures are taken from National Center for Health Statistics (NCHS) Growth Charts (1976), using as the range the 10th to 90th percentiles.

One can expect, from the same NCHS data, an average boy to gain approximately 9½ inches and 14½ pounds in the first year, 5 inches and 5½ pounds in the second year, 2½ inches and 5½ pounds in the sixth year, 2 inches and 6 pounds in the tenth year, 3

inches and 15 pounds in the fourteenth year, and ½ inch and 3 pounds in the eighteenth year. Girls will make similar gains in infancy, the preschool and early school years, but by 10 years they are gaining more than the boys (2½ inches, 6½ pounds). In the fourteenth year girls have passed their growth peak, gaining 1 inch and 9 pounds, and by the eighteenth year have stopped growing in height and are gaining less than a pound in weight.

Individual Differences

Individual differences in height and weight are apparent at birth and continue throughout the growing years and there is a considerable spread in the height figures for a given age. However, the degree of variability in height and weight changes from time to time. Individual differences in size tend to be greater as children grow older and especially during periods of more rapid growth. During the elementary years when growth is slower and during the college or late adolescent years when growth is tapering off, individual differences can be expected to be less than during the late elementary and early high school years.

A child's individual pattern of growth tends to become well established during the second to fourth years and to become regular during the years of steady growth in middle childhood. During the early adolescent years it may change for some. Some children are tall from a very early age and remain tall. Those children will be tall adults and achieve their mature height 2 or 3 years before their average peers. Some children are small throughout their growing years, mature slowly and reach small adult stature usually after 18 for girls and 20 for boys. Some, however, who are tall or short, merely because they are slow or fast maturers; and are not constitutionally large or small, may emerge from the adolescent growth spurt taller or shorter than might have been expected.

There are extensive differences in the timing and length of the adolescent spurt for boys. The onset of the puberal period can extend from 10½ to 14½ years and end anywhere from 14 to 17½ years. It can last anywhere from 2 to 4 years. Some boys have an early beginning, some a late one; some a short period, some a long one. During this period, growth for some is rapid and dramatic, for some moderately intense and long, for a few intense and long, and for another few neither intense nor long. Thus, boys have varied growth experiences during these years. Some early developers become short, some medium, some tall in stature. Some late developers also become short, some medium, and some tall in stature.

The majority of children, however, who begin their adolescent spurt earlier tend to grow faster and complete their growth earlier. At maturity they may not be taller than late maturing children. The late maturing children, on the other hand, tend to begin later and grow more slowly. They are not necessarily shorter at maturity. In fact, some are taller than those who mature early. Thus later maturing children may catch up eventually with their faster developing peers.

Growth of an individual child is dependent upon the interaction of heredity and environment. Heredity sets the potential for growth; health and environment, including nutrition, determine the degree to which that potential is achieved. These factors will be discussed in greater detail in Section 8 of the text.

GROWTH OF TISSUES

An examination of the growth of fat, muscle, and bone tissue provide useful insights for those interested in motor development.

Growth Curves for Different Tissues and Parts of the Body

Most body tissues follow approximately the growth curve described for height. Most of the skeleton and musculature grows in this manner, as do the internal organs such as the liver, spleen, and kidneys. But some exceptions exist: the brain and skull, the reproductive tissues, the lymphoid tissue of the tonsils, adenoids, and intestines, and subcutaneous fat.

These differences are shown in Figure 2.5, using the size attained by various tissues as a percentage of the birth-to-maturity increment. Height follows the general curve. The reproductive organs, internal and external, have a slow prepubescent growth, followed by a very large adolescent spurt. The brain, together with the skull covering it and the eyes and ears, develops earlier than any other part of the body and thus has a unique curve. There is little, if any adolescent spurt for the brain. A small but definite spurt occurs in head length and breadth, but all or most of this is due to thickening of the skull bones and the scalp and development of the air sinuses. The dimensions of the face follow a path somewhat closer to the general curve. There is a considerable adolescent spurt, especially in the mandible, resulting in the jaw becoming longer and more projecting, the profile straighter, and the chin more pointed. But, as always in growth, there are considerable individual differences, to the point that a few children have no detectable spurt at all in some face measurements.

The eye probably has a slight adolescent

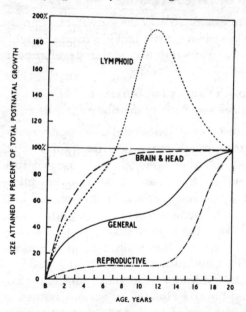

Figure 2.5. Growth curves for different tissues and parts of the body, showing the four chief types. All the curves are of size attained, and plotted as per cent of total gain from birth to 20 years, so that size at age 20 is 100 on the vertical scale. (Tanner, J. M. *Growth at Adolescence.* Second Edition, 1962, p. 11.)

spurt, although present data are not accurate enough to be certain. Very likely it is this that is responsible for the increase in frequency of short-sightedness in children during adolescence. Although the degree of short-sightedness increases continuously from at least age 6 to maturity, a particularly rapid rate of change occurs at about 11 to 12 in girls and 13 to 14 in boys, and this would be expected if there was a rather greater spurt in the axial dimension of the eye than in its vertical dimension.

The lymphoid tissue has quite a different growth curve from the rest of the body. It usually reaches its maximum before adolescence and then, probably due to sex hormone control, declines to its adult value.

Implications can be drawn from different growth curves for tissues and parts of the body. These are: (a) The general leveling off of growth curves for muscle, the skeleton, and height, during the elementary school years, probably helps to explain the steady progress in the attainment of physical skills that characterizes this growth period, (b) The rapid rise in growth curves for muscle, bone, height, and especially the reproductive system, in adolescence, represent tremendous growth changes. To some extent they help to explain adolescent unevenness in skill acquisition, and suggest the inappropriateness of demanding high levels of skill from some children during this period.

Bone

A good deal is known about bone growth. In the embryo, long bones are formed of cartilage. Ossification (hardening) of these bones begins at primary ossification centers located in the mid-portion of the bone. Usually, at birth, ossification has occurred to include the entire bone shaft. Cartilaginous epiphyseal centers develop at the end of the long bones. Secondary ossification centers appear in the epiphyseal areas. Between the secondary ossification center and the remainder of the bone shaft is a growth plate. Bone growth occurs in this area. When full growth has been completed, the epiphysis fuses to the rest of the bone shaft and the growth plate disappears.

The appearance of secondary ossification centers in the epiphysis and the time of closure of the growth plate differs for different bones, for both sexes, and for different individuals. Because of this it is possible to evaluate an individual's skeletal maturity. Ossification and growth plate closure of individuals can be examined, using X-rays, to determine how an individual is progressing in skeletal age.

Disturbances of bone growth generally involve the growth plate. The growth plate is made of cartilage cells which are dependent for nourishment on blood vessels. Growth disturbances can occur when the blood supply to these cells is lost or the cells have been damaged.

Just how much stress and strain can growing bone tolerate in physical activity and sport situations? It appears that mild degrees of stress act as stimulants and are absolutely necessary for normal growth, while severe degrees of stress result in bone inflammation and destruction.

Fat

The development of body fatness has a unique growth curve of its own and body fatness has important implications for the study of motor development. However, since this factor is considered to be one aspect of health related physical fitness it will be discussed separately in Chapter 17.

Muscle

From birth to maturity, muscle weight increases forty times. At birth, muscles make-up one-fifth to one-fourth of the body weight; in early adolescence, about one-third; and in early maturity, about two-fifths.

After birth muscles grow in size by increasing the length, breadth, and thickness of their component fibers. Muscles do not grow by increasing their number of fibers. Muscles change in composition with age and become more firmly attached to bones. They also gradually come under increased voluntary control. A more thorough coverage of muscle development is presented in Chapter 16 under the headings strength and muscular endurance.

BODY PROPORTIONS

In the process of growing, significant changes occur in body proportions. Characteristic sex differences in body form emerge and the unique physique of an individual presents itself.

Changes in Body Proportions

Differences in degree and timing of the growth of different segments of the body produce changes in body proportions with age for both sexes (Figure 2.6). The proportional growth of the head steadily diminishes; the legs grow relatively longer until about 15 years in boys and about 13 years in girls, after which sitting height increases proportionally more. The head changes from one-fourth of the total length at birth to about one-sixth at 6 years and about one-eighth at maturity. Legs change from about three-eighths of total length at birth to about half the total length at adulthood. Legs in-

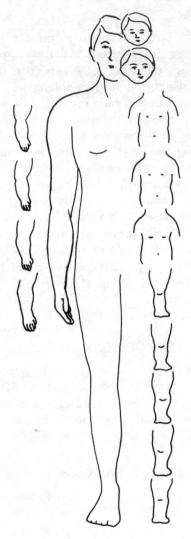

Figure 2.6. During a child's growth, the head doubles in size, the arms become four times as long, the legs five times as long, and the trunk three times as long

portional sex difference in width of shoulders and hips (they increase hip width relatively more than shoulder width). Boys, on the other hand, do not show any increase in relative shoulder width until 10 years. From approximately 10 years of age on, however, these sex differences consistently evidence themselves; girls develop proportionally broader hips and boys develop proportionally broader shoulders. During the adolescent spurt, growth in hip width is as great for males as for females, however males have greater adolescent spurts in shoulder width.

The proportions of body parts contributing to changes in stature during adolescence are different for girls and boys. For equal stature, adolescent girls have shorter legs than boys. For both boys and girls increase in leg growth is one of the earliest signs that childhood is ended. The maximum growth for sitting height, width of chest, shoulders and hips, all of which occur about the same time, follows leg length. While this is the pattern for most children, for some there is a different sequence. For girls, these increases generally come within a year preceding menarche. For boys the peak increments come within the period of maximum genital growth.

SUMMARY

The implications of physical growth for studying motor development are many. Certainly height-weight, growth of body tissues, and differences in body proportions affect the motor development of each individual. The growth factors discussed in this chapter should be kept in mind as the reader learns more about the various factors of motor development in the following pages. The interaction of these growth factors with motor development will be discussed later in the text, principally in Sections 7 and 8.

crease in lengh almost five times from birth to maturity; the head, twice; and the trunk, three times. As this occurs the center of gravity of the body drops, resulting in increased body stability.

During the early elementary school years, girls begin to evidence a characteristic pro-

Section 3

Motor Development:
Conception to Age 5

Importance of Studying Motor Development

3

William Hottinger
Wake Forest University

Movement is a fundamental function of life and is characteristic of the animal kingdom. It plays an important role in every facet of human development. If the reader is cognizant of the interaction of movement with other aspects of the child's development, he/she realizes that a treatise of motor development (development of movement) is to a large degree a study of the whole child.

While it takes somewhat over twenty years for the human organism to mature, child development authorities are in agreement that the early years, birth to age five, are the crucial years of one's life. The experiences that a child has during this period will determine to a major degree what kind of an adult the person will become. The NEA adopted a policy in 1966 which included the following passage. (Education Policies Commission, 1968, p. 5.)

Research shows clearly that the first four or five years of a child's life are the period of most rapid growth in physical and mental characteristics and of greater susceptibility to environmental influences. Consequently, it is the early years that the deprivation are most disasterous

in their effects. They can be compensated for only with great difficulty in later years, and then probably not in full. Furthermore, it appears that it is harder to modify harmful learnings than to acquire new ones. Finally, experience indicates exposure to a wide variety of activities and of social and mental interaction with children and adults greatly enhances a child's ability to learn . . . .

There is absolutely nothing that can offer as much hope to the future as the proper rearing of children. Hence, there is no task, no job, no responsibility as important as assuming a role in the molding of a human personality.

This section is concerned with the motor development of the child from conception to approximately age five. The prenatal period receives only cursory treatment. It is, of course, an important period and many factors, such as the emotional and physical condition of the mother, the habits of the mother, the period of gestation, and the conditions of the uterus all have a most significant effect on the emerging organism. The postnatal period is of greater concern here because it is during this time period that the readers of this text may have an opportunity to exert some influence on shaping the future behavior of the child.

While some of the material covered in the first chapters of this section can be found in any number of books dealing with the psychology of child development, the motor development aspect is often not given adequate treatment. The first chapter of this section is concerned with motor development; the latter part of the section deals with some of the implications of motor performance and its effect on the behavior of children from birth through the preschool years. In this section the writer's point of view is expressed in order to stimulate discussion concerning this important period within the life of the child.

For a long time, the preschool child did not receive very much attention from educators, but in recent years he has been the focal point of much study and research. Evidence has been accumulating which strongly states that the earliest years of a child's life are the most crucial in the development of future life patterns. Bloom (1965) suggests that 50 percent of potential intelligence is achieved by age four. Hunsicker (1963) claims that a child by the age of ten has the neuromuscular potential to master the skills normally taught at the college level. White (1975) feels that much of important development occurs by the age of three. It seems obvious that future research in these early years of child development will continue to reveal some startling and interesting information.

As a result of the research and studies which have provided new insight into the behavioral development of the child, many programs have emerged with the purpose of molding and shaping the child's behavior during these crucial early years. The programs are diverse in nature and include preschool programs developed for educational television, as well as federally funded, church sponsored and privately operated programs. Sudden new interest in any area results in diverse attempts to provide a solution and as can be expected considerable disagreement exists among interested and concerned parties. While almost universal agreement prevails that the preschool years are crucial in establishing life patterns, there seems to be little agreement as to the direction which should be taken to help the child attain maximal potential.

Research has uncovered some rather consistent predictable patterns of development in children. Some general principles have

been established defining these patterns. Becoming familiar with these principles of development will enhance the understanding of how the child's life pattern unfolds. Knowing what to expect of the average child at various stages of development can help parents and teachers plan and provide experiences which are usually appropriate.

MATURATION

Most of the early patterns of development are based upon maturation. While the concept of maturation is not defined alike by all psychologists, this chapter utilizes the concept to embrace the physical and behavioral changes which are primarily a product resulting from an innate process of growth rather than being influenced by direct experiences with the environment. Maturation and learning are so inextricably interwoven that it would be impossible to ferret out which changes are due to learning. In all likelihood both are involved in all areas of development and their influence is a matter of degree. It is not important for us to become highly involved with this problem. What we need to be aware of is that certain changes relatively independent of environmental influences do take place as growth proceeds. Since all human life is subject to this same basic process it is logical to believe that characteristics subject to the maturational process will be broadly predictable in all normal children.

CEPHALOCAUDAL DEVELOPMENT

The sequence of physical development has been found to be orderly and predictable; as physical growth takes place, the motor sequence seems to follow a similar pattern. In physical and motor development, two directional sequences have been noted.

The first of these is that growth tends to proceed from the head toward the feet or in a cephalocaudal direction. Both growth and function tend to follow this pattern. In the early stages of development the head forms first and arm buds form before leg buds. The nervous system also develops from the brain downward and therefore we can understand that in the early stages of motor response, the child gains control of the muscles which support the head before the muscles of the trunk. Likewise the child gains control of the trunk muscles before the muscles of the legs.

PROXIMODISTAL DEVELOPMENT

The second of the directional sequences is that growth proceeds from the center of the body to the periphery, or in a proximodistal direction. As with the first directional sequence, both growth and function tend to follow this pattern. The most rapidly differentiating cells in the embryo are those along the axis from head to tail. The cells in the head end show the greatest activity. Growth and function develop from this center axis toward the periphery. Control proceeds then from the trunk to arms, hands and fingers, and from the hips to legs, feet, and toes. Yet another principle is that growth proceeds from mass to specific. There will be control of gross muscle movements before fine muscle movements. In other terms, the movements will be simple and generalized at first and develop toward being more specific and refined.

INDIVIDUAL DEVELOPMENT

As a result of this developmental trend certain structural changes precede behavioral changes. This maturing, or maturation, is primarily a result of hereditary endowment, and while the developmental pattern is similar for the whole species, each child, because of his unique hereditary endowment, will follow this pattern at his own rate. This explains why all children are not ready for all the same experiences at the same time.

READINESS

While the maturational process is taking place with behavior changes that are independent of environmental factors, there are also behavioral changes occurring that are dependent upon environmental influences. These behavioral changes are learned and without the proper environmental conditions they may not appear. However, even with the proper environmental conditions they cannot appear until the child is ready (mature enough) for the behavior to be learned. Maturation must lay the foundation for the development of the behavior.

PHYLOGENETIC VS. ONTOGENETIC DEVELOPMENT

The behavioral changes that occur rather automatically with the maturing of the individual are referred to as phylogenetic behavior. It is sometimes said to be of racial origin rather than of individual or cultural origin. This type of behavior includes such activities as grasping, reaching, crawling, creeping, walking, and running. The behavioral changes that depend primarily upon learning are referred to as ontogenetic behavior. These changes will not appear automatically with the maturing of the individual but are learned, or acquired, through environmental experiences. Ontogenetic behavior includes such activities as swimming, skating, riding a tricycle, and driving a car.

References

Bloom, Benjamin S. *Stability and Change in Human Characteristics.* New York: John Wiley & Sons, Inc., 1967.

Education Policies Commission of the NEA and The American Association of School Administrators. "Universal Opportunity for Early Childhood Education." *Early Childhood Education Rediscovered,* Edited by Joe L. Frost. New York: Holt, Rinehart & Winston, Inc., 1968.

Hunsicker, Paul. "What Research Says to the Teacher." *Physical Fitness,* no. 26. Washington, D.C., Department of Classroom Teachers, National Education Association, 1963.

White, Burton. *The First Three Years of Life.* Englewood Cliffs, N.J.: Prentice-Hall, Inc., 1975.

Babyhood: Pre- and Postnatal Periods

4

William Hottinger
Wake Forest University

PRENATAL BEHAVIOR

A discussion of motor behavior must begin at conception since the patterns of development are set into play at the moment the egg, or ovum, is fertilized. The prenatal period is usually divided into three subperiods — the ovum, the embryonic and the fetal. The ovum period lasts about two weeks and consists of vast cell division. After the sperm and egg unite, the chromosomes are duplicated and two cells result, these cells divide making four, these divide making eight and so on.

The ovum attaches itself to the uterus about the second week and from this time to about the eighth week is known as the embryo. The embryonic period is one of cell differentiation where the apparently unorganized mass of cells formed during the ovum period undergoes a change which emerges into an identifiable structure with head, limbs, fingers, toes, brain, spinal cord, heart, lungs, and other vital organs and systems.

The embryonic heart becomes active about the third week but there is no other muscle movement until around the eighth week after conception and this marks the beginning of the fetal period — this period lasts until birth. Of particular importance to motor behavior is the development of the nervous system. Until the peripheral nervous connections are made there is no sign of movement. By the eighth week, however, connections between receptors and effectors are apparent and the human fetus has been found to respond to tactile stimulation. In accordance with the patterns of development the regions near the head are more sensitive than in areas farther away. By the third month some spontaneous movement occurs. The fetus begins to respond to tactile stimulation. The fourth month of prenatal life seems to be a very important period. Around this time numerous reflexes appear that approximate those of the newborn infant. Stimulation may now result in specific rather than generalized responses. Specific responses become more prevalent until at birth the baby has a wide variety of reflex actions. Near the end of the fifth month respiratory movements begin to appear and around the seventh month become established; the fetus could survive in the external environment if properly attended. By the eighth month most of the responses that are present at birth can be elicited. Some research is beginning to appear that concludes that the newborn has some cortical involvement but in general movement up to 12 to 14 weeks after birth is primarily an expression of brain stem, cerebellar and intersegmental spinal reflex mechanisms (Munn, 1965, Wyke, 1975).

Reflex Activity

The reflex system that evolves within the fetus is extremely important since it represents the most fundamental level of movement and ". . . normal motor coordination is based to a huge extent on the reflexes" (Easton 1972, p. 591).

While the human organism in the first year of biological existence is essentially a reflex machine the nervous system of the 12 to 14 week old baby undergoes a continuous process of neuromuscular functional maturation. The control of the systems evolving can be and are learned but ". . . an individual's control of his striated muscles remains dependent upon the background influences of the facilitatory and inhibitory reflexogenic mechanisms with which he was born . . ." (Wyke 1975, p. 27).

POSTNATAL BEHAVIOR

The postnatal periods include the neonate, from birth to one month; babyhood, one month to two years; and early childhood, two years to six years. These periods are designated only for convenience of discussion. There is, of course, no clear-cut demarcation from one period to the next.

The developmental process is a continuation of what has already been taking place in the prenatal period. The child must assume control over the own alimentary and respiratory functions but the basic patterns of development continue and behavior greatly expands. The environment in which the child has emerged is more complex and variable, and he/she is less restricted. While maturation continues to be a dominant force in the motor development of the child, learning also becomes an important factor in development as the child interacts with the environment. As has already been pointed out it is difficult to determine which developments are due to maturation and which to learning.

THE NEONATE

The full-term baby is approximately twenty inches long and weighs about seven and one-half pounds. The head is disproportionately large in comparison with the rest of his body; it is about one-fourth of the total length; at full maturity it is approximately one-eighth of total height. The lower extremities are small. Obviously the rate of growth cannot be the same for all parts of the body from birth to maturity. (The cephalocaudal trend which was reported earlier as a predictable pattern of growth reverses itself after birth.)

When the child is born he/she already has a large number of motor responses. A brief summary of these responses is presented in Table 4.1.

The activity reported in Table 4.1 from Dennis's survey is abridged. Nevertheless, it does show that the reflex responses of the newborn are quite extensive. It is believed that the cerebral cortex does not influence behavior to any significant extent until sometime after birth. Some attempts have been made to condition responses but such efforts at this level have not met with great success (Hurlock 1964).

In a short time, however, the infant becomes capable of making voluntary movements. Since this happens gradually and is sometimes difficult to determine if the movement is reflex or voluntary activity, an exact time of cortical involvement cannot be given. It does, however, occur within a few months after birth.

Some of the more common reflexes that may be observed in the neonate are the Moro reflex, commonly referred to as the startle reflex. This involves throwing the arms outward from the body, followed by bringing them together. This is a response to stimuli that may startle the infant such as

TABLE 4.1
Responses of the Newborn Infant

Eyelid responses. Opens and closes eyelids; this appears spontaneously and in response to a variety of external stimuli.

Pupillary response. Pupils contract and expand in response to light. The pupils tend to be consensual (when one is stimulated, the other eye also responds).

Ocular response. There are pursuit movement, and saccadic movements which are quick, jerky movements used later in reading.
There is coordination of the eyes, with convergence being rare. Eyes in sleep are up and sideways like the adult.

Tear secretion. Tear secretion is unusual in the newborn but has been observed during crying and with nasal irritation.

Facial and mouth response. Opens and closes mouth; lips move in response to touch; sucking occurs either spontaneously or in response to tactual or taste stimuli; smiles; yawns; frowns; wrinkles forehead; grimaces.

Throat responses. Crying is usually accompanied by activity of arms and legs. Swallowing occurs in all newborn infants, vomiting may occur, hiccoughing may occur, sneezing may occur, and holding the breath has been reported.

Head and neck responses. Moves head upward and downward and turns face to side in response to some stimuli. As early as two days of age the baby can balance his head in response to changes in bodily positions.

Head and arm responses. Closes hand in response to tactual stimulation of fingers and palm. Arm flexion can be elicited with pricking the hand or a tap on the hand. Rubs his face, and moves his arms. The startle response is evident—throws arm outward if startled.

Trunk reactions. Arches back—can be produced by pinching the nose.
Twisting—head rotates one direction, shoulders and pelvis in the opposite direction.
Abdominal reflex—draws in stomach in response to needle stimulus.

Sexual responses. Cremasteric reflex—raising of testes to stimulation of inner thighs.
Penis erection.

Foot and leg responses. Achilles tendon reflex is present in most newborn babies.
Flexion of leg—this action is accompanied by plantor flexion of the foot.
Kicking consists of a pedaling action and a simultaneous flexion and extension of both legs.
Stepping movements occur when the child is held upright with its feet touching a surface.
Toe phenomena consists of spreading the toes when the sole of the foot is stroked.

Coordinate responses of many body parts. Resting and sleeping position—the legs are flexed, fists closed, upper arm straight out from the shoulders with forearms flexed at right angles so they are lying parallel with the head.
Opisthotonis position—this is a strong dorsal flexion from head to heels, often occurs in crying.
Backbone reflex—this is a concave bending of a side that is stimulated with a stroke or a tickle.
Lifting head and rear quarters simultaneously.
Fencing position—this occurs when the baby's head is rotated to one side, the arm toward which the head is rotated will extend and the opposite arm will flex.
Springing position—this occurs when the infant is held upright and inclined forward. The arms extend forward and the legs brought up.
Startle response—this response consists of throwing the arms apart, spreading the fingers, extending the legs and throwing the head back. It sometimes occurs with no apparent stimulation but is usually a response to stimuli which could frighten it such as noise, falling or other sudden occurences.
Mass activity—general unrest and crying.
Creeping—this may occur when newborn is placed in a prone position. The legs and arms are drawn under the body and the head lifted. The legs push and the arms become more active.
Nursing posture—if an infant is hungry and given a nipple, it begins to nurse and at the same time it flexes its arms so they are pulled across the body with the fists toward the chin. The legs and toes are raised. The position relaxes as the child's hunger subsides.

Abridged from Wayne Dennis. "A Description and Classification of the Responses of the Newborn Infant." *Psychological Bulletin* 31 (1934):5-22. Copyright 1934 by the American Psychological Association, and used by permission.

a loud noise, falling, or a flash of light. The Moro reflex disappears around four months, although a startle pattern continues to exist in adults. The grasping reflex occurs when the palm of the infant is pressed and causes a closing of the fingers. This grasp may be strong enough to allow the infant to support its own weight. This reflex can be elicited as early as the third or fourth month of prenatal life and continues through the first few months of postnatal life. The Babinski reflex is an extension of the big toe and extension and fanning of the other toes when the sole of the foot is stroked. This reflex can be elicited by the fourth or fifth month of prenatal life and disappears several months after birth. The rooting reflex occurs when the hungry infant is touched on the face. The infant will respond with quick jerky movements bringing the mouth toward the source of stimulation.

The neonate period is usually considered a period of adjustment and by the end of one month the infant has made considerable progress. The body functions are under control, and all of the senses are operating and will continue to improve with maturation and practice.

BABYHOOD

Babyhood covers the period from one month to two years. It is a period of extremely rapid change, and the development that occurs in this period provides a basis for some of the most significant accomplishments that will take place in the child's lifetime. (Two very obvious accomplishments are upright locomotion and speech.) This chapter deals with the former, and with various motor functions associated with this period of life.

From the neonatal period to about six weeks there is a general improvement of reflexes but little learning, per se, takes place during this time. At about six weeks, things begin to happen. White (1971) refers to the period from six weeks to three and one-half months as the dawning of awareness and voluntary action. Intelligence is still considered to be in the primitive stage but there is some evidence of cortical control. In discussing the infant during this eight week period White states that

. . . he will discover and gain at least partial mastery over the use of his hands, fully develop the capacity to maintain clear focus on objects moving nearby (visual accommodation), increase his periods of alertness from less than ten minutes per hour to almost half the daylight hours, enter into a period of social smiling guaranteed to endear him to any but the coldest of adult hearts, acquire the tendency to blink at approaching visible targets, overcome the restrictive influence of the grasp reflex which in the neonatal period kept his hands mostly fisted, overcome the influence of the tonic neck reflex which has restricted his visual range and subordinated the motion of his limbs to the position of his head, acquire the capacity to hold his head vertically for several minutes when placed prone, begin to assimilate experiences which will lead to the construction of a world of objects (himself included) (Piaget 1952), exhibit the capacity to sustain interest in a spectacle (his own hands) for up to thirty minutes at a time, begin to exhibit the ability to imitate sounds, distinguish familiar social figures, make many fine sensory discriminations, form dependable conditioned responses, etc. (White 1971, p. 85).

White further points out that ". . . in spite of the impressive changes, until the infant acquires the ability to use his hands to reach for and examine objects, all he can do to explore the external world is to either lie on his back and stare or, if prone, he can with increasing skill raise his head and peer about (White 1971, p. 86)."

One of the most important occurrences, therefore, after three and one-half months, is the development of the ability to reach. Reaching, grasping and manual manipulation is referred to as prehensile behavior. When the infant is born, and for the first few months, he/she has a strong grasp which is a reflex action. This reflex grasp gradually disappears and is replaced by prehensive grasping which gradually comes under voluntary control. Halverson (1931) studied prehension cinematographically. He identified ten stages in the development of prehension. These stages appear in an orderly sequence from no contact at 16 weeks to superior forefinger grasping at 52 weeks. The sequence of stages proposed by Halverson are (1) no contact — 16 weeks; (2) contact — 20 weeks; (3) the primitive squeeze — 20 weeks; (4) the squeeze grasp — 24 weeks; (5) hand grasp — 28 weeks; (6) palm grasp — 28 weeks; (7) superior palm grasp — 32 weeks; (8) inferior forefinger grasp — 36 weeks; (9) fore-finger grasp — 52 weeks; (10) superior forefinger grasp — 52 weeks. Early attempts at reaching for an object are backhanded. This method gives way to a forward circuitous approach that becomes increasingly direct until at about fifty-two weeks at which time the child can reach directly for an object. Initial grasping efforts do not involve the thumb. The thumb becomes part of the grasp between six and eight months. The child becomes progressively more proficient until by eighteen months the entire act of reaching, grasping and manipulation is relatively smooth and automatic.

Another motor development of interest is that of handedness. The basis of handedness remains somewhat controversial. One opinion is that it has a neurological base.

One hemisphere of the brain is the seat of motor control for the opposite side of the body; if interference with the child's handedness is made it is thought by some that there will be interference of speech and other fine motor movements. Another opinion is that hand dominance is a cultural trait. Our culture is oriented toward right handedness and therefore right handedness becomes a matter of learning and habit. In either case most investigators agree that there is no hand preference during the early months of life (Munn 1965). The critical period for establishing handedness is from three to five years of age (Hurlock 1964). Before age two the child shifts from one hand to the other, but may show some slight preference. Most educators agree that while right handedness should be encouraged in our culture, it should never be forced.

One of the most important motor functions of the maturing infant is the attainment of the upright position leading to walking, running, and other skills. Achieving the upright position is the culmination of a long complex sequence of progressive skills. The progressive pattern proceeds in accordance with the patterns of development discussed earlier, and evidence (Shirley 1933) shows that the pattern does indeed follow a predictable sequence. The changes that occur appear to follow, or are closely associated with, maturity of the central nervous system. The infant must initially gain control of the muscles of the head and neck. Many infants can lift their heads for a short period within the first month and by four months most babies can turn their heads from side to side and hold their heads up for awhile if they are in the prone position. By six months, the infant has considerable control of the neck and trunk. At about this same time, the child has tried, or soon will try, to make some forward progress. While the sequence of events is similar, the specific methods and rates of progress may differ greatly from child to child. Ames (1937) describes the fourteen stages of prone progression which are presented in Table 4.2.

While this development is taking place the lower trunk has been growing stronger allowing the child to be able to sit alone with support at four months and alone by seven months. Around seven to nine months the child begins creeping, an act which greatly expands the environment. Some babies become highly proficient creepers and many times will revert to creeping after they learn to walk because, at the moment, it is a more proficient means of locomotion. Between seven and ten months a baby's trunk and legs have developed to the degree that allows him/her to stand with support and the child begins to pull erect by holding on to the furniture. Soon the child begins to

TABLE 4.2
Stages of Prone Progression

1. Knee and thigh forward beside body	28 weeks
2. Knee and thigh forward, inner side of foot against the floor	28 weeks
3. Pivoting	29 weeks
4. Attaining inferior low creep position	30 weeks
5. Attaining low creep position	32 weeks
6. Crawling	34 weeks
7. Attaining high creep position	35 weeks
8. Retrogression	36 weeks
9. Rocking	36 weeks
10. Creep—Crawling	36 weeks
11. Creeping	40 weeks
12. Creeping, near step with one foot	42 weeks
13. Creeping, step with one foot	45 weeks
14. Quadrupedal progression	49 weeks

From Louise Bates Ames. "The Sequential Patterns of Prone Progressions in the Human Infant." *Genetic Psychology Monographs* 19 (1937):409-60.

walk around the furniture or walks with the aid of parents. The average age of independent walking seems to be somewhere between thirteen and fourteen months. There is a wide range however, covering the span from seven to eighteen months — all considered normal. Walking usually receives enthusiastic encouragement from the parents and while many feel that they are responsible for teaching their child to walk, a child can and will walk when ready; that is, when muscular and nervous systems mature to the degree which allows the child to engage in this new motor act. Walking is a tremendous milestone in the child's life. It increases the environment immensely and makes the possibilities for exploration almost unlimited. It frees the hands from the locomotive act and the child can now use them for manipulation. Parents are usually delighted when their child learns to walk, but it marks a time when great demands are made upon their patience. A great deal of learning goes on during this period provided the environment offers exploratory opportunities and the parents are not overly restrictive.

The baby's initial style of walking is jerky and steps are uneven. The feet are spread and the toes turned outward. The arms are held up for balance and the child weaves about when walking. Falls are frequent. As muscles grow stronger and balance improves the walking pattern becomes more mature. By the time the child is 24 to 30 months old he/she usually walks quite well but Gutteridge (1939) concludes that on the average the art of walking is not perfected until fifty months.

The pattern used in running is similar to that of walking. Running requires more strength since the body must be propelled off the ground for a short period of time. Additional coordination and balance are other factors that the child must also master. Initially the run grows out of a fast walk but improves steadily and the child of four who has had ample opportunity to practice can be observed to run with good form.

Prehension and the upright position serve as the basis for the development of a myriad of motor skills. Feeding one's self, scribbling with a pencil, block building and various other kinds of play and manipulation are all part of the child's repertoire by the age of two. By this time the child has also developed and is in the process of refining a number of motor skills such as smiling and speech. Several scales of motor development have been devised to measure the motor achievements of children at various ages. A scale often referred to by writers was devised by Nancy Bayley. Her classification of the various motor achievements is presented in Table 4.3.

In addition to this scale, Gesell's (1954) statement of the trends of behavior development make a good summary for this age period:

In the first quarter (4-16 weeks) of the first year the infant gains control of his twelve oculomotor muscles.
In the second quarter (16-28 weeks) he comes into command of the muscles which support his head and move his arms. He reaches out for things.
In the third quarter (28-40 weeks) he gains command of his trunk and hands. He sits. He grasps, transfers, and manipulates objects.
In the fourth quarter (40-52 weeks) he extends command to his legs and feet; to his forefingers and thumb. He pokes and plucks. He stands upright.
In the second year he walks and runs; articulates words and phrases; acquires bowel and bladder control; attains a rudimentary sense of personal identity and of personal possession (Gesell 1954, p. 339).

TABLE 4.3

Development of Motor Abilities

.2 months —	crawling movements
.5 months —	lifts head at shoulders
1.7 months —	arm thrusts in play
1.9 months —	head erect—vertical
2.6 months —	dorsal suspension—lefts head
2.9 months —	head erect and steady
3.4 months —	turns from side to back
3.5 months —	sits with support
4.1 months —	beginning thumb opposition
5.0 months —	turns from back to side
5.4 months —	effort to sit
5.7 months —	sits alone momentarily
6.2 months —	pulls to sitting position
6.2 months —	sits alone 30 seconds or more
7.0 months —	rolls from back to stomach
7.6 months —	complete thumb opposition
8.5 months —	sits alone with good coordination
9.2 months —	prewalking progression
9.3 months —	fine prehension with pellet
9.4 months —	raises self to sitting position
10.5 months —	pulls to standing position
10.6 months —	stands up
11.6 months —	walks with help
12.5 months —	stands alone
13.0 months —	walks alone
16.5 months —	walks sideways
16.9 months —	walks backward
20.3 months —	walks upstairs with help
24.3 months —	walks upstairs alone—marks time
24.5 months —	walks downstairs alone—marks time

Abridged from Nancy Bayley, "The Development of Motor Abilities During the First Three Years." *Society for Research in Child Development,* Monograph No. 1 (1935):1-26.

References

Ames, Louise. "The Sequential Patterns of Prone Progressions in the Human Infant." *Genetic Psychology Monogram* 19 (1937): 409.

Bayley, Nancy. "The Development of Motor Abilities During the First Three Years." *Society for Research in Child Development, Monograph* no. 1: 1, 1935.

Easton, T. A. "On the Normal Use of Reflexes." *American Scientist* 60 (1972): 591-99.

Gesell, Arnold. "The Ontogenesis of Infant Behavior." *Manual of Child Psychology*, edited by Leonard Carmichael. New York: John Wiley & Sons, Inc., 1954.

Halverson, H. M. "An Experimental Study of Prehension in Infants by Means of Systematic Cineman Records." *Genetic Psychology Monogram.* 10 (1931):107.

Hurlock, Elizabeth. *Child Development*, 4th ed. New York: McGraw-Hill Book Company, 1964.

Munn, Norman. *The Evolution and Growth of Human Behavior*, 2d ed. Boston: Houghton Mifflin Company, 1965.

Shirley, Mary M. "The Motor Sequence" of *Readings in Child Psychology*, edited by Dennis Wayne. Englewood Cliffs, N.J.: Prentice-Hall, Inc., 1963.

White, Burton. *Human Infants, Experience and Psychological Development.* Englewood Cliffs, N.J.: Prentice-Hall, Inc., 1971.

Wyke, Barry. "The Neurological Basis of Movement—A Developmental Review." *Movement and Child Development.* Edited by Kenneth Holt. Philadelphia: J. B. Lippincott Co., 1975.

Early Childhood 5

William Hottinger
Wake Forest University

Early childhood, from two to six years, is a significant learning period. Most of the fundamental movement patterns develop to a fairly high level provided the environment furnishes ample opportunity. Also, during this period, there is a rapid development of speech. Many of the motor skills that will be perfected at this stage actually have their beginnings before the age of two. Walking, for example, is basic to the development of other movement patterns such as running, jumping, hopping, galloping and skipping.

CLIMBING

Climbing is an outgrowth of creeping and many babies can climb up steps before they can walk because these movement patterns do not deviate too much from creeping except that the child usually leads with one side. When the child reaches the top, he/she initially tries to come down head first. It requires some experimenting until the child discovers it is best to descend backwards. After the child learns to walk, attempts will be made to climb up and down steps in the upright position, usually marking time on each step in early attempts. This means that the child goes up one step at a time leading with the same foot. The child also uses the mark time method when descending the steps. Eventually he/she alternates the feet when climbing, this pattern appearing sooner in ascending than in descending. Wellman (1937) studied the climbing ability of children in an effort to determine the ages at which various levels of climbing could be achieved. Her tests consisted of a short and long flight of steps and a ladder with rungs spaced six inches apart and another with rungs twelve inches apart. She found that by the age of twenty-four months children could ascend both a step and ladder using a mark time pattern. They could negotiate the long flight of steps in alternating fashion by forty-one months of age. Ascending both the steps and ladders was easier than descending, the latter pattern following in four to five months. By sixty-two months the child could descend the ladder with the large rungs. Gutteridge's (1939) observations revealed that children's climbing ability was well established for half of them by three years of age. After that, a gradual increase occurred until by six years of age 92 percent were proficient climbers. Many factors determine which climbing skills will become proficient. Opportunity to practice is a prime factor but the slope of the incline of the steps or ladders and the distance between the risers and the rungs are also considerations. When children learn to climb poles, ropes and other obstacles will depend to a large degree on whether or not they are provided with this type of equipment.

There has been a dearth of research and publication on the development of climbing with the exception of steps and ladders. The author, however, includes inclined boards, poles, and an assortment of ropes and rope ladders in addition to steps and ladders in his early childhood motor development program. It is his opinion that climbing is a particularly important early childhood activity because not only does it have utilitarian value but nearly all children have a natural affinity for climbing. In addition, it is an excellent movement exploration activity and the wide variety of conditions that can be established make a success oriented situation almost always possible. Climbing is also an excellent activity for developing confidence and upper body strength, and has proven to be one of the best activities for developing social skills. (See illustration)

In general, there is little difference between preschool boys and girls in their ability to climb; descending is more difficult than ascending, higher heights may cause children to revert to an earlier climbing pattern, and there is wide variation in ability at all ages.

JUMPING

The first attempts at jumping are usually an exaggerated step from an elevated level. Greater strength is required for jumping than running since the body must be propelled upward. As the child increases in strength and general growth, jumping proficiency becomes greater each year. Jumping has many variations. At around twenty-four to thirty months jumping occurs from elevated levels and this precedes jumping with both feet simultaneously and jumping over barriers. Bayley (1935) places the ability to jump with both feet at about twenty-eight months and jumping for a distance of 36-60 cm at about forty months. Jumping over a barrier seems to be more difficult. Gutteridge (1939) judged that 42 percent of children at three years of age

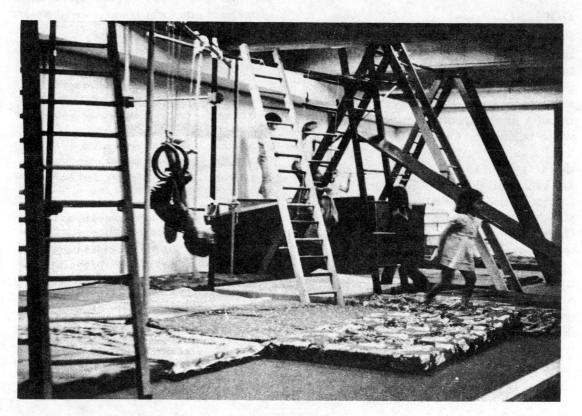

were able to jump well and by five, 81 percent were reasonably proficient.

Jumping is an excellent activity for movement exploration and can be easily promoted simply by structuring the environmental setting. While the trampoline is undergoing some harsh criticism, the author has found it to be an excellent piece of equipment for children between eighteen months and six years. Young children do not know the concept of front and back sommersaults and are happily content with controlled jumping, seat drops, and other elementary skills. Children have a natural affinity for jumping and delight in jumping from elevated heights in a well padded pit, over hurdles, and across "alligator infested rivers".

HOPPING

Hopping is a skill similar to jumping but more difficult in that it requires a one foot take-off and landing on the same foot. Hopping requires a higher degree of strength and greater balance than the two foot landing of a jump. According to Bayley (1935) static balance on one foot is not achieved until about twenty-nine months. She states that it is about fifty months before the average child can hop up to two meters on the right foot. Breckenridge and Vincent (1956) state that children are six years old before the majority can hop skillfully. There is a wide range of ability, however, for children have been observed to hop 100 feet or more by five years of age. Girls generally become more proficient hoppers at an earlier age than boys although, again, there is wide variation in the ability to perform this skill with both sexes.

GALLOPING

Galloping combines walking and leaping and has several variations. Three-year-olds seldom practice galloping but four-year-olds begin to practice and by five do fairly well. It is not until about six and one-half years of age that most children are considered to be really skillfull (Breckenridge and Vincent 1956).

SKIPPING

Skipping appears a little later than galloping. Some children can skip at four years of age and the numbers increase until by six most children can skip, but even then there is wide variation in ability (Gutteridge 1939, Breckenridge and Vincent 1956). Bayley's scale (1935) of the development of motor abilities which was referred to earlier is continued in Table 5.1.

TABLE 5.1
Development of Motor Abilities

28.0 months —	jumps off floor with both feet
29.2 months —	stands on left foot alone
29.3 months —	stands on right foot alone
30.1 months —	walks on tiptoes
32.1 months —	jumps from chair
35.5 months —	walks upstairs alternating forward foot
27.1 months —	jumps from height of 30 cm
37.3 months —	distance jump—10-35 cm
39.2 months —	distance jump—36-40 cm
41.5 months —	jumps over rope less than 20 cm high
48.4 months —	distance jump—60-65 cm
49.3 months —	hops on right foot less than 2 cm
50.0 months —	walks downstairs alternating forward foot

Abridged from Nancy Bayley. "The Development of Motor Abilities During the First Three Years." *Society for Research in Child Development*, Monograph No. 1 (1935):1-26.

THROWING

Another skill which derives its beginning in early childhood is throwing. The earliest crude throwing pattern occurs when a child releases an object from a jerky movement. Analysis of a study done by Wild (1938) revealed four distinct patterns of throwing. The throw that is demonstrated by two- and three-year-olds shows that the ball is thrown primarily with a forearm extension with no footwork or rotation of the body. The second pattern, demonstrated by three and one-half-year-olds involves more body rotation and greater arm range. The third pattern demonstrated by five- and six-year-olds introduces a forward step with the right foot as the ball is delivered with the right hand. The fourth sequence demonstrated by boys six and one-half and older shows a mature form of throwing with the weight transferred to the right foot during the preparatory phase with the trunk rotating to the right. A forward step by the left foot is followed by rotation of the hips and trunk as the elbow swings horizontally forward and is followed by an extension of the forearm.

One can expect a wide variation in the throwing pattern. Cultural opportunities and expectation play a major role resulting in this variation. Girls in our culture often have difficulty in learning to throw correctly. However, females who practice can achieve mature throwing form as is evidenced by skillful female softball teams. Many men who live in countries where ball throwing is not emphasized often lack mature throwing form. This merely demonstrates that throwing is a learned skill and will not evolve to any mature degree as the result of maturation alone.

CATCHING

By the time a child is two years old he can handle stationary objects with relative proficiency but to grasp a moving object presents a more complicated task. [This requires a good eye-hand coordination and develops a child's perception of time-space relationships.] Stopping a rolling ball is usually the earliest attempt at catching. Catching an aerial ball requires greater skill. The first attempts are usually awkward with the arms held stiffly out in front of the body. As with throwing, one can expect wide variation in catching skills throughout the entire age range and between the sexes.

BALL BOUNCING

There have not been many studies concerned specifically with ball bouncing. The range of ability is large and depends of course on the time the child spends practicing. It has been observed that some two-year-olds are proficient in bouncing (dribbling) a ball but, on the other hand, many five- and six-year-olds have not mastered the skill. Ball bouncing is an excellent hand-eye coordinating skill and is of such a safe nature that ample opportunity should be given to it and other related ball skills.

SWIMMING

Swimming is another skill that can be learned at an early age but many adults have never learned to swim and the majority cannot be classified as proficient swimmers. The age at which children should learn to swim is a subject of debate. Children can become reasonably proficient by the age of five if given the opportunity. Johnny, the experimental twin in McGraw's study

(1935), was able to swim 12 to 15 feet by seventeen months. Margaret Mead (1958) in describing the Manus tribe of New Guinea states that children are expected to swim by three and that all children can swim well by age five. There are swimming programs available in this country for children as young as three months (Life 1971).

The number of activities that can be learned by the child from birth to the age of six is almost unlimited. There probably is no motor act that a child cannot learn, at least to some degree, by the age of six. Tricycles can be manipulated by two-year-olds. Bicycles are sometimes mastered by four-year-olds and the majority can ride by six if given the opportunity. Roller skating can be learned by age three but perhaps five to seven is a more realistic time to expect the majority of children to develop this skill.

A consistent fact to note throughout this discussion has been that wide variation of motor skill and performance is evident at an early age. This variation can be explained by a number of factors some of which are hereditary endowment, opportunity to experiment and practice, attitude of parents toward motor performance, and the number of siblings and peers with which the child has to interact. Hereditary endowment is decided, of course, before the child is born, but after that event parents and other adults have considerable control over other factors which determine the levels of achievement which will be attained.

References

Bayley, Nancy. "The Development of Motor Abilities During the First Three Years." *Society for Research in Child Development, Monograph* no. 1 (1935):1.

Breckenridge, Marian and Vincent, Lee. *Child Development,* 3rd ed. Philadelphia: W. B. Saunders Co., 1955.

Gutteridge, Mary V. "A Study of Motor Achievements of Young Children." *Archives of Psychology* 244 (1939):1.

LIFE. "Water Babies" Volume 71, No. 6. August 6, 1971.

McGraw, Myrtle. *Growth: A Study of Johnny and Jimmy.* New York: Appleton-Century-Crofts, 1935.

Mead, Margaret. *Growing Up in New Guinea.* New York: New American Library of World Literature, Inc., (A Mentor Book) 1930, 1958.

Wellman, Beth. "Motor Achievements of Preschool Children." *Childhood Education* 13 (1937):311.

Wild, Monica R. "The Behavior Pattern of Throwing and Some Observations Concerning Its Course of Development in Children." "*Research Quarterly* 9 (1938).

Early Motor Development: Discussion and Summary

6

William Hottinger
Wake Forest University

DISCUSSION

Understanding factors related to childhood behavior is important because it allows adults to be realistic in their approach to guiding the child toward optimal development. Behavior begins in the prenatal period and little outside influence can be exerted in shaping the child's growth during this stage. Even the mother has little influence over the developing organism. The most she can do is take good care of herself physically and emotionally and consult an obstetrician before ingesting drugs or other chemicals. The next question, therefore, is what influence can adults exert on the organism after it arrives? As already pointed out, the infant arrives on the scene already capable of a number of motor responses. These are reflex in nature and the infant's capacity to learn is quite limited. The sense organs at birth, or shortly thereafter, can respond to some degree of stimulation. While the nature of learning remains theoretical, all theories agree that the child must interact with his environment in order to learn. Learning occurs by receiving sensations through the sense organs which results in some kind of information processing. Initially, of course, the sensations received by the infant can have little meaning since there have been no past experiences with which to attach these impressions. Gradually, however, meanings or associations become attached to these incoming sensations. Learning then depends upon sensory stimulation, even though the exact process of how this occurs remains conjectural. Currently there is great concern among psychologists and educators regarding the kinds of early experiences that will result in the optimal development of each child. There is a relatively consistent view that early experiences are of paramount importance in influencing future development. What is not so consistent regards the nature of the early experiences. How much experience, what kind of experience and when the experience should begin are the bases of these concerns.

Critical Periods

One of the concepts which provides some guidance in determining how the child's behavior can be influenced is that of "critical periods of learning." McGraw (1939) in her work with children concluded that there are critical periods when any given activity is susceptible to modification through repetition of performance. The critical period is the time following the age when the child is first capable of performing the act effectively. Scott (1968) concludes that the critical period is one in which rapid organization is taking place. This appears consistent with the concept of maturation. Research shows that trying to teach children acts that they are not maturationally (the nervous and muscular system are not mature enough to allow the act to be performed) ready to accomplish results in little learning. Combining this idea with the critical period concept suggests that as soon as the child is maturationally ready (the internal processes have organized) is the best time to learn that particular act. Present information regarding the optimal time for learning motor skills is sparse.

Environmental Effects

If learning takes place most readily during the certain critical periods, then it follows that conditions must be present which allow the learning to occur. This raises the subject of the effects of early experiences on behavioral development. Studies have been done with both animals and children to determine the effects of environments restricted and enriched in sensory stimulation.

Scott (1968) reports several studies conducted with different kinds of animals which show how normal behavior is altered when the animal does not go through the normal experience for its species. Dennis (1963) in studying institutionalized children aged one-year/to four-years in Iran found that children who were not provided with specific kinds of learning opportunities were retarded in normal locomotive development. The majority of children in one of the institutions did not learn to creep but rather locomoted by scooting prior to walking. Scott also reports on studies where enriched environments were provided. These studies indicate that an enriched environment produces positive results. Another interesting point regarding sensory stimulation or early experience is that it must be timed or matched with the organizing process going on at the time (Scott 1968).

Experiences beyond the maturational level of the child cannot be expected to produce positive results. Brazelton (1971) pointed out the need for a stimulating environment. As he puts it, a baby needs proper nutrients for physiological growth and needs stimulation for emotional and intellectual growth. Lack of stimulation can interfere with development. However, he has two concerns: (1) that the stimulation be appropriate for each baby, and (2) that there is not overstimulation. Babies, according to Brazelton (1971), have the ability to tune out or reject stimuli and this might occur when the stimulation is excessive or inappropriate. What constitutes a good environment? The exact answer cannot be given to this question yet, but from the limited information that is available there are some logical conclusions which may be drawn. Learning can only occur when there is sensory stimulation, but the right kind of stimulation is important. The kind of sensory stimulation the child needs will depend upon the child's present stage of development. As the child develops, the nature of the sensory stimulation will change and requires that the environment become more varied. Parents, child psychologists, and educators can contribute greatly to the child's developmental process by structuring an optimal learning environment.

To pursue this task when we do not fully understand the learning process is a bit frightening but, nevertheless, we are obligated to do the best we can with the information available. There will inevitably be a lot of disagreement, as there already is, on the form of such an undertaking. One practical procedure is to provide a rich varied environment and let the child choose from among the stimuli rather than try to impose the environment on the child.

Providing Environmental Opportunity

While there is not too much research to draw upon there are some rational approaches to providing sensory experiences. Perhaps the most important task of a child in the first two years of life is to gain sensory control over the environment. Naturally, the attitudes, creativeness and insight the parent has during this period are particularly important. There are a number of things that can be done soon after birth to help stimulate the child's senses and start him on the road to learning. To be sure, a parent must be sensitive to the needs of the child but supplying sensory experiences is, essentially, a matter of learning to follow the child's lead. The parent in observing the child attempts to provide the kind of stimulation to which the child can respond at a particular age. Most parents are capable of doing this once they realize that parenthood is more than meeting biological needs of the child. Soon after a baby is born, studies have shown that it can tell light from darkness and, in fact, can distinguish between different patterns. At this time, therefore, pictures of different designs, shades and colors can be attracted to the sides of the crib so that the child can focus on them during brief waking periods. This can be followed shortly by mobiles with objects of various sizes and colors at different distances from the child. This can keep the child in focus and practicing visual pursuit. Talking with the baby and providing other sounds will also help to heighten the auditory mechanism. By three months the baby will exhibit some voluntary control and will reach for and slap objects that are close by. A bar can be placed across the crib with various objects hung from it. These objects can be balls of different colors and sizes, large rings, bells and other kinds of objects of various shapes and textures. Draw attention to the objects but let the baby respond in his/her own time. Between three and six months the baby will be able to use the hands in grasping and manipulating. The child will place objects in his/her mouth as a part of learning about them. This is a time for teethers of various sorts and others objects the child can manipulate. Between six and nine months the child's world expands greatly. Prehension abilities increase immensely if the child is provided with objects that can be manipulated and controlled. The child in this period becomes aware that things have permanency. If you hide an object in your hand the child may look for it; he/she enjoys peek-a-boo games. During this time the child may begin to imitate sounds.

When the child first appears strong enough to move his/her body, a firm surface that can be pushed against should be provided. A child at this time should also be permitted to kick and splash in the bathtub. As the baby begins to crawl, it marks another of an expanding phase. The child is stronger now and ready for a variety of toys that can be manipulated and pushed on the floor. This is a period of exploration of objects and space using the eyes, ears, fingers and mouth. There are many kinds of sensory experiences that can be offered to a child at this age. The main thing is to provide toys or objects that will help him/her to discover. Don't be impatient and don't anticipate how a child will react to a toy. The child will react to it in his/her own way and time.

In the next few months the child will progress from creeping to walking. This is one of life's most significant events and opens up a whole new world to be explored. Up to this point, most of the things the child has reacted to were presented by the parent and while this continues to be important, the child if given some freedom to explore has a real opportunity to develop the senses. The attitude of the parent in this period is of utmost importance. The baby in most cases becomes an avid explorer and will be into everything. It is important to "babyproof" the home and make it stimulating but safe. Objects should be put aside that cannot be easily replaced because of personal or monetary value and a check should be made to see that items cannot be reached which might be harmful to the child. This period can be a trying time for parents and is certainly one that will test their patience. The child, if permitted, will not leave anything unexplored. A baby may unravel the toilet paper and splash in the toilet bowl, pull all the contents out of the drawers, remove the pots and pans from the cabinets, pour out the soap chips and the salt, manipulate the T.V. controls and may soon be writing on the walls and in the books with crayons, pens and pencils. It is a hectic period but can be a fascinating time depending upon the attitude of the parent. Life is much simpler at this stage if the movements of the baby are restricted. It is easier to place the child in a playpen, lock the doors and scold or ignore his/her urges to explore. However, this period in the child's life is too important to ignore and there is ample research to show that a restrictive environment may be the cause of a child's motor, social, emotional or intellectual retardation. The child's freedom to explore and move at his/her own pace expands the capacity to respond to varied stimuli. It is through exploration and movement that perception is developed. A child gradually becomes aware of and can descriminate between size, shape, weight, distance, color, and texture; these concepts serve as a foundation for symbolic learning.

There is, of course, concern among parents and disagreement among psychologists as to the desirable degree of freedom in the environmental setting. The idea just expressed could lead the reader to believe that the infant should have complete and total reign. That was not the intention, for the child must also learn to become a sociable being and part of the family structure. Parents who are cognizant of the total development of the child will probably be able to decide the limitations without too much trouble.

After the child can walk, pull-type toys can help increase proficiency, and a toy that also makes a sound as it is being moved adds to the novelty.

During the second year, there is a refinement of motor skills. The child becomes more aware of the environment and can begin simple matching tasks starting with a simple form board puzzle. The child may repeat simple tasks over and over again. During this year the child will understand the permanency of objects. He/she realizes that when things are out of sight they have not vanished permanently. As the child progresses through the second year, perceptual awareness expands greatly. The opportunities for exploring and manipulating continue to be an important part of development. Toys should be selected for their ability to lead the child toward understanding concepts as big, little, up, down, in, out, on, off, over, under and should be those which can be manipulated and mastered.

By the age of three the child has left the infant world. Provided a normal environment in which to grow, the child has gained a sensory control over the surroundings. In two years the world has expanded greatly, and into the third year it will continue to expand and become even more diverse. The child now has two years of past experiences upon which to build. The child's world will become more physical. It will be a time of refining the motor skills already in progress and a time to add new skills. At this stage of development it becomes difficult to be specific in suggesting what experiences to provide for children in general. There is considerable variation among children at this age and the motor and sensory experiences provided for any particular child will depend upon the child's background. The child should be observed closely and provided with challenging experiences which can be mastered. The parents should give their approval and encouragement to the child's efforts, but at the same time parents must be careful not to become too ambitious or overenthusiastic. Placing too great an emphasis on the child to succeed could result in the child becoming anxious and possibly even withdrawing from the activity.

Early Environmental Conditions

Research is showing that the preschool years are the years of most rapid growth in physical and intellectual development and that the nature of the environment plays a vital role in shaping the child. Since parents are the first teachers of children and continue this role until the child goes to school, there is need for concern about the optimal environment in the preschool years. The child needs maximal opportunities for movement experiences, physical activity and play. These represent natural childhood activities. In fact, the first responses of an infant are motor responses and his progress through early life is measured in terms of movements; even intelligence is determined by motor responses. Movement then, seems to be the essence of childhood. Later symbolic understanding is a process of building on perceptions formed through the child's movement world. Opportunity for a child to learn and develop through activities that are self-initiated and self-enjoyed are the ones through which he/she is going to benefit most readily. As pointed out by Godfrey and Kephart (1968), the activities "which contribute to the exploration of his environment are of greatest significance for education. The young child gains his initial information about the environment around him through exploration. Such exploration involves movement through space and the manipulations of objects. Both of these aspects are dependent upon motor activities and the ability to control motor responses."

The concept that motor development is an essential foundation to all aspects of learning and development is not new. The idea of learning through discovery, learning by doing and learning through movement has been proclaimed through the ages by educators like Socrates, Locke, Rousseau and Dewey. There are many psychologists and educators who are also presently promoting this concept. Piaget (Flavell 1963), the Swiss psychologist, perhaps the foremost authority on intellectual development of this century, has developed a theoretical framework of successive stages of intellectual growth that a child passes through on the way toward mature intelligence. The four major stages are the sensory motor stage, the preoperational stage, the concrete operational stage, and the formal operational stage. There are subdivisions within these stages. No exact time period can be assigned to these stages, but the sensory motor stage covers approximately the period from birth when the child is capable of only reflex activity, to the age of eighteen months or two years, when the child is capable of thought. The preoperational stage follows until about age seven and the concrete operational stage follows until about age twelve. The formal operational stage extends from twelve onward. Although these periods represent a progressively developing intellect, movement and movement experiences are particularly important in the first three stages, or from birth to age twelve.

Marie Montessori (Orem 1965) has also had an impact on childhood education. Her concepts are similar to those of Piaget in that she recognizes a sensory motor period and recognizes this period as the base to subsequent stages of intellectual development. The Montessori method emphasizes freedom of movement. She realized that the acquisition of motor skills is a crucial ingredient in the young child's understanding of and adjustment to the world of persons, things and ideas.

Getman (1964), an optometrist who became interested in academic performance because of his interest in vision, has a similar view. He believes that 80 percent of what is learned is learned visually. The program that he proposes includes a background of movement experiences which form a basis for symbolic learning.

Barsch (1965, 1967, 1968) has done some pioneer work with an educational theory called movigenics which deals with the origin and development of movement patterns leading to learning efficiency. Here

again we see the concept that the basis of learning is rooted in movement experiences.

Frostig (1970), an educational psychologist, also relies heavily on movement as the basis of her program. Through movement she develops sensory motor skills, creativity, body awareness and other facets related to learning.

Kephart (1971) has done extensive work with slow learners and brain damaged children. He believes that movement is the basis for learning. His theories embrace the development of body image, laterality, directionality, and perceptual-motor matching all of which are developed or enhanced through movement experiences.

There are also several authorities of child learning who employ movement skills directly in teaching concepts. Frostig uses whole body movements in teaching mathematics, reading, and other subjects. Both Humphrey (1965) and Cratty (1969) have promoted the idea of teaching reading, writing and number concepts through games.

The number of authorities who recognize the importance of early motor experiences — play and acquisition of skills — is by no means exhausted in the few examples presented. They, however, represent a central theme which should give insight to the order of learning. Learning is an active process and exploration, play and motor skills should be of primary concern in the early years. Through these concrete experiences, the child develops the concepts necessary for abstract thinking.

An effort has been made here to develop the relationship between motor development and the cognitive process. Motor development has long been accepted by parents and teachers as being important in itself and as being essential to physical, social and emotional development. This, however, has not brought any great demand to have motor development accepted as an intricate part of the curriculum. In general, parents and school board members see the primary function of the school in terms of intellectual development rather than total self-realization.

Movement experiences and motor skill learning are a preschool and elementary school function. By the eighth grade the child should have competency in a wide variety of motor activities. The ability to learn motor skills comes early. As pointed out earlier, Hunsicker (1963) states that research shows that a child by the age of ten has the neuromucular potential to master the skills normally taught at the college level. Adjustments may be necessary in the size and weight of some of the equipment but the child possess the capacity to learn.

While we know that children can learn early, we still do not know the best time to teach specific skills. Children are probably capable of far more than we suspect. Although norms are available on a number of motor skills, they merely tell us what the average child can do, not what he/she might be capable of doing if given the opportunity, guidance, and encouragement. The author conducted a study of climbing skills of kindergarten children. He tested 146 children on a variety of climbing items and found what could be expected of the average five-year-old (at least in the group he tested). During the study a two-year-old boy had daily access to the climbing equipment, and at twenty-seven months of age could far exceed the average climbing skill level of the kindergarten children tested. There was nothing mysterious about this, the child just had an opportunity to climb not afforded most of the other children. His climbing ability nevertheless was a bit surprising. It is likely that we will have many surprises just as soon as we give our children an opportunity to learn. It would be interesting to know the best time to teach a child to swim. There are swimming programs available for children as young as three months. Children are born with a swimming reflex and the idea of these programs is to take advantage of the reflex before it disappears. Whether this is a sound procedure or not remains to be decided. We have already seen that children of the Manus tribe can swim by the age of three. It appears logical that in America we should have swimming in our nursery school programs or at least in early elementary grades. In most cases today a gymnasium is not a part of the educational complex, let alone a swimming pool.

It appears that one of the primary tasks of educators is to change the traditional thinking concerning the time when movement experience should be taught. In light of what is now known concerning the importance of motor movement, fundamental skill development and sensory motor experience for early childhood development it is absurd that our best physical education programs are still at the college and high school level. Including movement education or physical education as an integral part of the preschool and elementary school program should receive prime consideration in the search for new approaches toward helping the child attain his optimal potential.

Key Principles for Establishing a Motor Development Program

There are a number of principles that act as guidelines in establishing an environmental setting for early childhood development.

The author lists and briefly comments on the key principles used in the motor development program at Wake Forest University.

1. A positive self-concept is essential to positive learning.

   Attention given to self-concept is one of the initial steps in dealing with children attending the motor learning laboratory. Children are continually recognized and complimented for themselves and for their achievements. The better the child begins to feel about himself or herself the faster the responses to the challenges presented in the laboratory.

2. Opportunity to learn is essential to learning.

   This principle is so obvious that it is often overlooked. If the readers review the past several pages, they will see a reference made to "opportunity" many times. For learning to occur, other ingredients are important besides opportunity, but without opportunity learning cannot occur.

3. Learning is best achieved by providing information or experiences just beyond what is already known or experienced.

   The task, mental or physical, that the child undertakes, or is asked to undertake, must be only slightly removed from what the child already knows or has experienced. The new material will more readily be assimilated if it is associated with similar knowledges or experiences the child has in his or her repertoire.

4. The environment should be child oriented, offering a wide range of movement possibilities of varying degrees of complexity.

Provide the child with the opportunity to seek challenges within known competency levels. The environment should provide opportunities for experimentation, exploration, and problem solving. The parent or teacher should provide encouragement, understanding, and some guidance. In this way the child will meet with success and grow in confidence. Learning should be a positive, enjoyable experience.

SUMMARY

This section deals first with the changes that a child undergoes in the developmental pattern from conception to age six. The last part of the section encompasses some of the implications these changes have for learning.

All human organisms follow a rather consistent predictable pattern of development. Two directional patterns of development are that growth tends to proceed from the head to the feet or in a cephalocaudal direction and that growth proceeds from the center of the body toward the periphery or in a proximodistal direction. Behavioral changes evolve as a process of both maturation and interaction with the environment.

Behavior begins in prenatal life. Movement occurs about the eighth week after conception. Initial movements are reflex activities which become more complex until by birth the baby has quite a repertoire of motor responses. These motor responses are all reflex or subcortical. There is no evidence of cortical control until several weeks after birth. By six weeks the baby begins to respond voluntarily to its environment. At first it can only explore visually but soon after three months the baby begins using the arms and hands for exploring. Attaining the upright locomotive position is one of the major motor functions of the maturing infant, and involves a long complex sequence of skills. There is a wide variation among children in learning to walk, ranging from seven to eighteen months, but the average is around thirteen to fourteen months. The walking pattern serves as the base for many other skills like running, jumping, hopping, galloping, and skipping. By the age of six the child will have learned a number of motor skills if given the opportunity.

Understanding the growth pattern and capabilities of children at different ages helps parents and teachers establish realistic experiences for them. Helping children develop is mainly a matter of offering stimulation and challenging stimuli to which they can respond. Research has shown that an environment rich in sensory stimulation has led to positive behavioral changes whereas environments restricted in sensory experiences have resulted in retardation of social, motor and intellectual development. The proper environment then is being sensitive to the varying sensory experiences which are appropriate to the child as he/she grows.

Whether nursery school and prenursery schools are necessary depends upon the ability of the parents to provide an environment conducive to optimal development of the child. An environment based upon motor development, opportunity for exploration and object manipulation, play, and fundamental motor skill development seems to be appropriate for developing the concepts upon which later cognitive processes are formed. Sensory and motor experiences are a function of the developmental years and opportunity for their occurrence should be abundant. In light of what is now known, move-ment education and/or physical education should be a part of the preschool and elementary school program.

References

Barsch, Ray H. *Movigenic Curriculum*. State Department of Public Instruction, Bureau for Handicapped Children, Bulletin No. 25, Madison, Wisconsin, 1965.

———. *Achieving Perceptual-Motor Efficiency*. (Volume 1 of a Perceptual-Motor Curriculum). Seattle: Special Child Publication, Inc., 1967.

———. *Enriching Perception and Cognition*. (Volume 2 of a Perceptual-Motor Curriculum). Seattle: Special Child Publication, Inc., 1968.

Brazelton, Berry. *"Are There Too Many Sights and Sounds in Your Baby's World?"* Redbook. Volume 137, No. 5. September 1971.

Caldwell, Bettye, "What is the Optimal Learning Environment for the Young Child" Early Childhood Education Rediscovered, edited by Joe L. Frost. New York: Holt, Rinehart & Winston, Inc., 1968.

Cratty, B., and Sister Margaret Mary Martin. *Perceptual-Motor Efficiency in Children*. Philadelphia: Lea and Febiger, 1969.

Dennis, Wayne. *Readings in Child Psychology*, 2d ed. Englewood Cliffs, N.J.: Prentice-Hill, Inc., 1963.

Frostig, Marianne. *Movement Education Theory and Practice*. Chicago, Illinois: Follett Educational Corporation, 1970.

Flavell, John H. *The Developmental Psychology of Jean Piaget*. Princeton, N.J.: D. Van Nostrand Company, Inc., 1963.

Getman, G. N. and Kane, E. R. *The Physiology of Readiness. An Action Program for the Development of Perception for Children*. Minneapolis, Minnesota: P.A.S.S., Inc., 1964.

Godfrey, Barbara and Newell Kephart. *Movement Patterns and Motor Education*. New York: Appleton-Century-Crofts, 1969.

Humphrey, James. *Child Learning Through Elementary School Physical Education*. Dubuque, Ia.: Wm. C. Brown Company Publishers, 1965.

Hunsicker, Paul. *Physical Fitness. What Research Says to the Teacher No. 2.* Washington, D.C., Department of Classroom Teachers, National Education Association, 1963.

Kephart, Newell C. *The Slow Learner in the Classroom.* Columbus, Ohio: Charles E. Merrill Publishing Co., 1971.

McGraw, Myrtle. "Later Development of Children Specially Trained During Infancy." *Child Development* 10(1939):1.

Orem, R. C. *A. Montessori Handbook.* New York: G. P. Putnam's Sons, 1965.

Scott, John P. *Early Experience and the Organization of Behavior.* Belmont, California: Brooks/Cole Publishing Company, Inc., 1968.

Section 4

Fundamental Motor Skills: Learning and Refining

Motor Skill Developmental Analysis: An Introduction

7

Michael J. Stewart
Kansas State University
Karen DeOreo
Kent State University

The purpose of this section is to examine the basic components of key fundamental skills. The emphasis is on the "how" of the performance, rather that the "how much" of the performance. Though there are many skills which could be included, only the basic skills of walking, running, jumping, kicking, and throwing are included. For ease in discussion these are divided into locomotor skills including walking, running and jumping, and non-locomotor skills including kicking and throwing.

Most children have some degree of proficiency in the fundamental motor skills by the time they enter school. The degree to which these skills have been refined depends in part on the enrichment programs or experiences to which the child has been exposed (see Sections III and VIII). Therefore, one would expect to see a variety of developmental levels among children of elementary school age. This is not only supported by the research, but can easily be seen by casual observations of children at play.

Corbin (1976) has suggested that the elementary school years (prior to the age of 12) are the skill learning years, and the years after age 12 are the skill refining years. However, a closer analysis indicates that for many, the elementary years are actually the skill refining years for fundamental motor skills. The acquisition of fundamental skills seems to occur in two phases, skill learning and skill refinement. In fundamental skill learning children progress through various levels of performance. The child first makes beginning attempts at the skill, followed by an immature performance, then a more mature or advanced level of performance. In Chapters 8 and 9 the beginning attempt (Level 1), the immature performance (Level 2), and the more mature performance (Level 3) for each skill will be described. By the time the child is able to perform a skill at Level 3, it can be said that the skill is "learned." The basic ingredients of a mature performance are present. However, it is clear that the performance of the skill may still be far from that of an athlete or highly skilled adult. For optimal performance to occur the skill must be refined.

The child actually begins to refine performance of fundamental skills from the very first time the skill is attempted. However, when we refer to skill refinement we are generally speaking of the improvement of skilled performance which occurs *after* Level 3 has been achieved. For skill refinement to occur at least minimum levels of strength are a prerequisite. With practice the skills become more refined but only if the practice takes into account the important underlying mechanical principles of movement. In Chapters 10 and 11 some of the mechanical principles necessary for skill refinement are described. Also included are Developmental Analysis Checklists for each of the skills. These lists may be used to evaluate motor performance or as lists of factors important to learning and refining fundamental movement skills.

WORDS OF CAUTION

As previously noted each child progresses differently, and for this reason one may learn a fundamental skill at a different age than another. Some may never really *learn* to perform the fundamental skills; that is, they may never perform at Level 3 for the skills described in Chapters 8 and 9. Others will *learn* the skill but never *refine* them and therefore never achieve optimal performance levels. Depending on the ability and current performance of an individual, regardless of age, the emphasis will either be on *learning* or on *refining*. For those who are still learning, attention should focus on progressing through the three Levels of Performance described at the end of each section of Chapters 8 and 9. After skills have been learned at Level 3 the emphasis should shift to skill refinement and the information included in the Developmental Analysis Checklists should be emphasized. *To emphasize skill refinement before relatively mature performance is present may be counterproductive.*

References

Corbin, C. B. *Becoming Physically Educated in Elementary School,* 2nd ed. Philadelphia: Lea and Febiger, 1976.

Fundamental Locomotor Skills

8

Michael J. Stewart
Kansas State University

In this chapter the locomotor skills of walking, running, and jumping will be discussed. At the end of the discussion of each skill a summary of three levels of performance is provided. Level 1 represents the early or beginning attempts, Level 2 represents immature but improved performance, and Level 3 represents a mature but unrefined movement performance. These levels can be useful in trying to identify the current performance level of children and also to help children learn to perform the skill effectively.

WALKING

Walking is defined by Broer as ". . . a matter of distributing the mechanical equilibrium of the body, pushing the body forward, and forming successive new bases by moving the legs forward alternately" (Broer 1973, 145). Walking then, is a fundamental motor task which is characterized by a rotary movement of the legs which moves the leg as well as the body forward in a linear motion. Furthermore, the entire action takes place without a period of nonsupport. One foot is always in contact with the walking surface.

Walking usually follows crawling. As the infant crawler becomes increasingly more curious about the environment, an upright bipedal locomotive type of motor task, walking, is attempted. Although the new fundamental motor task presents some learning difficulties, not to mention bumps and bruises, the infant soon discovers the numerous advantages of upright locomotion.

As any other type of fundamental motor task which is new to an individual's repertory of movement, walking is at first difficult. Before an infant can walk, he/she must first attain enough strength and maintain enough balance to stand. The developmental sequence of walking passes through a series of levels, beginning at the immature level with very jerky, unstable movements, and progressing to the mature level which is a free flowing, integrated movement.

In Shirley's classic research (1931) in which she studied the postural and locomotive development of the infant during the first two years of life, she identified four stages of development in the walking process. They were: 1) knees straight stepping, 2) standing with help, 3) walking when led, and 4) walking alone. This chapter will begin with Shirley's fourth stage, walking alone. It will discuss the developmental sequence from the time an infant takes the first step alone, until he or she is performing the fundamental motor task at a mature level.

Footwork

Although some infants show signs of "dancing," or walking on their toes (Shirley, 1931), in the initial stages of walking, flat-footedness is characteristic. In a study by Burnett and Johnson (1971) in which the gait of 28 children was studied to determine its development, it was reported that occasionally infants would place their heels down first, but the development of the heel strike was inconsistent in beginning walkers. Toeing out seems to be a general characteristic during first attempts at walking (Shirley, 1931), and although some infants demonstrate a pigeon-toed walking behavior, it is considered abnormal (Engel and Staheli, 1974). The width of the step during initial attempts is somewhat wide, but does narrow as the infant becomes more proficient at this fundamental motor task (Burnett and Johnson, 1971). Soon after the infant becomes proficient at walking, placement of the foot comes within the lateral dimensions of the trunk and narrows very little after the initial adjustment (Scrutton, 1969).

Hip Action

As mentioned in the beginning paragraphs of this chapter, the rotary movement of the leg at the hip enables the legs to alternately swing forward, which allows the infant to move forward in a linear motion. In the initial attempts at walking, the infant demonstrates hip and knee flexion with the lower extremity externally rotated or abducted. As the gait of the infant becomes more mature, a decrease in hip and knee flexion during the swing phase and an increase in hip, knee, and ankle extension in the propulsive leg is demonstrated (Statham and Murray, 1971). Pelvic tilt, as well as pelvic rotation are evidenced during the initial stage of walking and increases as the fundamental motor task becomes more mature (Burnett and Johnson, 1971).

Arm Action

Arms of the infant walker are abducted, and in the elbow-flexed position. This position is often referred to as the "on guard" position and derives its name from the fact

that the infant is actually preparing for the many falls that are characteristic during this unstable period of the infant's life. As stability increases in the infant, the arms are held at the side and swing alternately in a vertical arc in opposition to the legs. It was reported by Burnett and Johnson (1971) that this behavior seems to accompany the narrowing of the stance, as described in the area of footwork. The arm swing tends to be directed toward the midline of the body, but for the most part is in the antero-posterior plane. During the normal walking pace, the forward movement of the arm is approximately twice that of the backward movement when observed from the resting position.

Summary of the Development of Walking

Level 1. The individual walks with exaggerated hip and knee flexion and places the forward foot down in a flatfooted and abducted fashion. There is little evidence of extension in the hip, leg, and ankle of the propulsive leg. Arms of the individual are held in an on-guard position and are used primarily for protection. A wide step is utilized to provide a stable base of support.

Level 2. Hip and knee flexion of the individual is decreased and arms are held to the side and swing alternately in opposition to the legs, but seem to cross the midline of the body. There is a narrowing of the stance and the abduction of the foot is decreased.

Level 3. Hip and knee flexion of the individual continues to decrease and the arms are held to the side and swing in a vertical arc in opposition to the legs. Arm swing is increased with the forward movement of the arm approximately twice that of the backward movement. The stance, or base of support comes within the lateral dimensions of the body with the heel striking the surface first. The hip, leg, and ankle of the propulsive leg are fully extended.

RUNNING

Running is a fundamental motor task which is utilized in almost all sport skills and for that matter, in the everyday behavior of many individuals. Whether the individual is participating in a low organized game, a highly specialized sport, or a backyard game, the nature of activity usually requires the individual to run.

Running possesses many of the characteristics of walking. The major difference distinguishing a run from a walk is the period of non-support in the run. As pointed out earlier in the discussion concerning walking, at least one foot is always in contact with the ground, whereas in the run, there is a brief moment when the body is in flight. This period of non-support could be described as a series of leaps, or as Slocum and James defined it, "Running is really a series of smoothly coordinated jumps during which the body weight is borne on one foot, becomes airborne, is then carried on the opposite foot and again becomes airborne" (Slocum and James 1968, p. 98). As one can imagine, an improvement in the ability to balance and an increase in leg strength is required before the infant can perform a true run.

Footwork

Since many infants begin to run before they reach the mature level of the walk (Broer, 1973), the footwork of the run is quite similar to that of the walk in its initial stages. Those infants who have developed mature patterns of walking often revert to the immature pattern of locomotion in first attempting to run (Burnett and Johnson, 1971). For example, the foot of the running infant is placed on the running surface in a flatfooted fashion rather than in a toe first fashion as Deshon and Helson (1964) and Slocum and James (1968) describe the mature sprinter. Infants usually stand with a wide base of support to insure stability in the lateral plane and this behavior is often seen in the running infant. With increased maturity, the infant runner narrows the width of the base of support as balance has improved with maturation and practice. But as Scrutton (1969) pointed out following his study of 97 clinically normal children, out toeing is often demonstrated in infant runners to increase lateral stability. In out-toeing, the infant is able to use dorsi flexors and plantar flexors to assume some of the responsibility for lateral stability. During the beginning stages of running, the forward foot can be observed striking the ground well beyond the center of gravity. As the running behavior of the infant matures, the relative distance of the forward foot striking the surface ahead of the center of gravity is decreased. With the forward foot striking the surface directly under the center of gravity, the infant no longer lands with obvious flatfootedness.

Leg Action

In initial attempts at running, the infant can be described as bouncing and seems to be exerting more effort upward than forward. This behavior is due in part to the lack of extension of the propulsive leg. With increased maturity, the extension of the propulsive leg is increased and contributes to a lessening of upward movement of the body during the run. This increase in the extension of the propulsive leg also contributes to the increase in length of stride of the infant runner, thus increasing the period of non-support and ultimately the speed of the runner.

The infant runner also demonstrates very little knee lift during the immature stage. Bunn (1955), Fenn (1930), and Cureton (1935) describe the mature runner as having a very high knee lift at the end of the forward leg swing. It is also characteristic of mature running behavior to demonstrate maximum flexion of the recovery leg at the knee on the forward swing of the recovery leg. In other words, as the infant runner becomes more proficient in running behavior, during the forward leg swing of the recovery leg, the heel of that foot comes closer to the buttocks. The knee of the recovery leg also tends to swing outward in the immature stage, but as the runner becomes more proficient, the outward swing becomes progressively less.

Arm Action

Arm action of the fundamental motor task of running is an area which has not received nearly as much attention as the areas of footwork and leg action. Although arm action is important in walking, it is by no means as important as it is in running. Since running is a forceful action, the movement of the arms are thus forceful and seem to travel through a wider range of motion than when an individual is walking.

As in walking, the arms swing in opposition to the legs. In the immature stages of running, the infant seems to carry the arms flexed and in the on-guard position as in the beginning stages of walking. This position, if one recalls, is purported to be for protection should the infant fall. In the early stages of running, there does not appear to be much rotary movement of the arms at the shoulder, thus causing the arms to move with the rotary movement of the trunk. With this action the hands cross the midline of the body as the infant runs. This action is often referred to as "hooking of the arms." This action, of course, tends to cause the arms to "loop" outward during the backward swing. As the runner becomes more proficient, the mature stage is characterized by less "hooking" and more anteroposterior swing of the arms. On the forward swing the hand swings nearly shoulder level and on the backward swing, the elbow reaches almost as high, with the hand passing the hip posteriorly. Wickstrom (1977) points out that the angle of the elbow changes during the different positions of the arm swing. In other words, the angle of the arm at the elbow of a mature runner is near a right angle at the highest point of the upswing and increases during the downswing. As the arm passes the hip posteriorly the angle of the arm at the elbow is decreased and once again is at a near right angle, but this time during the backswing.

Summary of the Development of Running

Level 1. The individual has a very short period of non-support. The foot lands upon the surface well beyond the center of gravity in a flatfooted fashion, with a toeing out of the forward foot. Arms of the individual are carried in an on-guard manner. The individual demonstrates a "bouncing" motion as the body is propelled forward.

Level 2. The period of non-support is increased and the foot strike is placed nearly under the center of gravity. Less toeing out is evidenced and the arms are used more, but a hooking toward the midline of the body is demonstrated. Very little elbow flexion is demonstrated. There seems to be less bouncing of the body during the run, and there is an increase in the knee lift of the forward leg and an extension of the hip, knee and ankle of the propulsive leg.

Level 3. For sprinting or very fast running the foot strike is toe first and directly under the center of gravity. The period of non-support is maximal. Toeing out is not evidenced and hip flexion of the striding leg is maximal. Hip, knee, and ankle extension of the propulsive leg is increased. The arms of the individual swing in opposition with the legs in an anteroposterior motion, and are in an elbow flexed position.

JUMPING

Jumping is a fundamental motor skill which can be observed in many different forms. For example, the high jumper, the long jumper, the hurdler, as well as the triple jumper are performing a type of jump. A jump can be defined as leaving the ground from one or two feet and landing upon both feet simultaneously. The simultaneous two-foot landing is the characteristic which distinguishes a true jump from a leap and hop.

Jumping of many forms has been researched for four decades. Jumping from an elevated area to a lower surface area has been studied by Bayley (1935) and McCaskill and Wellman (1938). Poe (1976), and Martin and Stull (1969) have studied the vertical jump to attempt to describe the components of age related characteristics and manipulate experimental conditions to elicit improved performance. The characteristics of the running long jump have been researched by Cooper and Glassow (1976). This study was concerned with process or "how to" components rather than the product components (how much) of the running long jump.

The section will address itself to the standing long jump. It differs from the vertical jump in that it represents a change of direction in which the jump takes place, and from the running long jump in that there is not a preliminary run to the jump. In the initial stages, the standing long jump and the vertical jump have many similarities as both appear to be vertical jumps. As the jumper becomes more proficient, the jumps become more distinguishable due to the angle of propulsion — the vertical jump closer to 90 degrees and the standing long jump closer to 45 degrees. Figure 8.1 illustrates the developmental sequence of long jumping. The Hellebrandt, et al. (1961) study of the standing long jump, describes subjects as performing a behavior similar to a bipedal hop rather than a jump for horizontal distance.

Footwork

Although the standing long jump is characterized by a simultaneous two-foot take-off and two-foot landing, first attempts at the standing long jump do not follow this

Level 1

Level 2

Level 3

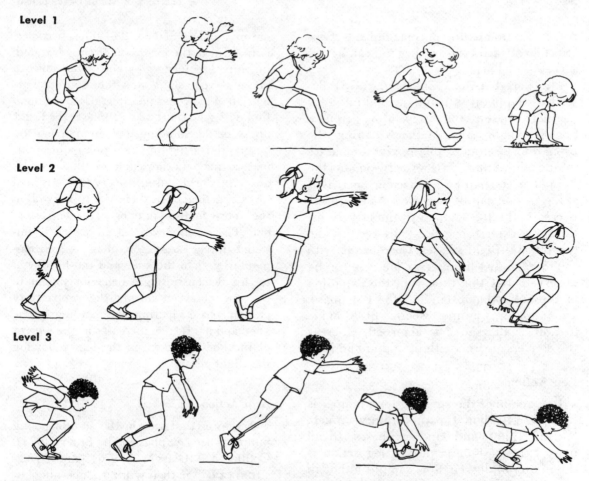

Figure 8.1 The developmental sequence of the standing long jump. (From McClenaghan, B. and Gallahue, D., *Fundamental Movement: A Developmental and Remedial Approach.* Philadelphia: W. B. Saunders Company, 1978. Redrawn with permission.)

pattern. Hellebrandt, et al. (1961) noted that infants demonstrated jumping patterns long before they were strong enough to propel themselves into space. Children at this stage can be observed as using the preliminary leg crouch, the trunk flexion, and the arm movement utilized in the standing long jump, yet when all body parts are extended, the feet do not leave the ground. After the child has gained enough strength to propel his or her body into space, the standing long jumper can be observed taking off with one

foot, then the other, and landing in a similar manner. During these immature stages the take-off point and the landing point are the same. Wickstrom (1977) suggested that a more mature pattern is characterized by a thrust in the horizontal plane rather than in the vertical plane. In other words, the standing long jumper does not land in the same place from which he or she took off, but rather at a location or distance in front of, and horizontal from the take-off position. Furthermore, as the standing long jump becomes more mature, a simultaneous two-foot takeoff and two-foot landing can be observed.

McClenaghan and Gallahue (1978) described the jump as being divided into four distinct phases: the preparatory crouch, takeoff, flight, and landing. During the preparatory crouch phase, the immature jumper shows very little ankle flexion. As the jumper becomes more proficient, increased ankle flexion can be observed. As the thrust is created by the immature jumper very little ankle extension can be observed in the takeoff and flight phases. Once again, with the more mature jumper, an increase can be observed, but this time with the extension of the ankle. Upon landing, the last phase, an immature jumper shows little ankle flexion as the shock is absorbed, whereas the converse is true with the mature jumper.

Leg Action

Leg action of the standing long jumper is best described in the preparatory crouch, takeoff, flight, and landing phases. In all phases the best descriptor of leg action is the matter of degree. For example, although knee and hip flexion is demonstrated in the immature jumper during the preparatory crouch phase, it is far less than the flexion demonstrated by the mature jumper. Cooper and Glassow (1976) noted that the thigh position of mature jumpers nears being horizontal during the preparatory crouch. Since the body must be lifted through the distance that it is lowered, the optimal distance of the preparatory crouch depends upon the strength of the leg muscles (Broer, 1973). Since there seems to be some relationship with leg strength and age, an increase in knee flexion is observed as the child gains leg strength.

During the takeoff phase, little extension of the knee and hip is observed in the immature jumper, but as the jump becomes more refined, the extension of the knee and the hip becomes apparent. The takeoff phase is very short, and therefore the extension of the knee and hip is also shortlived. Following the short takeoff phase, the flight phase of the standing long jumper can be observed. During the flight phase of the immature jumper, the extension that can be observed during takeoff (very little) is held for some time. The behavior observed in the more mature jumper is quite different. The complete extension which is initiated during the takeoff phase is held momentarily, then the knee and the hip begin to flex demonstrating a behavior similar to the one observed during the preparatory crouch phase. During the landing phase knee and hip flexion increases as the weight of the body is taken on the legs following the flight phase.

Arm Action

Action of the arms in the standing long jump has been emphasized by Broer (1973), Cooper and Glassow (1976), and Wickstrom (1977) in their writing concerning human movement. During the initial stages of attempting the standing long jump, the arms are used primarily for balance, rather than for an increase in momentum. Broer (1973) points out that the momentum of the arm swing is transferred to the upper body and, if timed properly with leg extension, adds to the force of the jump. Since the arm action during the initial attempts at the standing long jump is awkward and unnatural, it is apparent that the arm action does not contribute much to the force of the jump. As the jump becomes more refined, the arms are used more to propel the body forward than for maintaining balance. As the arm action becomes a propelling force, the arms can be observed moving in a sideward motion or path as opposed to a backward-forward motion or path which is characteristic of the mature jumper. During the **preparatory** crouch phase of the standing long jump the arms of the immature jumper can be observed moving backward and upward, but with little extension at the shoulder and oftentimes the movement between the two arms does not follow the same path or extend the same distance. As the jump becomes more refined the arm action becomes more bilateral in appearance. In the mature jump Wickstrom (1977) points out that as the arms travel backward and upward during the preparatory crouch, the arms reach a point well above the horizontal plane of the trunk. Furthermore, during the takeoff and flight phases, the arms are extended well above the head and in line with the trunk, acting as a long lever to react against the legs during the flight phase. During the landing phase, the arm action of the mature standing long jumper is basically the same as during the takeoff and flight phases; continuing to reach out and assist in bringing the center of gravity over the feet and to regain balance.

Body and Takeoff Angle

When distance is the purpose of the standing long jump, physical laws propose a projection of 45-degree angle is the most efficient. Initial attempts at the standing long jump (as indicated earlier) resemble a vertical jump which is closer to a 90-degree takeoff. As the jump becomes more refined, and arm action is employed, the jumper is more able to lean forward, thus shifting the center of gravity ahead of the feet at takeoff. This, of course, allows the angle of takeoff to be closer to the desirable 45 degrees. Jumpers which Zimmerman (1956) studied

demonstrated an average takeoff angle near 45 degrees. These jumpers were all classified as good jumpers. Therefore, one would suspect to see more mature jumpers approaching a 45 degree angle takeoff in the standing long jump.

Summary of the Development of the Standing Long Jump

Level 1. The individual jumps in a path more to a vertical than horizontal plane. There is little use of the arms in either the backswing or upswing. The feet normally do not leave or come back in contact with the surface simultaneously. Furthermore, there is very little preparatory flexion of the ankles, knees, or hips nor little flexion of those parts upon landing.

Level 2. The horizontal distance of the jump is increased and the vertical distance is decreased. The arms are used to some extent, but do not extend past the body in a backward motion during the preparatory phase. There is an increase in ankle, knee, and hip flexion during the preparatory and landing phases.

Level 3. Ankle, knee, and hip flexion is increased during the preparatory and landing phases and the angle of takeoff is decreased to approximately 45 degrees. There is a complete extension of the ankle, knee, hip, and arms during the takeoff phase. During the preparatory phase, the arms are extended at the shoulder backward and upward well behind the body.

References

Bayley, N. "The Development of Motor Abilities the First Three Years." *Monograph Social Research of Child Development* 1 (1935):1.

Broer, M. *Efficiency of Human Movement*, 3rd ed. Philadelphia: W. B. Saunders Company, 1973.

Bunn, J. *Scientific Principles of Coaching*. Englewood Cliffs, N.J.: Prentice Hall, 1955.

Burnett, C. N. and Johnson, E. W. "Development of Gait in Childhood, Part II." *Developmental Medicine and Child Neurology* 13 (1971):207.

Cooper, J. M. and Glassow, R. B. *Kinesiology*. St. Louis: C. V. Mosley Company, 1976.

Corbin, C. B. *Becoming Physically Educated in the Elementary School*, 2nd ed. Philadelphia: Lea and Febiger, 1976.

Cureton, T. K. "Mechanics of Track Running." *Scholastic Coach* 4(1935):7-10.

Deshon, D. E. and Helson, R. C. "A Cinematographical Analysis of Sprint Running." *Research Quarterly* 35(1964):451.

Engel, G. M. and Staheli, L. T. "The Natural History of Torsion and Other Factors Influencing Gait in Childhood." *Clinical Orthopaedics and Related Research* 99(1974):12.

Fenn, W. O. "A Cinematographical Study of Sprinters." *Science Monthly* 93(1930):443-62.

Hellebrandt, F. A.; Rarick, G. L; Glassow, R.; and Carns, M. L. "Physiological Analysis of Basic Motor Skills: 1. Growth and Development of Jumping." *American Journal of Physical Medicine* 40(1961):14.

Martin, T. P. and Stull, G. A. "Effects of Various Knee Angle and Foot Spacing Combinations on Performance in the Vertical Jump." *Research Quarterly* 40(1969):324.

McCaskill, C. L. and Wellman, B. L. "A Study of Common Motor Achievements at the Preschool Ages." *Child Development* 9(1938):141.

McClenaghan, B. A. and Gallahue, D. L. *Fundamental Movement: A Developmental and Remedial Approach*. Philadelphia: W. B. Saunders Company, 1978.

Poe, A. "Description of the Movement Characteristics of Two-Year-Old Children Performing the Jump and Reach." *Research Quarterly* 47(1976):260.

Scrutton, D. S. "Footprint Seauences of Normal Children Under Five Years Old." *Developmental Medicine and Child Neurology* 11 (1969):44.

Shirley, M. M. *The First Two Years: A Study of Twenty-five Babies, Volume 1, Postural and Locomotor Development*. Minneapolis: University of Minnesota Press, 1931.

Slocum, D. B. and James, S. L. "Biomechanics of Running." *Journal of American Medical Association* 205(1968):11, 97.

Statham, L. and Murray, M. P. "Early Walking Patterns of Normal Children." *Clinical Orthopaedics and Related Research* 79 (1971):8.

Wellman, B. L. "Motor Achievement of Preschool Children." *Childhood Education* 13 (1937):311-16.

Wickstrom, R. L. *Fundamental Motor Patterns*, 2nd ed. Philadelphia: Lea & Febiger, 1977.

Zimmerman, H. M. "Characteristic Likenesses and Differences Between Skilled and Nonskilled Performance of the Standing Broad Jump." *Research Quarterly* 27(1956):352.

Fundamental Nonlocomotor Skills

9

Michael J. Stewart
Kansas State University

The nonlocomotor manipulative skills of throwing and kicking will be discussed in this chapter. As with walking, running, and jumping a summary of the three levels of performance is provided for each of the skills discussed.

THROWING

As a result of the demands by various sports and activities, the fundamental motor skill of throwing comes in many different forms. For example, the bowler utilizes an underhand contralateral (with opposition) throw; the football quarterback a contralateral overhand throw; and the soccer player a bilateral overhead type of throw. The basketball player not only uses all of the previously listed throws, but also uses a two-handed sidearm throw, and a bilateral throw initiated at the chest.

From these examples, it would appear that the fundamental motor skill of throwing has a very broad definition and, thus, could very well create problems when conducting research, or even when discussing the term. In the developmental stages, one can observe a variety of throws also. There-fore, for the purpose of this discussion, the fundamental motor skill of throwing will be defined in its broadest sense as any unilateral or bilateral action of the arm or arms in an attempt to propel an object forward.

Due to the fact that throwing behavior requires the involvement of many other body parts, the acquisition of a mature throwing pattern is slow in its development. Despite the fact that the mature level of throwing is a long time coming for some individuals, and never achieved by many others, infants do perform very crude forms of throwing behaviors before they can even stand. The developmental stages of throwing are illustrated in Figure 9.1. Guttridge (1939) indicated that although infants can not control the direction of release of the object during the act of throwing, many children can throw from a sitting position as early as six months of age.

Probably the most in-depth study of the developmental sequences of throwing was conducted by Wild (1938) in which she studied thirty-two children ranging from 2 to 12 years of age. From her study, she concluded that many behaviors (those involving the arms, trunk, legs, and combined movements) are age-related. She hypothesized that children pass through four sequential stages. These stages have become so widely used that they are presented below:

Stage I is characterized by typical anteroposterior movements of which there is a preliminary incipient stage with no body movement. This stage can be assigned to ages two to three or possibly up to four and is described as follows: The reverse movement of the arm is either sideways-upward or forward-upward usually to high above shoulder elbow much flexed. With this reverse arm movement the trunk extends with dorsal flexion of ankles and carries the shoulders back. The trunk then straightens, carrying the shoulders forward, and flexes forward

Stage I (Level 1)

Stage II (Level 2A)

Stage III (Level 2B)

Stage IV (Level 3)

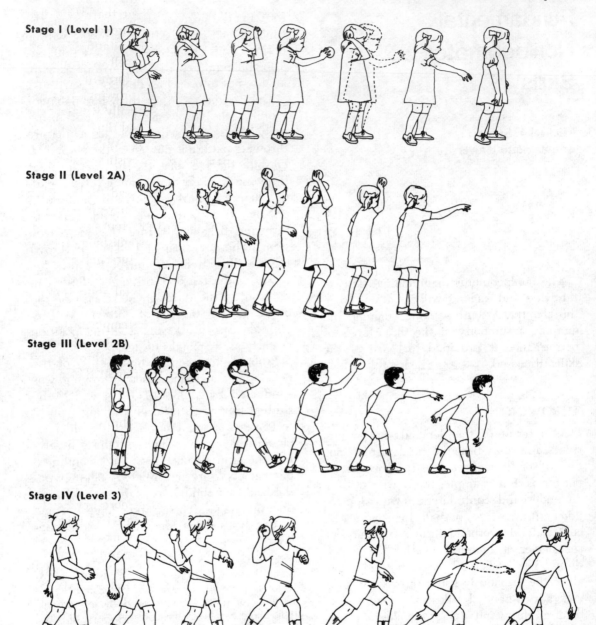

Figure 9.1. The developmental sequence of throwing. (Wickstrom, R. L., *Fundamental Motor Patterns*, 2nd ed., 1977. Philadelphia: Lea & Febiger, 1977. Redrawn from Wild, N., Research Q., Am. Assoc. Health, Phys. Ed., 1938.)

with plantar flexion of ankles as the arm swings forward over the shoulder and down in front. Elbow extension starts early. Movements of body and arm are almost entirely in the anteroposterior plane over the feet which remain in place; the body remains facing the direction of throw all the time; the arm is the initiating factor. There is trunk left rotation toward the end with the arm's forward reach.

Stage II is marked by the introduction of body and arm movement in the horizontal plane, as contrasted to the anteroposterior plane, and is assigned to ages three and one-half to five years. The whole body rotates right, then left above the feet; the feet remain together in place. The arm moves either in a high oblique plane above the shoulder or in a more horizontal plane, but with a forward downward follow-through. The elbow is much flexed; it may extend at once or later. The body changes its orientation and then reorientates to the throwing direction. The arm is the initiating factor.

Stage III marks the introduction of stepping; it is the right foot step-forward throw, assigned to age five to six. The weight is held back on the left rear foot as the spine rotates right and extends; the arm swings obliquely upward over the shoulder to a retracted position with elbow much flexed. The forward movements consist of a stepping forward with right foot, unilateral to the throwing arm, with spine left rotation, early turning of the whole body to a partial left facing trunk forward flexion, while the arm swings forward either in an oblique above-the-shoulder plane or in a sideways-around-the-shoulder plane followed by a forward downward movement of follow-through. Elbow extension does not start at once. This throw has both anteroposterior and horizontal features.

Stage IV is the left-foot-step-forward throw with trunk rotation and horizontal adduction of the arm in the forward swing. This throw is the mature form and all boys from six and one-half years up have it. The girls have, in most cases, attained the body and foot movements but incompletely developed forms of the arm movement. Others show decided regressions or retardations.*

*From Wild, Monica. "The Behavior Pattern of Throwing and Some Observations Concerning Its Course of Development in Children." *Research Quarterly*, 9 (3), 20, 1938. Used with permission.

It should be pointed out that Wild has associated the stages with chronological age, which of course, has its limitations. Many adolescent individuals as well as adults do not demonstrate a mature form in the fundamental motor skill of throwing. For example, many adults (especially women) do not step with opposition and thus would be classified in Stage III of Wild's (1938) scheme if all other characteristics were satisfied. Furthermore, many individuals, both men and women, do not lead the forward motion of the throwing arm with their elbow, which would be level four.

Probably the most distinguishing characteristics between an immature and mature thrower are trunk rotation, stepping with opposition, and the horizontal abduction of the arm in the forward swing. As Wild (1938) points out, initial attempts at throwing are characterized by anteroposterior movements. In other words, the thrower appears to be bowing by flexing at the hip as the object is propelled forward. A step either with the same foot as the throwing arm or the opposite foot of the throwing arm is not demonstrated in the initial stages. The arm is not extended in the reverse direction, and usually is extended much too early during the forward movement.

As the thrower becomes more proficient, trunk rotation is demonstrated but is not yet accompanied by any foot movement. As Wild (1938) points out, the arm moves either in a high oblique plane or a more horizontal plane, but with a follow through which is forward and somewhat downward. The arm is somewhat extended in the reverse direction, but is often kept extended during the entire throwing movement, giving the appearance of a catapult.

With increased trunk rotation, the addition of a step with the same foot of the throwing arm is typically demonstrated. The throw has progressively developed from an anteroposterior plane to one which has horizontal characteristics as well. Weight distribution has also progressed through some change, as now the weight of the body is shifted from the center of the body to the rear foot and back through the center, to the front foot as the forward, unilateral step is taken.

The mature throw, or Stage IV, of Wild's (1938) progressive stages is characterized by maximum trunk rotation; a shifting of the weight from forward, to back, to forward; extension of the arm in the backswing and flexion of the arm as the forward motion is initiated with the elbow leading the hand causing a whipping action upon extension of the arm and release of the object, and a step with the foot opposite the throwing arm. This contralateral movement not only provides increased stability, but also enables the thrower to complete a greater range of horizontal hip rotation as the object is thrown forward. As the object is released, the thrower "follows through" across the body with the throwing arm.

Summary of the Development of Throwing

Level 1. The individual throws almost entirely with the arm in the anteroposterior plane. In preparation for the throw the arm is brought back sideward and backward, but not behind the body. The throwing arm is flexed and a hyperextension of the back is observed. The throw consists of rapid extension of the arm in a forward and downward motion. The trunk is flexed as the throw is executed. There is no rotation of the body and the feet remain stationary.

Level 2A. The individual begins to show signs of horizontal rotary movement. Preparatory movement is characterized by a rotation of the trunk to the right (for right-handed throwers) with the arm swing sideward and backward behind the head. The movement of the arm during and after the throw does not change much from the previous level. There is still no action of the feet.

Level 2B. Increased preparatory and follow-through rotary movement of the trunk is demonstrated by the individual. The elbow is fully extended upon releasing the object and the follow-through is in a forward and downward movement. A forward step with the same foot as the throwing arm initiates the throw. A shifting of the weight forward during the step adds to the forcefulness of the throw.

Level 3. Maximum trunk rotation in preparation for the throw and during the follow-through are demonstrated by the individual. Shifting of the weight to the back foot during the preparation and to the front foot during the throw is more evident. The throwing arm is swung backward and upward in preparation, and the elbow leads the arm movement in a horizontal plane during the throw. The elbow is fully extended upon release of the object. A forward step with the opposite foot of the throwing arm is executed and is followed by rotation of the hips and trunk. The follow-through of arm is in a forward and downward path across the midline of the body.

KICKING

There are basically two types of kicks: the punt and the place kick. The punt is a type of kick which is used to a great extent by American and Canadian football players as well as soccer players (goalies). It can be defined as a kick in which the object being struck is held or dropped by the hands and struck by the foot before it reaches the ground. The place kick, on the other hand, is a kick in which the foot is used to apply a force upon an object as it rests or travels upon the ground. A very common example is the kick-off or field goal in American and Canadian football and dribbling in soccer. Both types of kicks are similar in that they are a form of striking in which the foot becomes the implement, rather than the arms, hands, or equipment. The place kick is probably the most widely used type of kick used by elementary school-aged youngsters. The reasons for this are two fold: (1) developmentally, this type of kick seems to be easier to master, and (2) many of the low-organized and lead-up games require this type of kick as a skill. For these reasons, the place kick will be discussed.

As compared to the other fundamental motor skills discussed thus far, the place kick is by far the least studied by researchers. Why this is true is beyond the scope of this discussion. However, due to its presence in so many childhood and adult games and activities it is a very important fundamental skill. It would seem that children would be able to attempt to place kick shortly after they could stand and maintain balance upon one leg for a very short duration. In fact, Gesell (1940) suggested that children are able to attempt a place kick shortly after they were able to run (hence, being able to balance upon one foot for a brief duration).

Probably the most thorough study of the place kick was completed by Deach (1950) in which she studied 83 children ranging in ages from two to six. Her study employed the use of a stationary ball in which the children stood directly behind and were instructed to kick.

Initial attempts at the place kick are characterized by a pushing or "nudging" motion of the leg of the kicker. There is very little use of the rest of the body parts except of a compensentory nature. For example, as the child nudges the ball with the foot there is some upward and outward movement of the opposite arm which enables the child to keep balance. Foot contact with the ball is inconsistent, as foot-eye coordination is not fully developed. As the neurological system develops and the child is exposed to practice, making contact with the object becomes more consistent. The nudging of the ball results from the lack of flexion at the knee. As the place kick matures, flexion at the knee becomes more pronounced prior to the kick. As one might suspect, as the place kicker develops the knee flexion behavior in the preparatory phase, knee extension is made possible during the striking phase and the follow through phase of the kick.

The early attempt at place kicking is also characterized by an upright position of the body prior to, during, and following the kick. As the behavior matures, the body can be observed as flexing at the trunk prior to the kick and extending simultaneously with the kick.

Summary of the Place Kick

Level 1A.   The individual demonstrates little forward movement of the lower leg with very little accompanying movement of the arms or trunk. There is very little knee flexion prior to the kick. Placement of the kicking foot upon the object is inconsistent during the initial attempts. There is very little backward lean as the object is struck with the foot.

Level 1B.   The kicking foot of the individual flexes more in preparation for the kick, but the kick itself is still characterized as kicking at the object, rather than kicking through it. Some compensatory movement of the opposite arm of the kicking leg is evidenced. There still seems to be little extension of the leg at the hip prior to the kick and little flexion at the hip following the kick.

Level 2.   A significant increase in the arc of the leg is demonstrated by the individual, which requires a compensating movement from the opposite arm of the kicking leg. There seems to be some backward lean upon contact of the object and an appearance of kicking through the object.

Level 3.   There seems to be a significant increase in all movements. A greater arc of the kicking leg, an increase in body lean, an increase in use of the arms as contributors to establishing balance and creating force, and a consistency at making contact with the object are all demonstrated by the individual. A preliminary step with the opposite foot of the kicking leg can also be observed.

References

Deach, D. "Genetic Development of Motor Skills in Children Two through Six Years of Age." Unpublished Doctoral Dissertation, University of Michigan, 1950.

Gesell, A. *The First Five Years of Life*. New York: Harper and Brothers, 1940.

Gutteridge, M. V. "A Study of Motor Achievement of Young Children." *Archives of Psychology* 1(1939):244.

Wild, M. "The Behavior Pattern of Throwing and Some Observations Concerning Its Course of Development in Children." *Research Quarterly* 9(3)(1938):20.

Refining Locomotor Skills 10

Karen DeOreo
Kent State University

In this chapter the refinement of the locomotor skills of running and jumping is discussed. Because refinement of walking is not a problem for most children and because the information provided in Chapter 8 is sufficient for aiding the refinement of walking, this fundamental skill is not discussed in the chapter. For each of the two skills discussed mechanical principles are presented which are important to refining the skill. Developmental Analysis Checklists for each skill are provided.

MECHANICAL PRINCIPLES PERTINENT TO THE SKILL OF RUNNING

There are many principles which bare in some way on running performance. Only the most pertinent ones were selected in order to help increase the reader's understanding of efficient running patterns. These principles are stated and explained below.

PRINCIPLE: Effects of Momentum—Momentum is the product of mass and velocity. Any increase in either component will result in increased momentum. The greater the momentum, the greater the resistance to change in direction or velocity.

EXPLANATION: In running, if the speed of the runner is increased, the runner will possess more momentum. The more momentum achieved, the harder it will be for the runner to change direction. This is why the running time for the shuttle run is so much greater than the running time for the dash. When the runner knows that a change in direction must be made, top speed can not be attained. If it is, change in direction is difficult due to a build-up of momentum.

PRINCIPLE: Transfer of Momentum — Momentum developed in a body segment may be transferred to the total body. The longer and heavier the body segment and the greater its speed, the greater will be its contribution to total body momentum.

EXPLANATION: The greater the momentum obtained by the thrust of the arms and legs during each stride, the faster the runner will be able to run. Careful attention should be given to the forward movements of the arms and legs. The limbs should be thrust forward in the line of direction in an attempt to increase the momentum. Any movement in a direction other than the line of direction will serve to decrease momentum. Because longer segments increase speed, the hands should be extended, not clenched. However, the elbows must be flexed to increase speed of movement through the joint.

PRINCIPLE: Acceleration: Proportional to Force — Acceleration is proportional to the force causing it, providing the mass is held constant.

EXPLANATION: A runner can increase acceleration by increasing the force applied backward and downward against the running surface. This can be achieved by pushing harder against the ground with the feet and legs.

PRINCIPLE: Body's Radius on Rotational Speed — When a body rotates, lengthening the radius slows rotation. Shortening the radius increases the rotation because the resistance against the rotating force is proportionately less.

EXPLANATION: A runner can increase stride, speed, and running efficiency by flexing the knees, elbows, and hip. This shortens the length of the legs and arms and increases the speed with which these limbs can be thrust forward.

PRINCIPLE: Direction of Counterforce — The direction of the counterforce is directly opposite that of the applied force. Applied force is most effective when it is perpendicular to the supporting surface.

EXPLANATION: When a person is running, it is important that the force the runner applies to the running surface be directly opposite the direction of desired movement. Fast running or sprinting occurs in a linear direction which is parallel to the ground. For this type running the body must lean forward so that the feet can "push" against the surface to propel the body forward. In slow running there is little or no body lean. If a runner assumes a too wide or too short of a stride, the forces will be directed poorly, causing inefficient movements and possible surface slippage.

PRINCIPLE: Total Force — A total force is the sum of the forces of each body segment contributing to the act, if the forces are applied in a single direction and in proper sequence with correct timing.

EXPLANATION: The total force in running is a combination of the force applied against the ground and the thrust of the arms and legs. How fast and strong these forces are applied will determine the resultant velocity of the runner. That is, if a person wants to run faster, he/she should push harder against the ground and swing the arms and legs faster. The force which is created is called the propelling force. Length of stride is also an important factor and cannot be overlooked when increasing the speed of running. However, lengthening the stride is effective only to a point. Reaching too far forward causes the foot to contact the ground ahead of the center of gravity which interrupts the forward momentum.

PRINCIPLE: Direction of Force Application — In general, all forces should be applied as directly as possible in line with the intended motion. Forces applied in other directions either retard motion in the desired direction or result in wasted energy.

EXPLANATION: It is important that all forces created by the runner be directed in the intended line of motion. For example, if the toes point outward during each stride, the force is not directed straight ahead. This reduces the effectiveness of the push of the foot. Or, if a runner moves the arms across the body toward the midline, instead of back and forth in line of direction, the efficient application of force is disrupted.

PRINCIPLE: Friction — The greater the friction between supporting surface and the body parts which come in contact with the surface, the greater the stability.

EXPLANATION: In order to run efficiently, it is important that the runner wear proper shoes. When there is lack of traction, forces that are applied to the ground must be applied more vertically than horizontally and desired speed is lost. That is why a person will run more "up and down" on a slippery or loose surface.

PRINCIPLE: Instability — The shorter the distance the center of gravity must move to clear the base of support, the more rapidly the body can be put into motion in that direction.

EXPLANATION: A runner who wishes to start quickly in a given direction should move the center of gravity close to the edge of the base of support in the direction of the intended movement. A track sprinter will assume a set position with the body weight shifted forward to start more quickly.

PRINCIPLE: Use of Gravity — Many locomotor activities depend upon deliberate loss of balance to enable gravity to combine with muscular forces to move the body.

EXPLANATION: In running, the center of gravity is shifted outside the base of support and a forward step must be taken to regain balance and establish a new base of support. Only one foot contacts the surface at a time; therefore, the base of support is provided by only one supporting limb. Because of this, running demands intricate timing of all moving parts. The runner must learn to utilize the force of gravity to help movement by continually shifting the center of gravity ahead of the base of support.

PRINCIPLE: Control of Momentum — To stop quickly or change direction when in motion, the performer should widen the base of support, lower center of gravity, and slow down to control momentum.

EXPLANATION: If, while running, the performer wishes to change direction or stop, this can be done by widening the base of support, (putting feet in wide apart position) lowering the center of gravity (stooping) and decelerating (stop pushing against ground and swinging arms and legs forward).

DEVELOPMENTAL ANALYSIS CHECKLIST
RUNNING

	Good	Fair	Needs Work

Position of Trunk

1. Upright except for slight lean as speed increases.

Movement of Arms

1. Elbows bent at 90°.
2. Arm action in opposition to leg action.
3. Arms swing in direction of movement.
4. Arms do not cross midline.
5. Arms swing as pendulum with pathway of hand extending from chin to buttock.
6. Hands and shoulder swing relaxed.

Movement of Legs

1. Relaxed stride.
2. Weight on sole of foot.
3. Feet and knees point straight ahead.
4. Center of gravity rides over support foot.
5. Support knee bends slightly (12°).
6. High knee lift.
7. Heel of rear foot near buttock.

MECHANICAL PRINCIPLES RELATED TO THE SKILL OF JUMPING

Several mechanical principles apply to various forms of jumping. Understanding of these principles will assist the reader in understanding the application of appropriate movements which will increase the effectiveness of the jump. These selected principles are stated and explained below.

PRINCIPLE: Continuity of Motion—When performing activities in which two or more consecutive motions contribute to movement in the same direction, there should usually be no pause between the motions. Any hesitation prior to the next motion will result in a loss of some or all of the advantage gained by the previous motion.

EXPLANATION: In jumping, the knees, arms, and trunk are extended in one continuous movement. If the jumper hesitates in extending any of these body parts, he/she will interrupt the flow of movement. The end result will be an inefficient jump lacking height or distance.

PRINCIPLE: Transfer of Momentum — Momentum developed in a body segment may be transferred to the total body. The longer and heavier the body segment and the greater its speed, the greater will be its contribution to total body momentum.

EXPLANATION: Momentum is transferred in three ways: a) from one body part to another, b) from entire body to a body part, c) from a body part to the entire body. In transferring from body part to entire body, the longer and heavier body segment and the greater its speed, the greater will be its contribution to the activity. Thus, the efficient swinging of the arms over the greatest available range of movement, as fast as possible, and with the arms extended is important. The addition of the rapid swinging of the legs forward in horizontal jumping contributes to the total momentum of the entire body.

PRINCIPLE: Acceleration Proportional To Force — Acceleration is proportional to the force causing it, providing the mass is held constant.

EXPLANATION: A jumper's height or distance is directly proportional to the force applied backward and downward against the supporting surface. The more force applied against the floor or ground, the more distance or height accomplished. The body can create more force by involving more and larger muscles of the body. This is the purpose of the preliminary crouch. By bending the hips, knees, and ankles the jumper is involving more muscles to push backward and downward, consequently creating more force.

PRINCIPLE: Direction of Counterforce — The direction of the counterforce is directly opposite that of the applied force. Applied force is most effective when it is perpendicular to the supporting surface.

EXPLANATION: In vertical jumping, the force must be applied downward because the counterforce is directly opposite the applied force. In horizontal jumping, it is important to push with the balls of the feet against the ground with the body in a 45 degree position or as close to it as possible. This means that it is important for the jumper to lean forward during the take-off stage.

PRINCIPLE: Total Force — A total force is the sum of the forces of each body segment contributing to the act; if the forces are applied in a single direction and in proper sequence with timing.

EXPLANATION: The forces created by the speed of the extension of each body part must be in sequence and should be applied in sequence as each previous force reaches its peak. The succession of forces should be extension of the legs, extension of the trunk, and extenion of the arms.

PRINCIPLE: Absorbing a Blow — A force from a blow can be diminished by distributing the force over either a greater time-distance, area, or both.

EXPLANATION: When a person lands after jumping, the shock absorbing joints of the legs eccentrically flex in order to distribute the force over a longer time and distance. Essentially, the landing force is absorbed by the bending of the hips, knees, and ankles. This lowers the body into a crouch or semi-crouch position which in turn distributes the force downward.

PRINCIPLE: Landing with Balance — The center of gravity must be kept above the supporting levers in order that each lever will make its greatest contribution. Each lever must bear weight as it moves through flexion.

EXPLANATION: During the vertical jump, the center of gravity is directly over the base of support which contributes to stability during the landing. During horizontal jumping, the center of gravity is usually behind the base of support and must be moved within or in front of the base of support in order to avoid falling backwards during landing. This means that the forward placement of the legs and feet during landing must be balanced with the forward lean of the trunk. If the feet are too far ahead of the trunk, balance cannot be maintained.

PRINCIPLE: Lowered Center of Gravity — Stability may be increased by lowering the center of gravity.

EXPLANATION: When landing, the legs are flexed not only to absorb the force of the blow, but to bring the center of gravity closer to the base of support, thus enhancing stability.

PRINCIPLE: Enlarged Base of Support — The larger the base of support, the more stable the body. (Center of gravity must be moved through a greater distance in order to disrupt balance).

EXPLANATION: The larger the base of support during take-off and landing, the easier it will be to maintain the center of gravity within that base of support. Placement of the feet during take-off and land-

ing is several inches (usually shoulder width) apart to promote stability. However, placement of the feet further apart reduces the propelling effect of the muscles and is not desirable for effective jumping.

PRINCIPLE: Friction — The greater the friction between supporting surface, the greater the stability and traction.

EXPLANATION: The use of tennis shoes on hard surfaces and the use of spikes on some surfaces will increase the stability and traction of the jumper.

PRINCIPLE: Instability — The shorter the distance the center of gravity must move to clear the base of support, the more rapidly the body can be put into motion in that direction.

EXPLANATION: In horizontal jumping, the center of gravity should be moved to the edge of the base of support in the direction of the jump. This will cause a forward lean of the body toward the desired take-off angle of 45 degrees. The straight arms should then moved forward and out in front of the body. This will move the center of gravity forward and thus create additional forward lean toward the desired 45 degree takeoff angle. In contrast, during vertical jumping it is desirable to have arms near to the body therefore maintaining the center of gravity closer to the body's midline and the desired 90 degree take-off angle.

DEVELOPMENTAL ANALYSIS CHECKLIST
STANDING LONG JUMP

	Good	Fair	Needs Work
Preparation for Take-Off			
1. Hips, knees, and ankles are flexed (approximately 90 degrees).			
2. Arms swing backward and upward.			
3. Trunk exhibits forward lean.			
Take-Off			
1. Arms swing downward and forward.			
2. Hip, knee, and ankle increase flexion as arms swing downward.			
3. Trunk continues to lean forward.			
4. Heels are pulled off floor as arms move upward.			
5. Take-off angle approximately 45 degrees (center of gravity).			
6. Hips, knees, and ankles extend placing body in straight line.			
7. Arms extend upward in line with body.			
Flight			
1. After take-off, lower legs begin to bend with heels moving toward buttocks.			
2. Hips flex bringing the thighs close to the trunk.			
3. Lower legs swing forward into landing position.			
4. Arms and trunk are brought forward.			
Landing			
1. Arms and trunk continue movement forward and downward.			
2. Legs forward with trunk close to thighs.			
3. As the feet touch the ground, there is a bending of the knees with body weight continuing forward and downward.			

DEVELOPMENTAL ANALYSIS CHECKLIST
VERTICAL JUMP AND REACH

	Good	Fair	Needs Work
Preparation for Take-off			
1. Hips, knees, and ankles bent (approximately 65-90 degrees).			
2. Trunk erect.			
3. Feet are parallel and shoulder width apart.			
4. Elbows slightly flexed along side of body.			
Take-off			
1. Arms moved upward to extend over head.			
2. Hips, knees, and ankles extend.			
3. Once airborne, non-reaching arm moves downward.			
Landing			
1. Ankles, knees, and hips bend to absorb shock of landing.			

References

Broer, M. *Efficiency of Human Movement.* Philadelphia: W. B. Saunders, 1973.

Jensen, C. R., and Schultz, G. W. *Applied Kinesiology.* New York: McGraw-Hill, 1977.

Wickstrom, R. L. *Fundamental Motor Patterns.* 2nd ed. Philadelphia: Lea & Febiger, 1977.

Refining Nonlocomotor Skills

11

Karen DeOreo
Kent State University

In this chapter the refinement of the non-locomotor manipulative skills of throwing and kicking is discussed. For each of the skills discussed mechanical principles are presented which are important to refining the skill. Developmental Analysis Checklists for each skill are provided. Similar analysis of other non-locomotor skills and similar checklists can be prepared to assist teachers and learners in refining such skills. The same general principles may be applied and the format presented may be used to prepare checklists for specific skills. Other skills of interest are striking and catching.

MECHANICAL PRINCIPLES RELATED TO THROWING

Forceful and accurate throwing demands the coordination of the upper and lower limbs with rotational trunk movement. Many mechanical principles come into play which govern body movement and the ultimate path of the ball. Selected principles which deal with throwing are stated and explained below.

PRINCIPLE: Continuity of Motion—When performing activities in which two or more consecutive motions contribute to movement in the same direction, there should usually be no pause between the motions. Any hesitation prior to the next motion will result in a loss of some or all of the advantage gained by the previous motion.

EXPLANATION: If a thrower hesitates during any part of the throwing sequence, the speed is lost.

PRINCIPLE: Transfer of Momentum—Momentum developed in a body segment may be transferred to the total body. The longer and heavier the body segment and the greater its speed, the greater will be its contribution to total body momentum.

EXPLANATION: All movement done by the body prior to the release of the ball is done in an effort to create a maximum culminating force in the throwing arm and ultimately the throwing object. The person throwing can utilize a run, hop, trunk rotation, and weight transfer to gain maximum body momentum to be transferred to the throwing object.

PRINCIPLE: Body's Radius on Rotational Speed — When a body rotates, lengthening the radius slows rotation. Shortening the radius increases the rotation because the resistance against the rotating force is proportionately less.

EXPLANATION: A thrower will flex the elbow of the throwing arm in order to shorten its radius. By doing so, the arm can be brought through its range of motion with greater speed and less resistance.

PRINCIPLE: Surface Contact While Applying Forces to Objects — In throwing, pushing, pulling, and striking activities, one or both feet should be kept in firm contact with the supporting surface until force is applied.

EXPLANATION: Surface contact is essential in applying force to an object. It is especially important as the weight of the object becomes greater. If surface contact is limited, there is a reduction in the maximum force that can be produced. However, the advantages of greater momentum that can be gained with the running approach cannot be overlooked. In order to maintain this momentum, compliance with the surface contact principle may be impossible, but in any case should not be ignored.

PRINCIPLE: Total Force — A total force is the sum of the forces of each body segment contributing to the act, if the forces are applied in a single direction and in proper sequence with correct training.

EXPLANATION: When the ball is released it is traveling at a velocity approximately equal to the sum of the velocities of all the body movements contributing at the time of release. Therefore, the greater the velocity created in each body movement, the greater the contribution at the point of release, if in proper sequence and timing.

PRINCIPLE: Distance of Force Application — If a constant force is applied to a body, the body develops greater velocity as the distance over which the force is applied increases.

EXPLANATION: The thrower should assume an open stance in the direction of the line of flight. This will create a greater distance over which to apply the force.

The greater the range of motion of each contributing body segment the greater will be the resulting velocity from that segment.

PRINCIPLE: Correct Muscle Selection — The performer must select (unconsciously) the muscles which are most effective for the task at hand. In a maximum effort, stronger muscles and more muscles are needed to be brought into action to produce greater force and limit muscle strain.

EXPLANATION: In throwing, approximately 50% of the force is initiated through hip and torso rotations. Therefore, it is important to note that these rotations are essential in achieving the most efficient throw and in eliminating muscle strain in the arm and shoulder.

PRINCIPLE: Initial Muscular Tension — The force of muscular contraction may be increased by increasing the initial tension of the muscle (putting the muscle on stretch).

EXPLANATION: The thrower will extend the arm backward in preparation for the throw. This preliminary movement will put the major contracting of the arm muscles into stretch. Putting these muscles into stretch will facilitate the greatest increase in muscular contraction and ultimately greatest force in the throw.

PRINCIPLE: Follow-Through — Correct follow-through eliminates the tendency to decelerate a throwing or striking action before its completion. Follow-through exists to 1) maintain balance, 2) to avoid boundary line violation, 3) to place the body in the ready position for movement, 4) to protect joints, muscles and connective tissues.

EXPLANATION: In throwing, the follow-through is absolutely essential for power and accuracy. If the follow-through is interrupted or eliminated, the result will be a decrease in final velocity. Lack of follow-through means the performer must decelerate the movement prior to the release of the ball. The consequences of this deceleration are a less forceful throw.

PRINCIPLE: Propelling Force — Certain effects produced by the propelling force depend upon its point and direction of application.

EXPLANATION: In order to gain the most distance it is essential to apply the propelling force through the object's center of gravity. This is why a curve ball will travel more slowly than a straight ball because part of the force is expended in producing spin necessary to curve the ball.

PRINCIPLE: Force of Gravity—The force of gravity diminishes the upward velocity of an object. When gravity overcomes the effects of the upward component of the projectile, the object will begin to descend.

EXPLANATION: There are factors which determine how soon gravity will cause an object to descend to the ground. These factors are the amount of force driving them upward, and the effects of air resistance.

PRINCIPLE: Angle of Projection — The optimum angle of projection with which to gain maximum distance is 45 degrees.*

EXPLANATION: If the angle is less than optimum, the projectile will not be in the air long enough to travel a maximum distance and if the angle is greater than 45 degrees, too much of the propelling force is wasted in vertical rather than horizontal flight.

PRINCIPLE: Effect of Spin on Flight of an Object — An object propelled without spin tends to waver because of air resistance.

EXPLANATION: A small amount of spin on an object produces a stabilizing effect which tends to hold it on its line of flight. Increased spin will cause an object to curve in direction of spin.

*Depending on the object and the height from which the object is thrown the exact angle of projection may vary, but in general this angle is best.

DEVELOPMENTAL ANALYSIS CHECKLIST
THROWING

	Good	Fair	Needs Work

Backswing

1. Ball held and thrown with fingers (not palm).
2. Weight on back foot.
3. Left side toward target (right handed throwers).
4. Throwing arm extended at side with elbow flexed.
5. Throwing elbow pointing away from target.
6. Wrist in cocked position (hyperextended).

Throwing Action

1. Weight is transferred to front foot.
2. Hips and torso rotate to face target.
3. Elbow leads the rest of the arm as it turns to face target.
4. Power comes from straightening the elbow and extending arm quickly.
5. The wrist snaps as the arm extends as if to throw the hand with the ball.
6. As arm extends bend front knee slightly.

Follow Through

1. Throwing arm continues forward motion after ball is released.
2. Back leg steps forward to establish new base of support as body rides over front foot.
3. Trunk flexes at hip as body movement continues forward.

MECHANICAL PRINCIPLES RELATED TO KICKING

Imparting force to an object by using a body limb as the striking implement requires unique timing and movement. Selected mechanical principles which apply to the kicking movement are stated and explained below.

PRINCIPLE: Continuity of Motion—When performing activities in which two or more consecutive motions contribute to movement in the same direction, there should usually be no pause between the motions. Any hesitation prior to the next motion will result in a loss of some of all of the advantage gained by the previous motion.

EXPLANATION: In order for the momentum of the entire body to be passed to the foot and to the object kicked, all prior movement must be continuous. Any interruption in the body sequence will result in a loss of kicking power.

PRINCIPLE: Transfer of Momentum — Momentum developed in a body segment may be transferred to the total body. The longer and heavier the body segment and the greater its speed, the greater will be its contribution to total body momentum.

EXPLANATION: In kicking, momentum is transferred from the entire body to the leg. Body momentum can be increased by taking a running start prior to the kick. The greater the speed of the total body the greater the momentum imparted to the ball.

PRINCIPLE: Body's Radius on Rotational Speed — When a body rotates, lengthening the radius slows rotation. Shortening the radius increases the rotation because the resistance against the rotating force is proportionately less.

EXPLANATION: During the backswing of the kicking leg, the kicker will flex the knee. This shortening of the radius of the leg makes it possible for the kicker to bring the lower leg and foot forward with greater speed.

PRINCIPLE: Counterforce of Striking Activities — The amount of force a striking implement imparts to an object depends on the combined momentum of the implement and the object at the moment of contact. Any give in implement or object at impact will reduce propulsive force.

EXPLANATION: It is important in kicking that the joints that are not actively moving be firm in their positions in order to reduce give. At ball contact, the knee of the kicking leg should be fully extended and firm.

PRINCIPLE: Surface Contact While Applying Forces to Objects — In throwing, pushing, pulling, and striking activities, one or both feet should be kept in firm contact with the supporting surface until force is applied.

EXPLANATION: It is necessary while kicking that one foot be in contact with the supporting surface until the kicking motion is complete. Otherwise, the maximum force of the kick is reduced.

PRINCIPLE: Total Force — A total force is the sum of the forces of each body segment contributing to the act, if the forces are applied in a single direction and in proper sequence with correct timing.

EXPLANATION: The total force contributing to the kick is a sum of all forces of each body segment. It is important that each force be applied at the peak of the previous force. Therefore, the force of the arms and the entire body should be transferred to the foot in proper sequence and with proper timing.

PRINCIPLE: Direction of Force Application — In general, all forces should be applied as directly as possible in line with the intended motion. Forces applied in other directions either retard motion in the desired direction or result in wasted energy.

EXPLANATION: The success and accuracy of the kick will depend on the ability of the kicker to apply the force with the foot on the side of the ball opposite to the direction he/she wishes the ball to go.

PRINCIPLE: Distance of Force Application — If a constant force is applied to a body, the body develops greater velocity as the distance over which the force is applied increases.

EXPLANATION: The greater the range of motion of each contributing body part, such as the greater the lean and leg backswing, the greater will be the resulting velocity from those body parts.

PRINCIPLE: Initial Muscular Tension — The force of muscular contraction may be increased by increasing the initial tension of the muscle (putting the muscle on stretch).

EXPLANATION: Backward lean of the kicker's trunk prior to kicking places the hip flexors and knee extensors on stretch enabling these muscles to flex the hip and extend the knee with greater force.

PRINCIPLE: Follow-through—Correct follow-through eliminates the tendency to decelerate a throwing or striking action before its completion. Follow-through exists to 1) maintain balance, 2) to avoid boundary line violations, 3) to place the body in the ready position for movement, 4) to protect joints, muscles, and connective tissues.

EXPLANATION: It is important for the kicker's foot to stay in contact with the ball as long as possible. This follow-through action is essential for both power and accuracy. Any break in follow-through would cause the kicker to discontinue force application sooner and the result would be a less forceful kick.

PRINCIPLE: Angle of Projection — The optimum angle of projection with which to gain maximum distance is 45 degrees (see note page 69).

EXPLANATION: If the angle is less than optimum, the projectile will not be in the air long enough to travel a maximum distance and if the angle is greater that 45 degrees, too much of the propelling force is wasted in vertical rather than horizontal flight. In order to acquire the greatest distance, the kick should be made at approximately a 45 degree angle.

PRINCIPLE: Friction — The greater the friction between supporting surface and body parts in contact with surface, the greater the stability.

EXPLANATION: Traction is vital when kicking because the base of support consists of one foot. Not only is force applied from the ground through that one foot, but it must also be able to offset the forces of the kicking foot which are trying to carry the kicker off balance. In order to withstand these forces, the supporting foot is dependent on sufficient traction with the supporting surface. This may be enhanced with cleated shoes.

DEVELOPMENTAL ANALYSIS CHECKLIST
PUNTING

	Good	Fair	Needs Work
1. Kicker takes several preliminary steps.			
2. Arms extended in front of body holding ball in line with kicking leg.			

Backswing

1. Kicking leg extended behind back with knee flexed and foot near buttock.			
2. Trunk leans slightly backward during backswing.			
3. Ball is dropped as support foot touches ground.			
4. Support leg slightly bent.			

Kicking Action

1. Ankle and knee extend as leg swings forward toward ball.			
2. Trunk bends forward at hip during ball contact.			
3. Arm opposite kicking leg extends forward in direction of kick.			
4. Arm on same side as kicking leg extends backward.			
5. During ball contact kicking leg completely extended.			
6. Support leg extends at contact.			

Follow Through

1. Leg extends along line of intended flight.			
2. Support leg extends so kicker is on sole of foot and eventually airborne.			
3. Kicker executes hop and both arms move upward.			

DEVELOPMENTAL ANALYSIS CHECKLIST
KICKING

	Good	Fair	Needs Work
1. Kicker takes at least two preliminary steps.			
2. Arms move in opposition to legs.			
Backswing			
1. Support leg is located behind and to the side of ball.			
2. Kicking leg extended behind back with knee flexed and foot near buttock.			
3. Trunk leans slightly backward during backswing.			
Kicking Action			
1. Ankle and knee extend as leg swings forward toward ball.			
2. Arm opposite kicking leg extends forward in direction of kick.			
3. Arm on same side as kicking leg extends backward.			
4. Trunk bends forward at hip during ball contact.			
5. Support leg slightly bent.			
Follow Through			
1. Leg extends along line of intended flight.			
2. Support leg extends so kicker is on sole of foot or possible airborne.			

References

Broer, M. *Efficiency of Human Movement.* Philadelphia: W. B. Saunders, 1973.

Jensen, C. R., and Schultz, G. W. *Applied Kinesiology.* New York: McGraw-Hill, 1977.

Wickstrom, R. L. *Fundamental Motor Patterns.* 2nd ed. Philadelphia: Lea & Febiger, 1977.

Section 5

Fundamental Motor
Skills: The
Performance of
Children

Performance of Fundamental Motor Tasks

12

Karen DeOreo
Kent State University
Jack Keogh
University of California,
Los Angeles

Great emphasis is placed on the fundamental motor tasks during the elementary school years because of their importance to the more complex movements of sports and recreational skills. Fundamental motor tasks including running, galloping, hopping, skipping, throwing, catching, kicking, striking, climbing, and balancing are all included somewhere within the vast array of the child's future sports and recreational skills: i.e., football, basketball, baseball, table tennis, skiing, etc. The greater the mastery of the fundamental motor tasks, the greater the ease with which the child will learn the activities of his/her choice.

The learning of fundamental motor tasks occurs during the preschool years and follows a definite developmental trend. As pointed out in the previous section, a three-year-old can throw, but the movement pattern does not resemble that of an adult. By the time the child is four-years-old the throwing pattern has changed and a few more elements of a mature pattern are seen. At age five, the child is developing a more mature throwing pattern. It is during the elementary school years that most children are learning and refining the fundamental motor tasks so that the overall movement approximates that of the skilled adult.

When the child enters school he/she can run, climb, gallop, and hop with some proficiency. Skipping is well on its way to being mastered as are throwing, catching, and kicking. Balancing is reasonably good. Most children can walk a low balance beam with no hesitation. Striking ability is somewhat weak unless the child has had opportunity to practice. At this point, it would seem appropriate to pose the following question. If the child possesses the fundamental motor tasks by age six, what then occurs in motor development between the ages six to twelve years? As noted in Chapters 10 and 11 this is a time of skill refinement. The need for skill refinement is quite easily seen when the performance of an adult is contrasted with the performance of a six-year-old child. Take, for example, the task of throwing. Even though the child's movement pattern looks quite similar to that of the adult, there is a marked difference in performance. The adult can throw much farther, demonstrating more power and speed in the throw. The throw is also more accurate, hitting targets the child cannot even approximate. Motor performance, then, during the ages six to twelve years, consists of refining and modifying fundamental motor tasks thus producing more diverse and complex movements. Changes in movement are more subtle and closely related to perfecting efficient movement mechanics such as proper timing of the movement of body segments, application of force, absorption of force, and many others. Also, the opportunity to practice and be coached definitely helps the child to improve motor skills. This frequently occurs in physical education class, in intramural experiences, youth sports programs, YMCA-YWCA activities, and other recreational events.

In this chapter the reader will find each of the fundamental motor tasks presented with a discussion of what is known about changes in performance with advancing age (five to twelve years). Differences in performance between sexes is highlighted. The following fundamental motor tasks will be discussed: running, hopping, galloping, skipping, jumping, throwing, kicking, striking and balance.

RUNNING

By the time the young child enters school, the overall running pattern appears very similar to that of the adult. However, results of running performance (speed over a prescribed distance) or still much poorer than those of the adult. Basic refinements in the running pattern will occur during the early school years which will result in continued improvement in running performance with advancing age. These refinements center mainly around growth and practice. With increasing age the child becomes bigger and stronger. Stride length will increase and the ability to exert muscular power will heighten. Opportunities to practice running will help the child to learn about the efficient ways to move in order to produce increased speed.

Studies of running performance in children have used basically three types of running tasks. One of the most common is the dash. This is an all out run for speed over a distance of 30 to 35 yards for the younger children and 50 to 60 yards for the older children. A second task that has been used is the shuttle run. This is a run over a pre-

scribed distance that incorporates one or more stops and/or changes of direction. The third task that has been used is the endurance run. The child is asked to maintain the running pattern for an extended period of time (3 to 10 minutes) or over a long distance (600 to 2,000 yards).

Results of the studies using dashes vary, of course, with the distance used. In order to provide a composite picture of running performance from 5 to 17 years of age, Espenschade (1967) used yards per second to graphically illustrate changes in performance of boys and girls with advancing age. During the elementary school years there is a linear increase in speed until age 11-12 when there is a sharp tapering off for girls and a gradual leveling for the boys. In other words, as boys and girls get older, they run faster. This is true until the age of puberty when this rate of improvement changes for both sexes. Speeds in yards per second reported by Espenschade (1967) ranged from approximately 3.75 yards per second at age five years to 6.0 yards per second at age eleven years. Improvement from year to year ranged from .25 to .50 yards per second. At all ages levels boys were faster than girls by approximately .1 to .2 yards per second.

Studies by Milne, Seefeldt, and Reuschlein (1975) and Glassow and Kruse (1960) both reported results of a 30 yard dash performed by elementary school children. In the Milne, Seefeldt, and Reuschlein study the means for kindergarten, first grade, and second grade boys were 6.29, 5.54, and 5.15 seconds respectively. For girls they were (in same order) 6.82, 5.85, and 5.64 seconds. In the Glassow and Kruse (1960) investigation, the means for six to twelve year old girls ranged from 6.37 seconds for the 6-year-olds to 4.60 seconds for the 12-year-olds. For both studies the mean improvement in speed with advancing age was approximately .2 to .3 seconds for all ages except kindergarten. These children improved their speed .7 to .9 seconds during the first grade year.

The shuttle run most commonly used is one that requires the child to run back and forth between two lines several times. The distance between the lines and the number of trips back and forth has varied from study to study. Generally, the total distance traveled has been from 40 to 60 yards and the number of trips has been from four to six. Milne, Seefeldt, and Reuschlein (1975) reported a 40 yard agility shuttle run administered to kindergarten, first, and second

grade children. The mean times for these children were 14.79, 13.42, and 13.00 seconds for males respectively. For the girls the mean times were 15.60, 14.06, and 13.76 seconds. Latchaw (1954) administered a 40 yard shuttle run to fourth, fifth, and sixth grade boys. The mean times for these grade levels, respectively, were 13.40, 13.00, and 12.40 seconds. A 60 yard shuttle run was given to boys aged 9 to 12 years by Clarke and Wickens (1962). The mean times of these children were 20.2, 20.3, 19.1, and 18.1 respectively. In order to contrast performance across age the data from these studies are shown in Figure 12.1. A conversion to

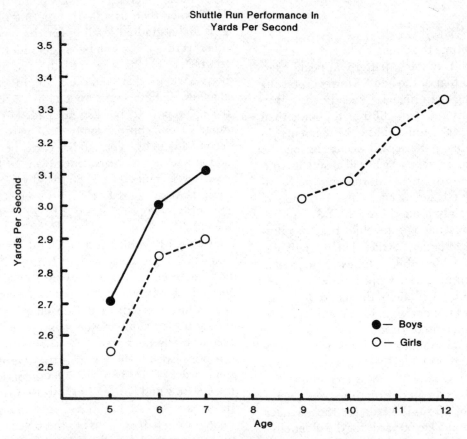

Figure 12.1. Shuttle run performance in yards per second. (After Milne, Seefeldt, and Reuschlein [1975], Latchaw [1954], and Clarke and Wickens [1962].)

yards per second was used. Again, as with the dash, boys and girls improved their speed with advancing age and girls were slightly slower than boys. Data is lacking for 8-year-olds and for girls 9 to 12. There seems to be a sharp change in speed from 5-7 years and then a leveling off from 7-9. The next three years, 9-12, show another decided change in speed.

For the endurance run, the child is asked to run for extended periods of time or to run over a lengthy distance. Milne, Seefeldt, and Reuschlein (1975) reported the results of a 400 foot run for kindergarten, first, and second grade children. The means for the boys were 50.77, 47.23, and 44.08 seconds respectively. For the girls the means were 53.06, 48.77, 46.15 seconds respectively. These means show a marked change in speed from age 5 to 7 years. Also, the boys are slightly faster than the girls.

Similar age and sex performance trends were found by Jackson and Coleman (1975) for 10-12-year-old children on a nine minute run. The mean distance covered by the boys was 1717, 1779, and 1841 yards respectively and the mean distance covered by the girls was 1514, 1537, and 1560 yards respectively. Gutin, Fogle, and Stewart (1975) reported data on distance running for 10-12-year-old children. These children ran 600 yards in 2.75 minutes, 1200 yards in 6.17 minutes, 1800 yards in 9.97 minutes and 1.3 miles in 12 minutes. No information on age and sex differences was reported. In order to contrast age level performance on the endurance run, these data were converted to yards per second and are shown in Figure 12.2. Age and sex trends are similar to those seen on the dash and shuttle run with boys being faster than girls and marked decreases occurring in speed with advancing age.

In comparing performances on the three different runs, a marked difference in each is seen through a decrease in speed. Performance on the dash is the fastest as it is straight running with no interruptions over a short distance. The shuttle run takes more time to complete due to the stops, starts, and changes of direction. Shuttle run performance in yards per second are .2 to .3 yards per seconds slower than the dash scores. The slowest run is logically the endurance run. Longer distances are covered and the ultimate fatigue factor operates to slow performance. However, in comparing the shuttle run and endurance run, the scores are relatively similar with an approximate .1 yard per second difference at ages 5-7. The older age group show markedly similar performances.

The similarities in performance of the three runs are readily apparent when viewing changes that occur with increasing age. All three runs show marked changes in speed from ages 5-7. There seems to be a slight decrease in speed from 8-10 years on the dash and a relatively constant performance for shuttle and endurance runs for this same age period. From ages 10-12 years there is a decided increase in running speed for all three runs.

HOPPING, GALLOPING, SKIPPING

There are a number of motor tasks stressing the proper sequencing of foot movements, while either remaining in place or moving in space. Hopping is such a motor task where a child may hop in place or while moving forward skip for speed. This summary of footwork is limited to the tasks studied by Keogh (1970).

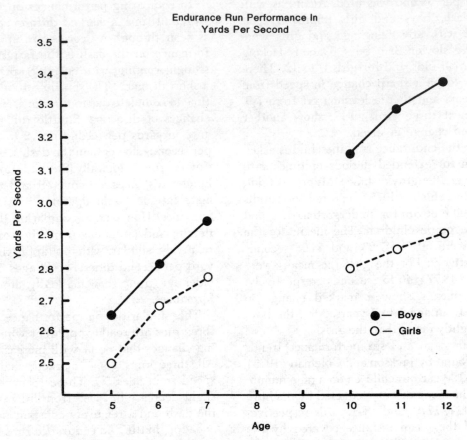

Figure 12.2. Endurance run performance in yards per second. (After Milne, Seefeldt, and Reuschlein [1975], Jackson and Coleman [1975], and Gutin, Fogle, and Stewart [1975].)

Girls perform better than boys on hopping, galloping, and other footwork tasks. This is seen in the ability to perform the complete task at an earlier age and in the quality of movements. These observations are limited to the early school years, since performance on these tasks cannot be measured well beyond the time of basic acquisition of the movements. Most children are able to gallop at age four and to skip at age six. But girls generally learn to skip and gallop sooner than boys. Similar boy-girl differences have been noted for ability to hop on one foot. Many observers have described girls as hopping more gracefully in contrast to boys who seem more forceful and flat footed. Girls also perform better when hopping alternately from one leg to the other, and when hopping forward for speed (50 feet) or control (within squares marked on a mat). Control of foot movements can further be examined in alternate tapping of feet and in foot movements out-and-back or back-and-forward (leg movements of a jumping-jack). Both boys and girls show marked improvement in such tasks from age five to seven, but girls perform better than boys.

It is an important generalization that girls acquire control of foot movements at an earlier age than boys. It is not possible to explain this difference in term of girls' preference for play activities like hopscotch since these activities follow in time the acquisition of more basic foot skills. Cultural factors may influence these boy-girl differences, but there is no evidence to indicate how this occurs. Girls are generally more mature biologically than boys of the same chronological age, and advanced biological maturity must be considered as a factor for boy-girl differences in control of foot movements. As might be expected, young girls also perform better in arm movements requiring sequential control (tapping and clapping), which further indicates earlier control by girls of limb movements.

JUMPING

The ability to jump encompasses several movement patterns. The young child most commonly learns to jump through space in a series of jumps and to jump "down" — as from stairs, chairs, bed, etc. Occasionally the child will attempt to jump "over" something, but this is rare. On most occasions, it is not until a child enters school that he/she will experience jumping "up", jumping "over", and jumping "far". The most commonly found studies of jumping performance deal with jumping for distance which is usually called the standing long jump. There is also a running long jump, but this is not used much before junior high school age when track and field events are studied. Investigations of vertical jumping and high jumping (also called hurdle jumping) in the elementary school child have been conducted but are less numerous than the standing long jump.

Since the standing long jump has been used the most extensively, our discussion of jumping performance in the elementary school child will begin with the results of these investigations. Glassow and Kruse (1960) in a study of the motor performance of 6-14-year-old girls administered the standing long jump to 125 children. The range of distance jumped varied from 40.5 inches for the 6-year-olds to 69.7 inches for the 14-year-olds. The average increase in distance jumped for each year of age was approximately four inches. Children in kindergarten, grade one, and grade two (N=533) were given a standing long jump as one item among a motor performance battery (Milne, Seefeldt, and Reuschlein, 1975). Differences between males and females were contrasted. The means for the girls in kindergarten, grade one, and two were 34.78, 41.37, 46.41 inches respectively. The means for the boys in kindergarten, grade one, and two were 33.73, 38.05, 41.42 respectively. Changes in performance over each year showed that boys increased their jumping distance five to six inches while girls increased their jumping distance to three to four inches.

Between 1960 and 1968, Keogh collected data in seven studies on standing long jump performance of children ages 7 to 17. A composite of these data are shown in Figure 12.3. Increased performance with age and group differences between boys and girls are illustrated graphically on the composite curve. From the graph mean points in Figure 12.3, it can be seen that group performance on the standing long jump increases three to five inches per year for both boys and girls from age seven to age eleven. These yearly increases are similar to those reported by Glassow and Kruse (1960) and Milne, Seefeldt, and Reuschlein (1975) for children from age five to seven. Also, group

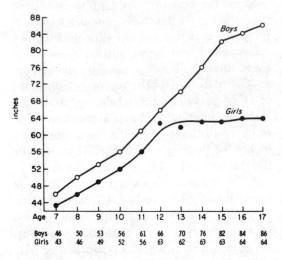

Figure 12.3. Standing long jump performance based on data from seven studies (Keogh).

performance for boys at each age during these years is three to five inches better than group performance for girls. The overlap in distributions, standard deviations of six to eight inches, is great enough that it is not unusual for some girls to perform better than many boys of the same age nor is it unusual for some boys to perform poorer than many girls of the same age. The same is true when comparing distance jumped among individual children who differ one or two years in age. All of this is another reminder that graphic and tabular summaries portray group (average) performance and that such summaries are not predictive of individual expectancies. Although boys have a consistently higher mean score at each age, both boys and girls increase approximately 30 percent in mean performance from age seven to age eleven. Comparable figures from age seven to age fifteen are 78 percent for boys and 47 percent for girls. Performance data are not as abundant for earlier years, but the increase from age five to age seven appears to be as large or larger than increases at later two

year intervals, and boys also have slightly higher mean figures than girls.

Other studies that have reported mean data for standing long jump performance show that these means are very close in comparison to the means of the Keogh data. Clarke (1971) obtained results from standing long jump performance of Oregon boys almost identical to mean points in Figure 12.3. Espenschade (1960) in a summary of earlier studies on standing long jump prepared a graphic composite of male and female performance from age five to seventeen years. The pattern for her composites matches quite closely the pattern in Figure 12.3.

Espenschade (1960) also prepared a similar summary for performance on the vertical jump by five to seventeen-year-old children. The scores ranged from 2.5 inches for five-year-old boys to 12.2 inches for twelve-year-old boys. For girls the scores ranged from 2.2. inches to 11.2 inches. The average yearly increase in jumping height was 2.0 inches for boys and 1.6 inches for girls aged five to ten. Between ten and twelve years the average increases dropped to .6 inches for boys and .4 inches for girls.

Data for hurdle jumping is quite limited. However, Cowan and Pratt (1934) conducted an extensive study of this jumping ability in 540 children aged three to twelve years. The approximate means ranged from 5 inches in three-year-olds and 28 inches in twelve-year-olds. There was a linear increase in height jumped with advancing age. Between the ages of three and five, yearly gains were approximately 4.5 inches. Between five and seven years, these gains dropped to 1.5 inches. Ages seven to nine years showed a rise in yearly increase of jumping height of 3 inches per year, followed by a return to 1.5 inch increases for ages ten to twelve. No information was reported on differences in performance between boys and girls.

THROWING

By the age of five the child has mastered the basic gross pattern of throwing. During the elementary school years throwing becomes more proficient. This proficiency occurs through growth and increased strength, opportunity to practice, and gradual learning of the principles of efficient movement. Measures of throwing performance most commonly used by investigators have been primarily those of distance throwing. Some studies have investigated accuracy throwing or target throwing, but there is wide variation in procedure and cross study comparisons are difficult to make.

Espenschade (1960) has presented a compilation of the results of various studies using a distance throw for children aged five to seventeen years. These studies show that boys throw farther than girls at all ages. The difference between sexes in distance thrown ranges from approximately nine feet at age five to forty-five feet at age twelve. Mean performance figures for boys in early years generally are equal to girls who are two or three years older. There is little overlap in test distributions for boys and girls of the same age, particularly during adolescence when boys have mean performance figures more than twice as large as mean performance figures for girls.

In spite of marked sex differences in throwing for distance, both boys and girls increase mean performance more than 100 percent from age seven to age eleven. These are large proportional increases compared to 20 percent and 30 percent increases for running and standing broad jump during the same ages. Throwing power increases with age at a more rapid rate than muscle strength, thus indicating an increase in coordination of body movements to produce such proportionately large increases. The lack of boy-girl differences in throwing power (distance) in some studies of European children is indicative of cultural effects upon the level of performance achieved in this motor task.

Studies have been conducted to investigate throwing accuracy in children by several investigators. Latchaw (1954) used a target throw task in her study of motor skills in fourth, fifth, and sixth grade children. The target was an 8' x 4' wall target placed three feet above the floor. The child, standing four feet away, tried to hit the wall target with a ball as many times as possible in 15 seconds. The mean number of hits reported for fourth, fifth, and sixth grade boys was 15.85, 16.29, and 18.59 respectively. For the girls the mean number of hits were 13.50, 13.27, and 14.51 respectively. Dobbins and Rarick (1974) investigated the performance of eight-year-old boys on a target throwing accuracy task. The target was a six foot square area divided vertically into fifteen segments, 12.2 cm wide. The center vertical segment was painted red and designated as the area the children should try to hit with their throws. Placement of the target was 91 cm above the floor and 15 feet away from the thrower. The children were given 28 throws at the target as described above and then the target was rotated so that the segments ran horizontally and 28 throws were given again. The children's accuracy was scored by the distance of the deviations from the center target area. The mean deviation for the vertical target was 2.18 inches and for the horizontal target, 2.25. Sturtevant (1974) used three wall targets (25", 14", 7" in diameter) in a study of accuracy throwing performances of nine-year-old boys. The boys were given five tries to hit each target from a 25 foot distance. Thirty percent of the children could hit it once out of five tries. Throwing at the 25" target was more accurate as all boys could hit the target at least two out of five tries.

KICKING

If a ball is stationary the very young child can walk up to it and kick it reasonably well. However, difficulty is experienced in kicking a rolling ball because the child cannot coordinate the elements of visual tracking, speed of oncoming ball, and timing of the motor act. By the age of five the child has matured to the point that he/she can successfully kick both a stationary and a rolling ball. During the years six to twelve the child increases in ability to kick with force and accuracy. These increases are due to improved overall strength occurring through natural growth and maturation, gradual use of more efficient movement patterns, and opportunity to practice the skill of kicking.

Studies investigating the kicking performance of children have used distance kicking, accuracy kicking, and punt kicking as tasks to measure performance and to reflect changes over age and differences between boys and girls. Jenkins (1930) administered a soccer kick for distance to children aged five, six, and seven years. The mean distance kicked for the boys were 11.5, 18.4, and 25.4 feet respectively. For the girls the means were 8.0, 10.1, and 15.0 feet respectively. A soccer kick for distance was also used by Dohrman (1965) in a study of kicking skills of eight-year-old boys and girls.

The boys were able to kick the ball a mean distance of 31 feet while the girls kicked 22 feet. Williams et al. (1970) assessed kicking performance in five to nine-year-old children by using a distance kick with a utility ball. Results were recorded in feet per second. The scores for the boys ranged from 18.11 for five-year-old to 33.73 for nine-year-olds. For the girls the scores ranged from 13.06 for five-year-olds to 25.59 for nine-year-olds.

A graphic composite of the data from these studies is presented in Figures 12.4 and 12.5. The similarities are striking. There is a marked increase in kicking performance with each advancing age level. The yearly increases in kicking distance for boys are six to seven feet. For girls the increases are not so dramatic being two, five, and seven feet across age respectively. In feet per second, yearly increases are approximately two to three feet per second for both sexes except between years seven and eight, when the increases are five to six feet. At all ages boys performed better than girls. On distance kicking tasks respectively, the mean differences between boys and girls across age were 3.5, 8.1, 10.4, and 9.0 feet respectively. For the feet per second measure, the differences were 5.05, 4.32, 5.87, 7.21, and 7.14. The differences between male and female kicking performance increases as children get older.

Accuracy kicking was investigated by Latchaw (1954) by administering a target kicking task to fourth, fifth, and sixth grade children. The task was to kick a soccer ball into a wall target area as many times as possible within 15 seconds. The target area was 4' x 2½' in size and the child stood four feet away to perform the repeated kicking. The mean number of target hits for nine, ten, eleven, and twelve-year-old boys was 9.12, 9.98,

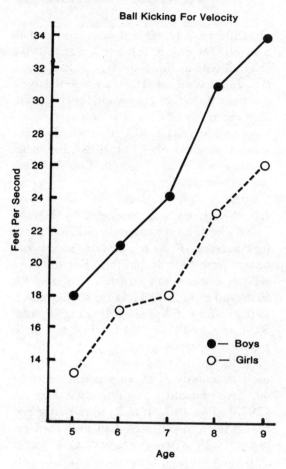

Figure 12.4. Ball kicking for velocity in feet per second (After Williams [1970], and Dohrman [1965]).

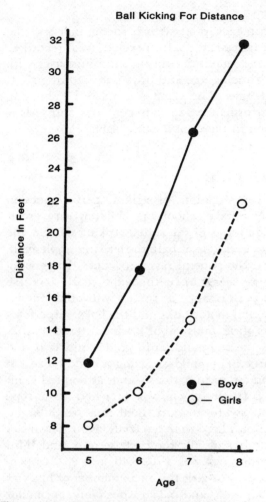

Figure 12.5. Ball kicking for distance in feet (After Williams [1970], and Dohrman [1965]).

10.31, and 10.90 respectively. Johnson (1962) also administered a target kicking task to children in grades one through six. The target area was marked on a wall space five feet high and ten feet wide and divided into two-foot vertical rectangles. Hits in the center rectangle were scored five points, the two adjacent rectangles three points, and the end rectangles one point. Each child was asked to kick a soccer ball three times into the target area from each of three distances 10 feet, 20 feet, and 30 feet from the

wall. The final score was the accumulation of points from the nine trials. Mean scores for the first through sixth grade boys were 22.56, 26.58, 29.62, 33.25, 34.40, and 32.88 points respectively. Mean scores for the girls were 22.39, 25.86, 25.08, 29.72, 30.92, and 32.73 points respectively.

The soccer punt was used as the kicking task in an investigation by Hanson (1965) of the motor performance of elementary school children. The children performed a drop kick punt with a soccer ball and the distance the ball traveled was recorded. Once again kicking distance increases with advancing age and boys outperform girls at all ages. The same age related increasing performance gap between boys and girls is seen in the punt kicking data.

STRIKING

Investigations of striking performance in elementary school age children vary greatly in terms of the actual striking motion, the size and type of ball, the striking implement, and the general task procedure. In general, there seems to be the same yearly increase in performance as found with other fundamental motor tasks and the boys outperform the girls. Seils (1951) administered a striking task to children in grades one, two, and three. The children using a child's size bat and a typical batter's stance attempted to hit a softball which was attached to a rope and swung toward them in a pendular fashion. There were ten trials given. The mean number of hits for first, second, and third grade boys was 4.70, 8.40, and 9.00 respectively. For girls the mean number of hits was 4.33, 4.46, and 5.33 respectively. A similar striking task was used by Johnson (1962) in a study of fundamental motor skills in elementary school children. Using a base, a batter's stance was assumed with bat in hand. Ten trials were given to hit a plastic ball swung over the plate. The number of hits were recorded. For the first through sixth grades, the means for boys were 2.67, 3.12, 3.07, 4.91, 5.69, and 6.24 respectively. Scores for the girls were 2.08, 2.12, 2.92, 4.21, 4.75, and 5.57 respectively.

Williams et al. (1970) used a two arm swing, similar to batting, in studying the striking performance of five to nine-year-old children. A tennis ball was suspended on a string. The object of the task was to strike the ball with as much force as possible with a badminton racket. The score was the average velocity in feet per second for five trials. The mean velocity for five to nine-year-old boys was 31.1, 34.1, 39.3, 41.3, 45.1 feet per second respectively. For girls the mean velocity was 21.5, 27.4, 31.6, 35.8, 36.7 feet per second respectively.

Striking performance in elementary school children was measured by Hanson (1965) with an underhand volleyball serve for distance. Five trials were given and scores were recorded in feet. For the boys serving distance ranged from 78.85 feet for first graders to 222.88 feet for sixth graders. Performances for the girls ranged from 50.02 feet to 161.00 feet for first and sixth graders respectively.

An actual softball batting situation was used in a study of striking performance of 40 five-year-old children by Skovran (1977). Two striking tasks were performed first with a seven inch ball and then repeated with a five inch ball. One was a stationary striking task where the ball was hit off a batting tee. The second was a moving striking task where the ball was tossed with an underhand pitch from a distance of ten feet and fifteen feet. The number of hits were then totaled to get a score for stationary striking (5" and 7" ball) and for moving striking (7" ball, 10'; 7" ball, 15'; 5" ball, 10'; 5" ball, 15'). The mean number of hits for stationary striking were 17 out of a possible 20. Performance dropped considerably on the moving striking task with children averaging 27 hits out of a possible 40. Information on sex differences was not reported.

Shope (1976) studied striking performance of five-year-old children on two tasks.

The first task was stationary striking using a batting tee, whiffle bat, batter's stance, and six inch ball. The same equipment was used for the second task which involved hitting a pitched ball which rebounded approximately 30 inches in front of the child and traveled up over the plate. The mean score for stationary striking was 20.30 feet per second and for moving striking was 17.08 feet per second.

Sheehan (1954) studied batting performances of boys aged seven to fifteen years. The evaluation situation was an actual baseball practice with batter and pitcher in appropriate locations on the diamond. The ball was pitched ten times and the batter attempted to hit it. Scoring was based on the type of hit, line drive, grounder, or fly, and the distance it traveled. A point system was used which assigned number values to each type of hit and the distance it traveled. The highest number of points that could be accumulated was 70. The mean score for the seven, eight, and nine-year-olds was 21.63 points and for the ten, eleven, and twelve-year-olds 27.43 points.

BALANCE

It is difficult to isolate balance, define it, and measure it because of its complexity. First, there is postural balance which occurs as our body's reflexive response to gravity. This type of balance allows us to maintain upright posture and to walk, sit, and move about in our world. No matter what type of movement in which the human body is engaged, this postural balance plays an important role. Another area of balance identified in the literature is called static balance. This has been defined as the ability of the body to maintain a particular body position without moving. Attempts to measure this type

of balance have used stabilometers, balance boards, dynabalometers, and stick balances. A third variation of balance has been referred to in the literature as dynamic balance. This is the ability of the body to maintain and control posture while it is moving through space. Most typically, dynamic balance is measured by walking balance beams. Fourthly, we have balance as it is performed by the gymnasts in skilled stunts and complex movement combinations. None of these balance variations is mutually exclusive of the other. All interrelate in some manner thus making measurement difficult. Regardless of the inherent problems involved, no one would dispute the important role of balance in all movement patterns.

Seashore (1947) studied dynamic balance performance in boys five to eighteen-years-of-age. He devised a beam walking test which was composed of nine 10 foot long beams each of progressively lesser width (4, 3½, 3, 2½, 2, 1½, ½, ¼ inches). These beams were placed 4½ inches off the floor. Each beam was marked in quarters and the child walked the widest to the narrowest beam until stepping off twice. At this point, the score was recorded to the nearest quarter. A perfect score would be 36 (9 beams x 4 quarters each). The mean scores for the five to twelve-year boys were 18.1, 18.1, 22.9, 24.0, 23.5, 25.3, 27.4, and 27.4 respectively. These scores show an increase of ten quartiles (25 feet) from age five to age twelve years. Williams et. al (1970) administered a beam walking test to children aged five to nine years. The size of beams and scoring procedure were similar to the Seashore study with the 2½ inch beam being omitted. A perfect score was 20 points (five beams divided into quartiles). The mean scores for the five to nine-year-old boys ranged from 13.3 to 24.6 points. For the five to nine-year-old girls the mean scores ranged from 14.8 to 28.9.

A similar beam walking test was given to children aged eight to sixteen years by Goetzinger (1961). He used the Heath Rail-walking Test which was composed of walking two 9 feet and one 6 feet long beams placed just off the floor. The three widths were 4″, 2″, and 1″ respectively and three trials were given to walk each beam. The distance to first step-off was recorded and added for the three trials. This was then multiplied by a difficulty rating factor of one for the 4″ wide beam, two for the 2″ wide beam and four for the 1″ beam. The

total points possible were 153. The means prepared by Heath (1943) for six to fourteen-year-old children were compared to those obtained by Goetzinger. Means were similar for both groups. Figure 12.6 illustrates the change in performances for boys and girls from six to twelve years of age.

Three 12′ long balance beams were walked by kindergarten boys and girls in a study of balance performances conducted by DeOreo (1971). The beams were placed one foot from the floor and varied in width being 4″, 3″, and 2″ respectively. The children were asked to walk each beam forward and backward for three trials. Distance to

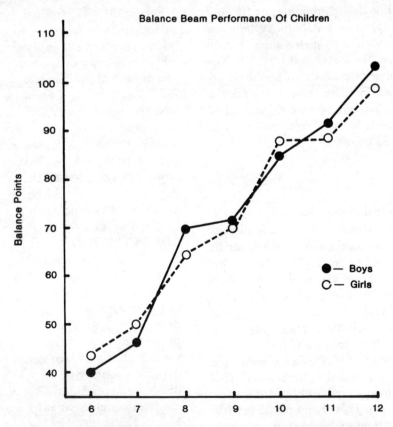

Figure 12.6. Balance beam performance of children. (After Goetzinger [1961] and Heath [1943].)

first step-off was recorded. For the walking forward tasks, the mean distance traveled on the 4″ beam was 12 feet for both boys and girls; on the 3″ beam, 11.5 feet for girls and 10 feet for boys; and on the 2″ beam, 5.5 feet for girls and 7.8 feet for boys. For the walking backwards tasks, the mean distance traveled on the 4″ beam was 11 feet for girls and 10 feet for boys; on the 3″ beam, 9 feet for girls and 6.5 feet for boys; and on the 2″ beam, 4 feet for girls and 3 feet for boys.

Even though the above studies vary in the length and width of beams, procedure, and scoring methods, it is interesting to note the similarities in results. Data from all studies indicate a steady increase in performance from ages five to twelve years as shown in figure 12.6. There does not appear to be the clear-cut boy-girl performance difference as seen for other fundamental motor tasks. Performance of boys and girls seems to be relatively similar with the younger girls out-performing the younger boys. All three graphs show a slowing down of increased performance around the ages of seven to eight years. This is especially true for the boys. This is then followed by a marked increase in performance for both sexes for ages eight and nine years.

Studies of balancing ability seem to be more numerous than those of dynamic balancing. Seils (1951) administered a static balance task to children in grades one, two, and three. The task involved standing on one foot lengthwise on a narrow piece of wood for as long as possible. The means for the first, second, and third grade boys were 5.02, 7.59, and 9.19 seconds respectively. For the girls the means were 5.17, 5.07, and 10.50 respectively.

DeOreo (1971) tested kindergarten boys and girls on a 14″ x 14″ balance board placed on rockers which placed the top of the board

8° off the floor. The children attempted to keep the board in balance for six 15 second trials in the lateral plane and in the anterior-posterior plane. The number of contacts with the base was also recorded. No significant differences were found between the performance of boys and the performance of girls. The mean time in balance for the lateral plane was 9.75 seconds and for the anterior-posterior plane 11.15 seconds. The number of contacts were 2.6 and 4.0 respectively.

Balance performance on a stabilometer of seven to nine-year-old children was investigated by Eckert and Rarick (1976). The apparatus consisted of a board mounted on a central pivot. Five trials were given to balance on the board and the score was recorded in work-adler units. These reflect the amount of rotation of the board during the 15 second trials. A low score reflects less movement and thus a more in balance trial. The mean scores for the seven to nine-year-old boys were 25.03, 22.17, 24.18 units respectively. For the girls the mean scores were 25.38, 24.37, and 23.48 respectively.

A dynabalometer was used by Williams et. al (1970) to measure static balance performance in children aged five to nine years. The apparatus consisted of a platform balanced on a trailer hitch knob which was attached to a base. Two 30 second trials were given. The mean time in balance for five to nine-year-old boys ranged from 8.01 to 12.99 seconds respectively. For the girls the mean time in balance ranged from 9.82 to 12.98 seconds respectively. The data which are plotted in Figure 12.7 show improved balance performance with increasing age. As in the dynamic balance data, there seems to be a similar slowing down of increased performance with age. As in the dynamic balance data, this is particularly true between the ages of seven and eight years.

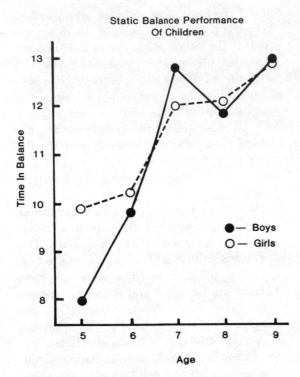

Figure 12.7. Static balance performance of children. (After Williams [1970].)

Bachman (1961) administered a stabilometer test to children and adults aged six to twenty-five years. The apparatus consisted of a rectangular board upon which the subjects stood with their feet 14″ apart. The board was mounted on a center pivot rod axle which allowed it to tilt laterally. Ten 30 second trials were given. There seemed to be a slight performance decrease from ages six and seven to eight and nine followed by a sharp increase in performance after age 9.

SUMMARY

Performance on fundamental motor tasks, in terms of group mean scores, increases throughout the early years, ages five to ten.

Beyond these years, it is a general expectancy that group mean performance for boys will continue to increase until seventeen or eighteen years of age, whereas group mean performance for girls may plateau at twelve to fourteen years of age.

Mean performance figures for boys and girls often are significantly different from each other at each age during early years of development, but overlap in score distributions tends to be sizable. The same is true for comparisons between age groups that are one or two years apart. This means that group performance differences are expected by age and sex during the early years, although many individuals may contradict group expectations. It is not unusual in an elementary school that individual children perform as well as older children or children of opposite sex in spite of group differences to the contrary.

References

Bachman, J. C. "Motor Learning and Performance as Related to Age and Sex in Two Measures of Balance Coordination." *Research Quarterly* 32(1962):123.

Clarke, H. H. and Wickens, J. S. "Maturity, Structural, Strength, and Motor Ability Growth of Boys 9 to 15 Years of Age." *Research Quarterly* 33(1962):26.

Clarke, H. H. *Physical and Motor Tests in the Medford Boys' Growth Study.* Englewood Cliffs, N. J.: Prentice-Hall, 1971.

Cowan, E. and Pratt, B. "The Hurdle Jump as a Developmental and Diagnostic Test." *Child Development* 5(1934):107.

DeOreo, K. L. "Dynamic and Static Balance in Preschool Children." Unpublished Ph.D. Dissertation, University of Illinois, 1971.

Dohrman, P. "Throwing and Kicking Ability of 8-Year-Old Boys and Girls." *Research Quarterly* 35(1965):465.

Dobbins, D. A. and Rarick, G. L. "The Performance of Intellectually Normal and Educable

Mentally Retarded Boys on Tests of Throwing Accuracy." *Journal of Motor Behavior* 9 (1977).

Eckert, H. M. and Rarick, G. L. "Stabliometer Performance of Educatable Mentally Retarded and Normal Children." *Research Quarterly* 47(1975):619.

Espenschade, A. S. "Motor Development, Science and Medicine of Exercise and Sports." Edited by W. R. Johnson. New York: Harper and Row Publishers, 1960, pp. 419-39.

Espenschade, A. A. and Eckert, H. M. *Motor Development.* Columbus, Ohio: Charles E. Merrill Publishers, 1967.

Glassow, R. B. and Kruse, P. "Motor Performance of Girls Aged 6 to 14 Years." *Research Quarterly* 31(1960):426.

Goetzinger, C. P. "Re-evaluation of Heath Railwalking 1951 to 1967." *Journal of Educational Research* 54(1961):187-91.

Gutin, B.; Fogle, R. K.; and Stewart, K. "Relationship among Submaximal Heart Rate, Aerobic Power, and Running Performance in Children." *Research Quarterly* 47(1975): 536.

Hanson, M. "Motor Performance Testing of Elementary School Age Children." Unpublished Ph. D. Dissertation, University of Washington, 1965.

Heath, S. R. "The Railwalking Test: Preliminary Motivational Norm for Boys and Girls." *Motor Skills Research Exchange* 1(1949):34.

Jackson, A. S. and Coleman, E. "Validation of Distance Run Tests for Elementary School Children." *Research Quarterly* 47(1975):86.

Jenkins, L. "A Comparative Study of Motor Achievements of Children of Five, Six, and Seven Years of Age." *Contributions to Education.* Teacher's College, Columbia University No. 414, 1930.

Johnson, R. "Measurements of Achievement in Fundamental Skills of Elementary School Children." *Research Quarterly* 33(1962):94.

Keogh, J. F. "Motor Performance Test Data for Elementary School Children." *Research Quarterly* 41(1970):600-602.

Latchaw, M. "Measuring Selected Motor Skills in Fourth, Fifth, and Sixth Grades." *Research Quarterly* 25(1954):439.

Milne, C.; Seefeldt, V.; and Teuschlein, P. "Relationship Between Grade, Sex, Race, and Motor Performance in Young Children." *Research Quarterly* 47(1975):726.

Seashore, H. G. "The Development of a Beam Walking Test and Its Use in Measuring the Development on Balance Beam in Children." *Research Quarterly* 18(1947):246.

Seils, L. "The Relationship between Measures of Physical Growth and Gross Motor Performance of Primary Grade Children." *Research Quarterly* 22(1951):244.

Sheehan, F. "Baseball Achievement Scales for Elementary Junior High Boys." Master's Thesis, University of Wisconsin, 1954.

Shope, G. N. "Relationships Between Striking Skills and Various Perceptual Components in Five-Year-Olds." Unpublished Master's Thesis, Kent State University, 1976.

Skovran, S. K. "The Relationship Between Visual Information Processing and Motor Proficiency in Five-Year-Old Children." Unpublished Master's Thesis, Kent State University, 1977.

Sturtevant, S. B. "An Investigation of the Role of LA and Task Complexity as Evidenced in Throwing Performances of Eight and Nine-Year-Old Boys." Unpublished Paper, Kent State University, 1974.

Williams, H.; Clement A.; Logsdon, B.; Scott, S.; and Temple, I. "A Study of Perceptual-Motor Characteristics of Children in Kindergarten through Sixth Grade." Unpublished Paper, University of Toledo, 1970.

Fundamental Motor Task Development: A Discussion and Point of View

13

Jack Keogh
University of California,
Los Angeles
Karen DeOreo
Kent State University

The preceding six chapters have described many different aspects of fundamental skill learning. Details for learning and refining these fundamental skills as well as normative data which provide insights as to the "typical" performances of children of different ages and sexes were presented. This chapter offers some general discussion and commentary which may be useful to those interested in the analysis and teaching of fundamental skills.

PERFORMANCES OF THE INDIVIDUAL WITHIN THE GROUP

Much of the information presented in the previous chapters deals with "normative" or group data. But what of the individual within the group? Is the child who is a good performer at grade one still the best performer at grade 6? Is the child who is good at one task likely to be good at all of the fundamental skills? To answer these questions we must take a look at "group stability" or the relative position of a child in the group from year to year and "individual stability" or the ability of the child to perform well on different tests and different items within a test.

Group Stability

The best way to determine group stability is to measure the performance of children on a given task and repeat the measurement some time later, usually months or years later. If there is group stability, the same people retain their relative position in the group over time, and there should be a high correlation coefficient between the results of the first measurement and the results of the second.

This discussion of individual change is limited to information from three studies and three motor tasks — jumping, running and throwing. Glassow and Kruse (1960) reported correlations on jumping, running, and throwing for Wisconsin girls tested at one year intervals while in elementary school. Rarick and Smoll (1967) tested a group of Wisconsin boys and girls on the same motor tasks from grades one through six and again when the children were in grade eleven. A group of California boys and girls were tested by Keogh on jumping, running, and throwing at six month intervals during four years when the children were in elementary school.

Interested readers should consult two other reports not included here, simply because the information and analyses do not fit the limited approach taken in this discussion. Glassow, Halverson, and Rarick (1963) studied improvement in motor performance as related to instructional programs, with detailed mechanical analyses of performance changes. Clarke (1971) recently reported the results of a twelve-year longitudinal study involving physical and motor tests of boys from ages seven through eighteen.

There is general agreement among the three studies that performance on the standing long jump generally has a high group stability, as measured by correlations of .6 to .8 for test sessions at several year intervals. Correlations between test sessions at three to four year intervals include many figures around .7. In the longest test of this generalization, Rarick and Smoll (1967) reported correlations of .60 and .56 for boys from ages seven to seventeen and seven to eighteen with comparable figures of .50 and .80 for girls. In marked contrast to jumping, correlations across time for running and throwing are generally not as high with considerable lack of agreement among studies. California boys had higher and more consistent patterns of correlations than California girls, but the opposite was generally true in the Wisconsin studies. It is important that additional longitudinal data be accumulated and studied to examine group stability in motor performance, since only the data for jumping are consistent among the available studies.

Individual Stability

The simplest and most direct way to examine individual stability is to plot a child's profile of several different fundamental skills tests. This approach was used in an examination of longitudinal data for California children (Keogh), and a brief summary of some findings will be given here. It must be remembered that these analyses of individual stability were drawn from a study where group stability was generally higher and internally more consistent than comparable group stability figures for children in the Wisconsin study of Rarick and Smoll (1967). It is likely that this will result in greater individual stability for California children.

Raw scores for each child were transformed to standard scores based on deviation of an individual score from the mean for the appropriate test session. A profile was made for each child on each task to describe performance over a four-year period in terms of relative position in the peer group. Ten standard score points on the profiles are equivalent to one standard deviation from the mean. Variability for each child, both for one or several tasks, can be counted in terms of the range of the standard scores. As an example, a child who had all of his/her standard scores for one motor task between plus eight and minus four would have a range of twelve. This means that his/her best score on this motor task was eight-tenths of a standard deviation above the mean and his poorest score was four-tenths of a standard deviation below the mean. Individual variability calculated in this manner does not designate level of performance, because a child with high scores and a child with low scores could have the same variability in scores.

Most children (74%) had most of their standard scores (seven of eight) within a personal range of 12 standard score points for individual motor tasks. Older boys (ages eight to eleven) were generally less variable in contrast to younger girls (ages six to nine) who were more variable on all comparisons. There were many children, (70%: excluding the younger girls) who had most of their standard scores (75%) for all motor tasks within a personal range or limit of 15 standard score points. It is up to the reader to decide the limits of individual variability that should be accepted as stable or unstable, and it is clear that we need standard techniques for analyzing individual change in order that comparisons may be made among studies. Many of the California children were quite stable, in the sense that a teacher or parent observing a child during the early school years would find the child at the same general level of performance within the peer groups. The child might occasionally perform higher or lower, but the overall evaluation would be "good", "fair", or "poor." It should be recognized that our evaluation of an individual child usually indicates a general performance level, such as good, fair, or poor, rather than a precise score.

Bloom (1964) presented some interesting analyses of individual change and stability for human characteristics, but we do not have such a summarizing analysis for motor performance. Based on the limited information available, it seems that many, if not most, individuals are quite stable in relative performance level on many motor tasks. If true to any marked extent, it is important to determine the factors contributing to the maintenance of performance stability as well as the disruption or change of stability. The understanding of individual change is basic to all who participate in an educational process.

NATURE OF THE CHILD VERSUS NATURE OF THE TASK

In testing young children we find far too often that investigators test the nature of the task rather than the nature of the child. Perhaps the simplest example is a motor task having a performance floor or ceiling. The task may be so difficult that few children can achieve any success (floor), or, somewhat the opposite, the task may be so easy that most children can perform it, which means that there is no way to register improved performance (ceiling). If a floor or ceiling effect operates over a several year age span, we do not observe a change in motor performance. We should not conclude that it is the nature of children not to increase in performance on this type of task when it is likely that we have done little more than identify a too difficult or too easy task. For example, Singer (1969) tested third and sixth grade children on an accuracy throw involving ten trials to bounce a ball into a box. All mean scores for boys and girls in this study were less than two. This indicates that this is a difficult task, but it does not help us examine the nature of motor development in accuracy throwing.

There are a number of other ways in which we might confuse the nature of the task and the nature of the child. Tapping tasks are frequently scored in terms of the child making a proper sequence of movements without regard for the speed or the timing (tempo) of the movements. Of greater concern would be the observation of a child's ability to control movements sufficiently to make a designated sequence of movements, rather than taking a count of how often the movements were made or requiring the movements to match a designated pace. Tapping for control should not be misinterpreted as tapping for speed and vice versa. It is important to recognize that test requirements or demands can be altered to change markedly the nature of the task. This brings up the point that speed and control are elements of most motor tasks, but they tend to be in conflict in the sense that an individual must make a "trade-off" in emphasizing one or the other. Tapping control may suffer if tapping speed is required, as throwing accuracy (control) may suffer if throwing distance (speed of body movements) is required. It is useful to think more carefully about the nature of a motor task before making a statement about the nature of motor development of a child.

POINT OF VIEW

A brief discussion of fundamental motor task development might well end here, since a general description with comments has been provided for development in fundamental motor skills. However, a point of view is offered here that might be useful for others in their study of motor development during early childhood. The first part of this final section is an argument for focusing upon control rather than maximum performance in assessing the motor development of young school children. The second part contains suggestions for improving one's ability to observe changes and differences in motor performance.

Motor Control

The earlier description of changes and differences in motor performance (Chapter 12) is almost completely based on maximum performance or achievement. This is probably true because it is easier to measure and compare motor performance in terms of maximum achievement. Consistent with the earlier remarks about altering the nature of the motor task, the emphasis upon maximum speed, force, or time may alter the meaning and interpretation of the achievement. It is more important in the early years (5 to 10) that movements be observed and studied from a point of view focused upon how much control a child has of his/her movements rather than how much effort can be mobilized. Increased control of a movement is basic to increased achievement, but it is inefficient to study the acquisition of control only in terms of maximum achievements.

Focus upon maximum achievement has restricted our view that acquisition of motor control should be a basic focus in the study of motor development (Keogh 1971b). Also preschool and early school age children view achievement and success in physical activities on a noise-and-energy basis rather than on an achievement basis. If a child displays sufficient energy and makes enough noise, he/she is readily accepted in play and games, and viewed as successful. Eventually, most children and adults adopt achievement — tag-escape, hit-miss — as the success goal.

The focus upon motor control requires a radical shift in thinking about motor performance, which can be appreciated only after some practice in this direction. One way to apply the concept of motor control is in developmental analyses of movements. If increased control of body movements is the basic concern, it is important to be able to observe such changes. Chapters 10 and 11 are presented specifically to aid the reader in observing these changes. The following comments offer some suggestions on how the Developmental Analysis Checklists might be used.

Observation of Movement Changes

Developmental Analysis Checklists can be used in several ways. One logical use is error detection. This consists of observing a child's performance and filling out the checklist. Another effective technique is to have the children use the checklist themselves to observe the movement of a partner.

Learning to watch and analyze someone else's movement helps the child understand his or her own movement patterns.

Several tips may be useful in observing the performance of children in various fundamental skills. First, it is important to watch the movements made by the child rather than watch the product of the child's movements. Do not watch the ball, watch the child; do not watch the game, watch the child. Second, begin by watching parts of the child's body rather than trying to see the total movement. Watching the upper or lower limbs is a good place to start. Position of head or trunk, movement of eyes, and action of hands and fingers are other body parts that tell a great deal about the movement. Look for similarities and differences in the way body parts are used. When a child is not performing the task adequately, it is important to note *what he/she is doing* rather than worrying only about what he/she is not doing.

Each motor task must be analyzed to determine what are important body parts to observe. The standing long jump is a good motor task for practicing observations, because the movements occur in a limited space and time. Begin by watching the legs to note that very young children will take a step rather than have both feet leave the ground at the same time. Also, legs will not be bent much nor will legs extend fully when taking off. When landing, a variety of leg movements will be observed, but a mature jumper will land with both feet together and knees moving forward. Arm movements are easily observed and indicative of jumping maturity. Children initially do not move their arms forward as they jump, keeping them to the side or rear. As the child learns to bring the arms forward in the jump, it may only be to place them as if

they are to resist or stop forward motion. It also is useful to watch head and body position, changing from "down" to "up" as the body becomes more extended.

Running is better observed by standing directly behind or in front of the child rather than at the side. Start by watching segments of one limb rather than a complete limb or a set of limbs. Hands, elbows, knees, and heels or toes will trace the general path of movement for the limb. After a little practice, the movement pattern for both limbs can be seen. Younger children will move their limbs around the vertical axis, their upright body, such that their limbs appear to rotate on their body. This will change to more movement in the path of their movement, arms and legs moving forward and back rather than horizontal and around the body.

Throwing also can be observed in terms of movements of body parts. Both shoulders initially remain in position, facing forward, but the shoulder of the throwing arms will be rotated back, then forward, in a more mature throwing motion. This indicates trunk rotation. The elbow of the throwing arm initially remains in front of the body, as the child pushes rather than throws the ball. A complex set of changes takes place as the child brings the ball backward before throwing. Watching the elbow will trace the path of the arm movement. As the throwing motion becomes better developed, follow the hand to note almost complete extension of the arm behind the back followed by flexion of the arm as the arm moves forward. It is also useful to look at the hand and fingers at the point of release and in the follow through, noting whether the fingers spread (less mature) or close (more mature) as the ball leaves the hand. This leads to watching the amount of hand or wrist snap. Leg-arm positions also are readily observable.

As noted in the checklists, there are many other movements that can and should be observed if one is going to examine the motor development of a child. The approach described here should be applicable. More important, it is hoped that this will divert attention from the movement outcome or product to the child and the development of movement control.

References

Bloom, B. S. *Stability and Change in Human Characteristics.* New York: John Wiley and Sons, 1964.

Clarke, H. H. *Physical and Motor Tests in the Medford Boys' Growth Study.* Englewood Cliffs, N. J.: Prentice-Hall, Inc., 1971.

Glassow, R. B.: Halverson, L. E.; and Rarick, G. L. "Improvement of Motor Development and Physical Fitness in Elementary School Children." Madison, Wisconsin: University of Wisconsin, 1963.

Keogh, J. F. "Comments on Singer's Study of Differences between Third and Sixth Grade Children." *Research Quarterly* 42(1971a): 96.

Keogh, J. F. *Motor Control as a Unifying Concept in the Study of Motor Development.* Motor Development Symposium, Berkeley, California: Department of Physical Education, University of California, 1971b.

Rarick, G. L. and Smoll, F. L. "Stability of Growth in Strength and Motor Performance from Childhood to Adolescence." *Human Biology* 29(1967):295.

Singer, R. N. "Physical Characteristics, Perceptual-Motor, and Intelligence Differences between Third and Sixth Grade School Children." *Research Quarterly* 40(1969):803.

Section 6

Physical Fitness: The Performance of Children

Physical Fitness Development of Children

14

Charles B. Corbin
Kansas State University

One important part of the total development of a child, more specifically, the motor development of the child, is physical fitness. While it is generally accepted that physical fitness is an important part of the normal development of a child, a general definition of the exact nature of physical fitness has not been universally accepted. For purposes of this discussion, physical fitness requires more than one definition. Since physical fitness is multidimensional, each aspect of it must be described separately. The emphasis of this section of the text will be on health related physical fitness, since other sections focus on the skill development of children. However, in as much as many of the standardized tests of physical fitness deal with more than one factor of physical fitness this discussion will involve some mention of skill related physical fitness factors.

SKILL VS. HEALTH-RELATED PHYSICAL FITNESS

For the purpose of this discussion, physical fitness factors have been grouped in two general categories, skill-related and health-related physical fitness (see Figure 14.1 for descriptions). The health related aspects are endurance or cardiovascular fitness, strength, muscular endurance, and flexibility. Body fatness can also be considered as a health related aspect of fitness (Corbin, 1978). These aspects are considered health related because people who possess them are less likely to suffer from such health problems as heart disease, back problems, obesity, and diabetes, to name a few. The skill related aspects of fitness include agility, reaction time, balance, coordination, and speed. These are considered skill related because people who possess them are likely to be skilled in games and sports as well in various vocational skills. Power is considered a combined aspect because is involves both strength (a health related aspect) and speed (a skill related aspect).

A HISTORY OF YOUTH FITNESS TESTING

Physical fitness testing has been carried on in one form or another for centuries. In the United States, Sargent, McCloy, Hitchcock, and Rogers were among the pioneers. Their work ranged from as early as 1880 to the late 1920s and early 1930s. More recently, it was the testing of Kraus and Hirschland (1954) which caused a great concern for the physical fitness of American children. The results of their research, reported in the *New York State Journal of Medicine* and later in the *Research Quarterly,* prompted the then-President of the United States, Dwight D. Eisenhower, to establish the President's Council of Youth Fitness in 1956. Since that time testing of American children, as well as the children of other countries, has become more widespread. Among tests most commonly used to assess the physical fitness of children are the Amer-

PHYSICAL FITNESS

Definition: Physical fitness is composed of many different aspects including health-related physical fitness aspects and motor fitness (skill-related) aspects. To function effectively in our society without undue fatigue and to have reserve energy to enjoy leisure time require adequate development of both the health-related and skill-related aspects of physical fitness. The important aspects of physical fitness are:

HEALTH-RELATED ASPECTS

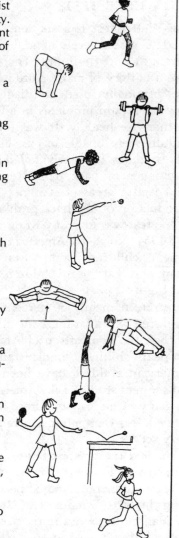

Cardiovascular Fitness. The ability to persist in numerous repetitions of an activity. Specifically, this aspect involves development of the respiratory and circulatory systems of the body.

Flexibility. The ability to move joints through a full range of motion.

Strength. The ability to exert force such as lifting a weight or lifting your own body.

Muscular Endurance. The ability to persist in numerous repetitions of an activity involving strength.

COMBINED ASPECT

Explosive Power. The ability to display strength explosively or with speed.

MOTOR-FITNESS ASPECTS

Agility. The ability to change directions quickly and to control body movements (total body).

Reaction Time. The ability to perceive a stimulus, begin movement, and finally complete a response.

Balance. The ability to maintain body position and equilbrium both in movement and in stationary body positions.

Coordination. The ability to perform hand-eye and foot-eye tasks such as kicking, throwing, striking, and the like.

Speed. The ability to move from one place to another in the shortest possible time.

Figure 14.1. The aspects of physical fitness. (From Corbin, *Becoming Physically Educated in the Elementary School.* **Second Edition, 1976, p. 54.)**

ican Alliance of Health, Physical Education and Recreation (AAHPER) test battery, the Kraus-Weber test, the Oregon Motor Fitness Test, and the California Physical Performance Test. The remainder of this chapter is devoted primarily to a discussion of the results of research using the Kraus-Weber and AAHPER tests.

THE KRAUS-WEBER TEST

The Kraus-Weber test is a six-item battery designed to assess levels of minimum muscular strength and flexibility. The test evolved from a battery of many more items which were originally used to diagnose potential low back pain problems in adults who were otherwise healthy. It was found that most adults were unable to pass all of the original test items. Those who failed had a higher incidence of back pain. Regular exercise for specific areas of weakness resulted in a reduction of low back problems. Ultimately, the test was given by Kraus and Hirschland (1954) to 4,458 American and 3,156 European children. Comparisons of the American and European children are presented in Figure 14.2.

The failure rate of nearly 60 percent for American children was a far more meaningful statistic than the comparison of American to European children. Similar failure rates for American children have been reported in subsequent studies. Like American adults, too many American children were found to possess less than minimal strength and flexibility scores.

Children showed the greatest failure rate on the hamstring flexibility item (toe touch), 59.4 percent of boys and 33 percent of girls failing the test (Kirchner and Glines 1957). American children did fairly well in back strength, but did not do so well on

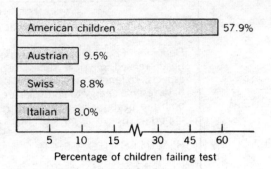

Figure 14.2. Comparison of American and European children on the Kraus-Weber Test. (Based on the research of Hans Kraus, and Ruth P. Hirschland. "Minimum Muscular Fitness Tests in School Children." *Research Quarterly* 25 [1954]: 178.)

other strength measures. Interestingly, girls made fewer overall failures and many fewer failures on flexibility. The boys showed superiority on strength items. Children show a lesser failure rate with age on strength items, but as age increases the failure on flexibility items increases.

It should be pointed out that there have been many objections to the use of the Kraus-Weber test as a measure of physical fitness (Phillips 1955). Included among the frequently voiced criticisms are the following: (1) it is limited in the areas of fitness which it tests; (2) it does not give partial credit for completion of test items; (3) it does not account of sex and age differences; (4) it is task specific to activities which are more related to the European than to the American culture; and (5) it samples only motor aspects of fitness.

Certainly there is reason for concern if the test is to be considered more than a test of minimal muscular strength and flexibility, and, of course, results of the test must be construed in a context which is consistent with the test's original purpose. If more comprehensive data on the physical fitness of children is desired, a more complete test would be appropriate. However, in view of the results of the studies reviewed above, it seems that typical American children were not meeting their potential for physical fitness development at the time of the study.

THE AAHPERD TEST BATTERY

The AAHPERD Physical Fitness Test, originally a seven item and now a six item test, was administered in 1958, 1965, and 1975. Items currently included in the test are the standing long jump, the 600-yard run, the shuttle run, the 50 yard dash, the bent knee sit up and the pull up (boys) or flexed-arm hang (girls). The softball throw, an item included in the test battery in 1958 and 1965 was eliminated in 1975. Also in 1975 the bent-knee sit up was substituted for the straight-leg sit up which was used previously.

For several years now, a special task force has been working to make further revisions in the AAHPERD test. The intent is to make the test one which truely emphasizes the health related aspects of fitness. A recent report of the task force (Falls, 1978) indicated that the test will be revised to include a longer distance run for cardiovascular fitness, a bent knee sit up or similar strength-muscular endurance item, a new test of trunk and leg flexibility, and probably a skinfold test of body fatness. The items from previous tests which measure skill related fitness may be included in a separate test. It should be noted that distance runs of 9 and 12 minutes are already available in the 1975 test manual as options for older children.

Results summarizing the three AAHPERD test administrations (1958, 1965, and 1975) are presented in Figure 14.3. All of these tests were administered to a national sample of children by Hunsicker and Reiff (1977).

The age-performance curves for the health related fitness tests, namely the 600-yard run-walk, pull-ups, and sit-ups, are similar in nature. Performance for boys increases as they grow with little improvement prior to age thirteen. Great increases occur with increased age until age sixteen or seventeen at which time performance again levels off. The post-pubescent increase can be attributed to increased muscle mass precipitated by the secretion of the male sex hormone. The leveling off at age sixteen or seventeen could be attributed to either lessened activity levels at those ages or to the fact that performances are near ceiling levels and improvements are unlikely.

Girls have virtually no increase in health-related physical fitness with age as measured by the pull up, sit up and 600-yard run performance. The increase in adipose tissue during and after adolescence, coupled with a more limited gain in muscle mass when compared to boys, can at least partially account for the lack of increases in performance with age. However, the fact that girls improved from 1958 to 1965 and then again from 1965 to 1975 on the 600 yard run suggests that girls have a potential for increased performance. Similarly girls increased in flexed arm hang performance from 1965 to 1975 for all except the older age ranges. Since the 1975 test includes a new sit up test, between year comparisons for it are not possible. Clearly these results show that girls do have a potiential for achieving health related fitness. Other laboratory test results which are not so affected by motivational level also show improved performance as girls grow older. A more complete discussion of the physical fitness performance of girls is included in Chapter 17.

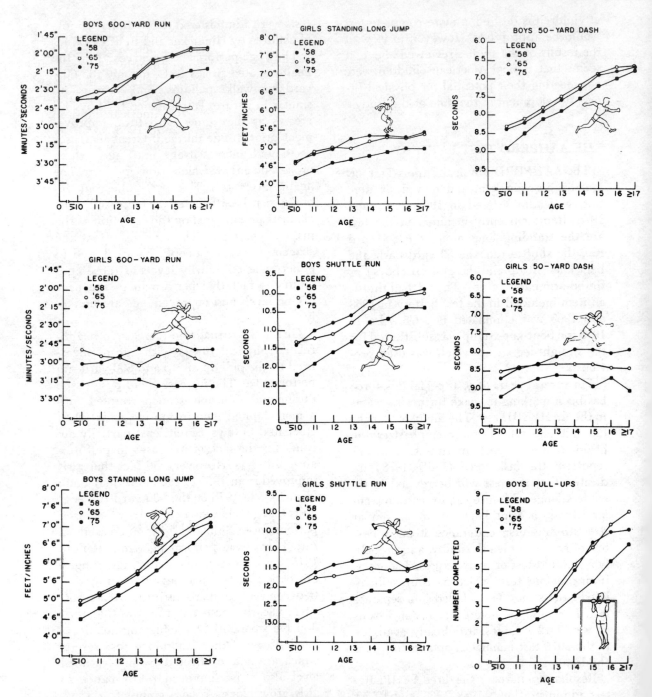

Figure 14.3. Comparative Mean Scores for AAHPERD Youth Fitness Test, 1958-1965-1975. (From Hunsicker, P. and Reiff, G. *JOPER.* 48: January, 1977, pp. 32 and 33.)

Age-performance curves for the skill-related fitness tests (shuttle run, 50-yard dash, softball throw, and standing broad jump) are somewhat different than for the health-related fitness tests discussed on the preceding pages.

For boys, age performance curves for skill-related fitness reflect increased performance with each year of age beginning at age ten. There is no lull in performance prior to age twelve, as there is for the health-related measures. Further, there is not always a leveling off or decrease in performance at age sixteen or seventeen for the skill-related measures.

Girls do not perform as well as boys on skill-related fitness tests at any age, but there is a near linear increase in performance with age. It is interesting that for both boys and girls the performance curves for skill-related fitness are linear. Performance curves for health-related variables are nonlinear as previously discussed. Possible differences in health-related and skill-related fitness curves are discussed in detail in Chapter 18.

Several other investigations have been conducted using the AAHPERD battery. Knuttgen (1961) tested Danish school children and the results were compared to the American AAHPERD standards. Both Japanese (Noguchi 1956) and British, (Pohndorf 1961) children have been tested. Results of all of the above studies indicated American children to be inferior to foreign children in all measures except ball throwing. The most significant implication of these studies is that the potential for physical fitness performance of American children exceeds that which is actually achieved. While foreign children do outperform American children, there is no reason to believe that their potential for performance is greater than

that of American children. Accordingly, it is suggested that a more active American youth would score significantly higher on tests such as those included in the AAHPERD battery. This opinion is also borne out by the fact that American children improved in fitness from 1958 to 1965. Though the increases from 1965 to 1975 were not as dramatic, it is significant that girls improved on the 600 yard run and the flexed arm hang, both tests proported to measure health related fitness. For the first time since the test was constructed, older girls had better scores on the 600 yard run than younger girls.

There are other test batteries which have been used in various states and countries to test the fitness of children. Because many of these use similar items they will not be discussed in this chapter. It should be pointed out, however, that several states such as South Carolina, Missouri, and Texas have already developed tests to measure the health related aspects of fitness similar to those currently being developed by the task force for the AAHPERD test.

References

Corbin, C. B.; Dowell, Linus; Lindsey, Ruth; and Tolson, Homer. *Concepts in Physical Education,* 3rd ed. Dubuque, Iowa: Wm. C. Brown Company, 1978.

Corbin, C. B. *Becoming Physically Educated in the Elementary School,* 2nd ed. Philadelphia: Lea and Febiger, 1976.

Falls, Harold. "Revision of the AAHPER Youth Fitness Test Battery." A paper presented to the National Conference on Aerobic Exercise, Tulsa, Oklahoma, October, 1978.

Fox, Margaret G. and Atwood, Janet. "Results of Testing Iowa School Children for Health and Fitness." *Journal of Health, Physical Education, and Recreation* 26(1955):20.

Hunsicker, Paul and Reiff, Guy. "Youth Fitness Report: 1958-1965-1975." *Journal of Physical Education and Recreation* 48(1977):32.

Kirchner, Glenn and Glines, Don." "Comparative Analysis of Eugene, Oregon, Elementary School Children Using the Kraus-Weber Test of Minimum Muscular Fitness." *Research Quarterlry* 28(1957):16.

Knuttgen, Howard G. "Comparison of Fitness of Danish and American School Children." *Research Quarterly* 32(1961):109.

Kraus, Hans and Hirschland, Ruth P. "Minimum Muscular Fitness Tests in School Children." *Research Quarterly* 25(1954):178.

Noguchi, Yoshiyuki. "Fitness Testing of Japanese Children." *Journal of Health, Physical Education, and Recreation* 27(1956):20.

Phillips, Marjorie et al. "Analysis of Results from the Kraus-Weber Test of Minimum Muscular Fitness in Children." *Research Quarterly* 26(1955):314.

Pohndorf, Richard H. "British Youth Take Fitness Test." *Journal of Health, Physical Education, and Recreation* 32(1961):75.

Cardiovascular Fitness of Children

15

Charles B. Corbin
Kansas State University

For operational purposes, cardiovascular fitness is defined as the ability of the human organism to supply oxygen to the working muscles and the ability of the muscles to utilize the oxygen to support work. This requires a heart muscle fit enough to pump oxygenated blood, a vascular system capable of carrying it, and a muscular system capable of utilizing the oxygen when confronted with demanding work situations. Cardiovascular fitness is roughly synonomous with the terms cardiorespiratory fitness, cardiovascular endurance, general endurance, stamina, and physical working capacity.

THE CHILD'S HEART MYTH

As early as 1879, Beneke warned of the dangers of repetitive work to the heart of the young child. He indicated that a child should refrain from vigorous exercise because of the "natural disharmony" between the development of the size of the heart muscle and size of the large blood vessels. Because he believed that the large blood vessels develop at a relatively slower rate than the heart muscle, he warned that the vessels would be unable to accommodate the blood flow created by the faster growing heart. He therefore warned of the "grave danger" to the exercising child who was predisposed to high blood pressure and accompanying circulatory problems (cited by Karpovich 1937).

Young (1923) perpetuated the child's heart myth. He suggested that the natural discrepancy in development between the heart and blood vessels, which becomes noticeable at age seven, continues to grow worse as children grow older.

It was not until 1937 that Karpovich (1937) reevaluated Beneke's theory. He noted a simple, but obvious, error in Beneke's calculations. Although the size of the artery was smaller in proportion to the heart in young children compared to older children, the blood carrying capacity was proportionate to heart development. The error was a mathematical one. Beneke had assumed that increases in blood carrying capacity were proportional to increases in the circumference of the blood vessel. In fact, the blood carrying capacity of the artery increases relative to the cross-sectional area rather than in a linear relationship to the circumference of the artery. In other words, what appears to be an artery growing relatively slowly, is one that is able to carry blood in proportion to a growing heart's ability to supply it.

In spite of Karpovich's finding, the child's heart myth is not entirely extinct. A relatively recent child growth and development text implies a danger for the child participating in vigorous exercise. This book states:

In the circulatory system there is an increase in the size of the heart and in the length and thickness of the walls of the blood vessels. The heart grows so rapidly that, in the seventeen or eighteen year old, it is twelve times as heavy as it was at birth. The increase in the veins and arteries during this time, by contrast, is only fifteen percent. By the end of adolescence, the ratio of the size of the heart to the arteries is 290 to 61 as compared with 25 to 20 at birth. This means that a large heart must pump through small arteries. Until this condition is corrected, late in adolescence, too strenuous exercise may cause an enlargement of the heart or result in valvular disease. Furthermore, tension in the arteries resulting from disproportion in the size of the heart and of the arteries, causes much of the restlessness of this age (Hurlock 1967, p. 47, 48).

Studies such as those by Boas (1931) now clearly show that fears for children in exercise are unfounded. Boas after studying children in exercise, concluded "that muscles will flag so that the person will collapse before the heart is called for its last ounce of effort." This study, and others which are reviewed in a later section of this chapter, indicate that children are capable of much greater cardiovascular performance than previously thought possible. In fact a recent position paper of the American Academy of Pediatrics (1978) suggests that many children with congenital and rheumatic heart defects who have been screened out of physical activity, are capable of "full and active" participation. The Academy indicates that for those who are free of hemodynamic impairments, it is likely that psychological harm due to limitation of activity far outweighs the risk of problems associated with permitting participation. Of course medical supervision and screening is important. However, many children previously thought to be "cardiac cripples" may, with medical supervision, participate fully in physical activity. In summary, the following statement by Corbin (1976) relative to the child's heart and exercise seems defensible. "Like any other muscle, the heart reacts to over-

load, and exercise stimulates heart growth in both size and function. *A healthy child* cannot physiologically injure the heart permanently through exercise unless the heart is already weakened or diseased (Corbin, 1976, p. 20).

MAXIMUM O_2 INTAKE OF CHILDREN

Maximum O_2 intake is generally considered the most valid method of assessing cardiovascular fitness. The most comprehensive study of maximum O_2 intake for children is that of Astrand (1952). Results of this study are presented in Table 15.1.

Absolute maximal O_2 intake values for children were less than for adult subjects. However, *when O_2 values were corrected for body size (ml/kg), children had scores equal to, or higher than, adult subjects, except for extremely young children.* Astrand suggests that the young child's poorer maximal O_2 may not be a result of real O_2 intake differences, but rather the willingness to "give up" before true maximal values are achieved.

It can be seen in Table 15.1 that oxygen intake is fairly linear up to age thirteen, but after that age the scores of men increase more rapidly than those of women. After this age, boys generally have significantly better performance than girls.

Like PWC, O_2 intake correlates well with physiological measures, particularly body weight. However, the relationship decreases for girls after age thirteen.

A recent study (Gilliam, Sady, Thorland, and Weltman, 1977) yielded similar results to those reported by Astrand. While Maximum O_2 intake increased with age, it did not increase with age when adjusted for body weight. O_2 intake develops in close

TABLE 15.1
Maximal O_2 Intake; Ages 4-33.*
Numbers Represent Means, Standard Error of
the Mean and Standard Deviations.

	Sex	Age Groups						
		4–6	7–9	10–11	12–13	14–15	♂ 16–18 ♀ 16–17	♂ 20–33 ♀ 20–25
Number of subjects	♂	10	12	13	19	10	9	42
	♀	7	14	13	13	11	10	44
Maximal O_2-intake	♂	1.01±0.05 0.14	1.75±0.05 0.17	2.04±0.06 0.20	2.46±0.12 0.50	3.53±0.22 0.69	3.68±0.17 0.49	4.11±0.06 0.37
	♀	0.88±0.03 0.07	1.50±0.05 0.16	1.70±0.05 0.17	2.31±0.07 0.25	2.58±0.12 0.39	2.71±0.09 0.29	2.90±0.04 0.25
Maximal O_2-intake per kg body weight (ml per min.)	♂	49.1±1.4 4.3	56.9±1.0 3.6	56.1±1.0 3.6	56.5±0.6 2.4	59.5±0.9 2.7	57.6±1.4 4.3	58.6±0.7 4.1
	♀	47.9±1.5 4.0	55.1±0.9 3.2	52.4±0.8 2.8	49.8±0.7 2.5	46.0±1.0 3.3	47.2±0.9 2.6	48.4±0.5 3.2
Maximal O_2-intake per m^2 body surface area (litre pr. min.)	♂	1.26±0.03 0.09	1.62±0.03 0.08	1.67±0.02 0.07	1.75±0.04 0.17	2.07±0.04 0.13	2.05±0.05 0.15	2.20±0.03 0.16
	♀	1.16±0.04 0.08	1.49±0.02 0.08	1.49±0.03 0.10	1.59±0.03 0.09	1.60±0.05 0.15	1.65±0.05 0.14	1.74±0.02 0.10

*Adapted from Per-Olaf Astrand, *Experimental Studies of Working Capacity in Relation to Sex and Age.* Copenhagen: Munksgoaard, 1952, used by permission.

proportion to increases in body mass. This study and those of Astrand support the potential for children in performing tasks requiring great cardiovascular fitness as long as performance standards are adjusted by differences in body size.

PHYSICAL WORKING CAPACITY (PWC) OF CHILDREN

Considerable research has been considered in recent years in an effort to shed some light on the actual physical working capacity of children. The following basic statements summarize the research concerning the physical working capacity of children.

First, and most obviously, the research indicates that children can perform considerable amounts of work. While absolute work load amounts are less than those reported for adults, the work loads are substantial. Secondly, it can be observed that PWC increases with age. In fact chronological age may be a better predictor of ability to do work than many of the physical fitness tests commonly used in schools.

Finally, girls do not achieve the PWC of boys at any age, either in the study of American or Swedish children. This sex difference becomes quite marked as children grow older. Readers are referred to the works of Adams et al. (1961a, 1961b), Cumming and Cumming (1963), Taylor (1960), Alderman (1969), Shepard (1971), Corbin (1972), Cunningham and Egnan (1973), and Bouchard, Malina, Hollman, and LeBlanc (1976) for further information concerning the physical working capacity of children.

HEART RATE RESPONSES TO EXERCISE

Early studies of the circulatory responses of children suggested that children should not be exercised at high heart rates. In fact early research by Wilson (1920) reported maximal heart rates of 174 beats per minute. The literature is now filled with research showing the capability of children for doing work at much higher heart rates. In fact the maximal heart rates of children exceed those of adults (see Table 15.2).

Observations of Table 15.2 allow several conclusions. First, it is obvious that young children can and do achieve high heart rates in maximal work. Second, maximal heart rates tend to decrease with age as do resting rates. Finally, it can be seen that there is little difference in maximal heart rates of boys and girls, though adult women tend to have higher maximal heart rates than men.

Other research using heart rate to assess capabilities for cardiovascular performance have been reported by Takacs (1971), and Hanson (1967). In each of these studies the electrocardiograms of children were monitored using biotelemetry apparatus. Takacs (1971) monitored the heart rates of children performing runs of 200, 400, 600, and 800 yards. He noted near maximal responses within 30 seconds, regardless of the length of the run, with average heart rates ranging from 190 to 200 during the runs. Recovery was nearly complete for all children within 90 seconds after completing the run. Takacs also noted that children were able to maintain a high steady state heart rate during the running. Heart rates in excess of 170 heart beats for the entire duration of running were not uncommon.

Unlike Takacs, who noted near maximal responses to running, Hanson (1967) found responses to playing baseball for children to be minimal. He did note that heart rates increased significantly when the child batted and attributed the increase in rate to emotional stresses. It is obvious that children are capable of work at high heart rates. Not only are children capable of working at high heart rates, but the research of Massicotte and MacNab (1974) suggest that children must work at heart rates relatively higher than adults if they are to improve in cardiovascular fitness.

CARDIOVASCULAR PERFORMANCE CRITERIA FOR CHILDREN

Evaluative criteria, other than Maximal O_2 Intake and PWC, have been used to determine cardiovascular fitness levels of children. The modified step test is one of many tests used to determine cardiovascular fitness of children. Early research by Gallagher and Brouha (1943) established a testing procedure, as well as a rating system for boys age twelve to eighteen. Montoye et al. (1965), tested an entire community using a three-minute step test. Results show heart rates before, during, and after exercise decrease with age from ten to twenty, with lesser decreases occurring between ages twenty and thirty-five.

TABLE 15.2
Maximal Heart Rates: Ages 4-33.*
Numbers Represent Means, Standard Error of the
Means, and Standard Deviations.

	Sex	Age Groups						
		4—6	7—9	10—11	12—13	14—15	♂ 16—18 ♀ 16—17	♂ 20—33 ♀ 20—25
Number of subjects	♂	10	12	13	19	10	9	42
Number of subjects	♀	7	14	13	13	11	10	44
Max. heart rate	♂	203±2.2 7.0	208±2.4 8.4	211±2.3 8.1	205±4.1 17.7	203±4.1 12.8	202±3.1 9.2	194±1.6 10.3
Max. heart rate	♀	204±5.0 13.2	211±2.0 7.5	209±2.5 8.8	207±2.8 10.0	202±2.0 6.6	206±2.5 7.7	198±1.5 9.9

*Adapted from Per-Olaf Astrand, *Experimental Studies of Working Capacity in Relation to Sex and Age.* Copenhagen: Munksgoaard, 1952, used by permission.

This and other modifications of the step test are still used today, but most practitioners interested in field tests of cardiovascular fitness have used run of various length. The 600-yard run-walk, for example, has been used by some as a measure of cardiovascular fitness. However, researchers have been unable to verify the validity of the 600 yard test. Though Doolittle and Bigbee (1968) reported moderately high validity coefficients for the test, Vodak and Wilmore (1975) found the 600 yard run to be a poor predictor of Maximal O_2 and Corbin (1972) found running times for the 600 yard run to be poor predictors of PWC.

With the new emphasis on health related fitness, several states have now included longer runs in their test batteries. These runs appear to be better predictors of aerobic capacity, as measured by maximal O_2, than the 600 yard run. Jackson (1978) suggests that the longer runs are necessary to sort out the speed or anaerobic capacity factors pre-sent in shorter runs. Recently, the 12-minute run has been used widely as a field test of cardiovascular fitness. Bigbee and Doolittle (1968) reported a .90 correlation between the 12-minute run and a maximal O_2 criterion in young boys. However, a similar study (Maksud and Coutts 1971) on a larger sample of young boys, reported a .65 correlation between the two variables. The authors of the study urged caution when attempting to predict aerobic capacity from 12-minute run times for children. In their research Jackson and Coleman (1976) found the 9 minute run or one mile run to be as good as the 12 minute or 1 and ½-mile run as a test of cardiovascular fitness for children. It was this research which was principally responsible for the inclusion of a 9 minute or one mile run for children ages 10-12 and a 12 minute or one and one-half mile run for children 13 and older in the 1976 revision of the AAHPERD Youth Fitness Test.

50th percentile scores for boys and girls based on norms from the 1976 revised AAHPERD Youth Fitness Test Manual are presented in Figure 15.1. Boys had better performance than girls at all ages. Both boys and girls improved with age though the increase from age 11 to 12 was more dramatic for boys than girls. For the 12 minute test (age 13 and over) 50th percentile scores are 1861 yards for girls and 2592 for boys. On this test boys had considerably higher scores than girls.

Though several recent attempts have been made to find a field test for measuring cardiovascular fitness of children less than ten years of age, none has been found.

Krahenbuhl, et al. (1977) found moderately high correlations between maximal O_2 and one mile run times for 8 year old boys but not for girls of the same age. It is increasingly apparent that motivation is a problem associated with using distance runs as test of fitness for young children. As Astrand has suggested, children tend to "give up" when asked to do all out performances. The findings of Stone (1978) further supports the contention that motivational factors may be responsible for the lack of a good field test of cardiovascular fitness for young children.

It also should be noted that even for older children (10 plus) the running performance of children does not equal that of motivated adults, even when adjusted for body weight. Children do have the potential to do work equal to adults (per unit of body weight). However, this does not mean that they should be expected to run distances at the same rate of speed as mature adults.

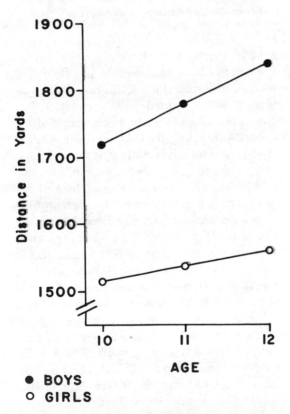

Figure 15.1. 50th percentile scores for the 9 minute run. (*AAHPER Youth Fitness Test Manual.* 1976 Revised Edition, pp. 44 and 52.)

OTHER FACTORS RELATING TO CARDIOVASCULAR FITNESS OF CHILDREN

Astrand (1952) has reported significant findings relevant to the cardiovascular performance of children. These findings are summarized as follows.

1. Children have, in relation to body weight, a smaller blood volume, but have a slightly higher maximal O_2 intake per liter of blood volume. Thus, as previously mentioned, children can achieve maximum O_2 values similar to adults when corrected for body weight.

2. While adults have an increased O_2 pulse with increased heart rate, children do not. This may explain the reason why maximal heart rates of children exceed those of adults.

3. Children are capable of lower maximal blood lactate levels during exercise. This might be a result of the child's "unwillingness to strain" in exhausting feats or a lower buffering capacity of younger subjects. If children were able to "persist," thus building greater maximal lactate levels, it would follow that they would be capable of greater maximal O_2 intake than possible for the average child.

References

Adams, Forest H.: Linde, Leonard M.; and Miyake Hisazumi. "The Physical Working Capacity of Normal Children, I." *Pediatrics* California 28(1961a):55.

Adams, Forest H. et al. "The Physical Working Capacity of Normal School Children, II." Swedish city and country. *Pediatrics* 28 (1961b):243.

Alderman, Richard B. "Age and Sex Differences in PWC 170 of Canadian School Children." *Research Quarterly* 40(1969):1.

American Academy of Pediatrics. "Cardiac Evaluation for Participation in Sports." *The Physician and Sports Medicine* 6(1978):102.

Astrand, Per-Olaf. *Experimental Studies of Working Capacity in Relation to Sex and Age.* Copenhagen: Munksgoaard, 1952.

Boas, Ernest P. "The Heart Rate of Boys During and After Exhausting Exercise." *Journal of Clinical Investigation* 10(1931):145.

Bouchard, C. et al. "Relationships between Skeletal Maturity and Submaximal Working Capacity in Boys 8-18 Years." *Medicine and Science in Sports* 8(1976):179.

Corbin, Charles B. *Becoming Physically Educated in the Elementary School.* (2nd Ed.) Philadelphia: Lea and Febiger, 1976.

———. "Relationships Between Physical Working Capacity and Running Performances of Young Boys." *Research Quarterly* 43(1972): 235.

Cumming, Gordon R. and Cumming, P. M. "Working Capacity of Normal Children Tested on a Bicycle Ergometer." *Canadian Medical Association Journal* 88(February 1963):51-55.

Cunningham, D. A. and Egnon, R. B. "The Working Capacity of Young Competitive Swimmers 10-16 Years of Age." *Medicine and Science in Sports* 5(1973):227.

Doolittle, T. L. and Bigbee, R. "The Twelve Minute Run-Walk: A Test of Cardiorespiratory Fitness of Adolescent Boys." *Research Quarterly* 39(1968):491.

Gallagher, J. Roswell and Brouha, Lucien. "A Simple Method of Testing the Physical Fitness of Boys." *Research Quarterly* 14(1943): 23.

Gilliam, T. B. et al. "Comparison of Peak Performance Measures in Children 6-8, 9-10, 11-13." *Research Quarterly* 48(1977):695.

Hanson, Dale L. "Cardiac Response to Participation in Little League Baseball Competition as Determined by Telemetry." *Research Quarterly* 38(1967):384.

Hurlock, Elizabeth B. *Adolescent Development.* New York: McGraw-Hill Book Co., 1967.

Jackson, A. S. "Biometric Characteristics of Distance Run Tests." *AAHPER Research Consortium Symposium Papers* 1(1978):63.

Jackson, A. S. and Coleman, A. E. "Validation of Distance Run Tests for Elementary School Children." *Research Quarterly* 47(1976):86.

Karpovich, Peter V. "Textbook Fallacies Regarding the Development of the Child's Heart." *Research Quarterly* 8(1937):33.

Krahenbuhl, G. S. et al. "Field Estimates of VO_2 Max in Children Eight Years of Age." *Medicine and Science in Sports* 9(1977):37.

Maksud, G. Michael and Coutts, Kenneth D. "Application of the Cooper Twelve Minute Run-Walk Test to Young Males." *Research Quarterly* 42(1971):54.

Massicotte, D. R. and MacNab, R. "Cardiorespiratory Adaptations to Training at Specified Intensities in Children." *Medicine and Science in Sports* 6(1974):242.

Montoye, Henry J.; Willis, Park W.; Cunningham, David; and Keller, Jacob, "Heart Rate Response to a Modified Harvard Step Test: Males and Females, Ages 10-69." *Research Quarterly* 40(1969):153.

Shepard, R. J. "The Working Capacity of School Children." In *Frontiers of Fitness*, edited by R. S. Shepard. Springfield, Ill.: C. C. Thomas, 1971.

Stone, W. J. "Running Tests for 7-9 Year Old Children." *AAHPER Research Consortium Symposium Papers* 1(1978):54.

Takacs, Robert F. *Heart Rate Response of Children to Four Separate Bouts of Training* Doctoral Dissertation, Texas A & M University, 1971.

Taylor, Henry L. et al. "Contributions of Physical Health." *Research Quarterly* 31(1960): 263.

Vodak, P. A. and Wilmore, J. H. "Validity of the 6-Minute Jog-Walk and the 600-Yard Run-Walk in Estimating Endurance Capacity in Boys, 9-12 Years of Age." *Research Quarterly* 46(1975):230.

Wilson, May G. "The Circulatory Reaction of Graduated Exercise in Normal Children." *American Journal of the Diseases of Children* 20(1920):183.

Young, E. *Hygiene of the School Age.* Philadelphia: W. B. Saunders Company, 1923.

Strength, Muscular Endurance, and Flexibility of Children

16

Charles B. Corbin
Kansas State University

Strength is defined here as the ability of a muscle to exert an external force. Muscular endurance is related to strength, but is a separate factor. Muscular endurance is the ability to repeat strength feats. The reader can see that muscular endurance is to a certain extent dependent upon prerequisite strength; however, those with great amounts of strength do not necessarily have high muscular endurance and visa versa. Flexibility is the range of motion available in a joint. It is a health related aspect of fitness and its development is important to proper programs for developing strength and muscular endurance. Since muscular strength is necessary for muscular endurance performance, a discussion of this factor will be considered first, followed by discussion of muscular endurance and flexibility.

STRENGTH

As early as 1899, a large number of children were tested for grip strength (Montpetit et al. 1967). A more comprehensive study of the strength capabilities of children was conducted later by Jones (1949). Though Jones' study was really a longitudinal growth and development investigation, which dealt with many different variables, it did report strength measures for grip (right and left) strength, the arm push, and the arm pull. More recently, Clarke (1971) and Montyoe et al. (1977) have published results of more comprehensive studies which include more detailed strength measurements. Much of the information presented in this chapter is based on the results of the Medford Project as summarized by Clarke and the Tecumseh Study as summarized by Montoye et al. The above mentioned studies are emphasized because they are truly investigations of strength performance. While many other studies have been reported, most of them involve tests like sit-ups, chin-ups, and other similar measures which are really measures of muscular endurance. Results of these studies will be included in the muscular endurance section of this chapter. A summary of research using the Kraus-Weber test as a test of minimal muscle strength and flexibility is presented in Chapter 14.

Strength as Measured by the Dynamometer

Strength as measured by the dynamometer is generally confined to four basic tests: (1) right hand grip strength; (2) left hand grip strength; (3) back strength; and (4) leg strength. For detailed testing procedures, the reader is referred to Clarke (1967). Longitudinal data from the Medford Growth Study (Clarke 1971) is now available and provides excellent information concerning the strength capabilities of boys. The reader is referred to this study for a complete discussion of strength and muscular endurance performance of young boys.

Generally speaking dynamometer tests show strength performance to be similar for prepubescent boys and girls with girls having slightly lower scores than boys. While data on girls is less available than that for boys, enough evidence is available (Monpetit et al. 1967; Tuddenham et al. 1954; Jones 1949; Metheny 1948 and Montoye, et al. 1977) to show that girls differ markedly from boys after age twelve or thirteen. Girls tend to level off in performance after this age (see Fig. 16.1) while boys become stronger. In fact, for boys the rate of increase for dynamometer strength measures is much greater after the onset of puberty than before. When body weight is considered, the strength differences between boys and girls are even more exaggerated (post pubescent). When corrected for body weight, there is virtually no increase in dynamometer strength in the post pubescent girl. Relative strength, on the other hand, increases dramatically after puberty for boys.

It can be summarized that as the child grows older and larger, the child grows stronger. The spurt in strength at puberty is easily explained by the increased hormonal secretions and accompanying increases in muscle weight and muscle fibers for both boys and girls. However, the female hormone which increases at puberty promotes fat development but relatively lesser muscle growth in girls, partially explaining the more gradual strength increases with age and the complete lack of relative strength increases with age for girls. The increases in body fat for girls at puberty are also reflected in the lack of increases in relative strength as girls grow older. It should be noted that there is a strong relationship

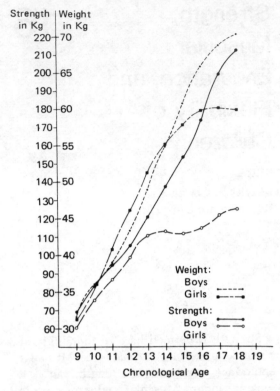

Figure 16.1. Growth and weight of boys and girls: 9-18. (From Read D. Tuddenham, and Margaret M. Snyder. *Physical Growth of California Boys and Girls from Birth to Eighteen Years.* Originally published by the University of California Press, 1954, p. 364; reprinted by permission of the Regents of the University of California.)

between strength of children and other physical growth measures (Clarke 1971; Jones 1949; Metheny 1948).

Strength as Measured by the Tensiometer

Clarke is credited with popularizing strength tests using the cable tensiometer. This type measurement is particularly valuable because it allows the measurement of many different muscle groups, as opposed to the dynamometer, which is generally limited to the basic four tests discussed earlier in this chapter.

Clarke, in the Medford study, administered a total of eighteen different cable tension tests. Four of the eighteen tests showed a high multiple correlation to the mean of all eighteen measures. However, Clarke summarizes cable strength based on the average of eleven different measures: elbow flexion, shoulder flexion, shoulder inward rotation, trunk flexion, trunk extension, hip flexion, hip extension, knee flexion, knee extension, ankle dorsal flexion and ankle plantar flexion. Average cable tension strength scores for boys are summarized in Figure 16.2.

When plotted graphically, the results of the cable tension measures showed similar growth curves to those for dynamometer measures. The most notable difference is the linear slope of the growth curve. Boys improved in cable tension strength each year before and after puberty. Dynamometer strength increases were relatively small each year prior to age twelve.

Results of the Tecumseh Study using a cable test of arm strength, provide information for making boy-girls comparisons for each year of age after 10 (see Figure 16.3). The top graph illustrates the ratio of arm strength to body weight and the lower graph arm strength in kg. of force exerted. The data are quite similar to the data for dynamometer strength. However, one point is illustrated in Figure 16.3 which is unique. At no age do girls achieve a ratio of arm strength to body weight equal to 1.00. On the other hand boys have a ratio greater than one for all ages except 10. Since these are 50th per-

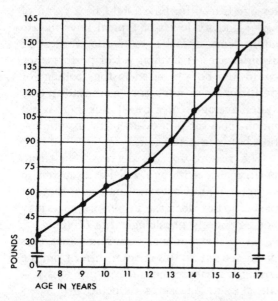

Figure 16.2. Cable tension strength for boys 8-18. (From H. Harrison Clarke, *Physical Motor Tests in the Medford Boys Growth Study*, © 1971, p. 189. By permission of Prentice-Hall, Inc.)

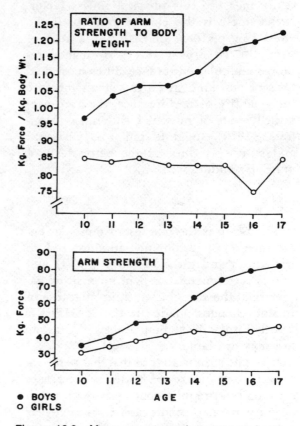

Figure 16.3. Mean arm strength scores and arm strength/body weight ratios for boys and girls. (Montoye, H. and Lampier, D. E. "Grip and Arm Strength in Males and Females, Age 10-69." *Research Quarterly.* 48: pp. 113 and 118.)

centile values, it is not hard to see why girls of all ages have a hard time with the chin up or pull up as a test of strength or muscular endurance. "Average" girls of all ages do not have the arm strength to lift their own body weight. Also 50% of all boys age 10 do not have the strength to lift their own body weight.

MUSCULAR ENDURANCE

Muscular endurance is the ability to persist in strength performance. Many of the tests commonly given to school children really measure this physical fitness factor. An example is the chin or pull-up. If the child can perform one, this is a feat of strength. To repeat this performance requires muscular endurance. Since most field tests of any kind given in schools measure the quantity of performance, they are necessarily tests of muscular endurance. Montoye (1970) suggests pull-ups, push-ups, and sit-ups as three of the better tests of muscular endurance.

Sit-ups

The sit-up is the one test of muscular endurance most commonly administered to both boys and girls. Montoye (1970) and others recommend the bent knee sit-up rather than the straight leg sit-up. Because of recent changes made in the AAHPERD Youth Fitness Test Bent Knee Sit Up data are now available.

It can be seen in Figure 16.4 that performance for boys increases with age. Increases are small in prepubescent years, with much larger performance increases with each year between twelve and fifteen. Muscular endurance performance levels off after ages fifteen. The performance for girls does not increase with age after ten as it does for boys.

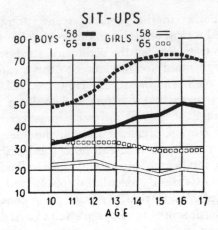

Figure 16.4. Sit-Up Performances of Boys and Girls 10-17. (From Paul A. Hunsicker, and Guy G. Reiff. "Youth Fitness Report: 1958-1965-1975." *Journal of Physical Education, Recreation* 48 (1977):33, used by permission.)

The upsurge in the performance of boys after adolescence can be explained, as with strength increases, by the increase in muscle mass in adolescence. The slight decrease after age fifteen for boys might be a result of lesser activity levels of typical boys in late adolescence, or lack of motivation for testing at older ages. A leveling off of performance could also be attributed to the "ceiling" of performance on a test such as the sit-up test. When average scores are 40-plus there is not much room for improvement or discrimination between performers.

The reasons for the decreases in sit-up performance with age will be discussed in Chapter 17, but note here and now that the basis for this decrease in performance may not be entirely physiological in origin.

All of the muscular endurance measures discussed within this chapter differ from the strength measures considered previously — the strength measures reflected gross performance without correction for body size. Because the nature of muscular endurance tasks, such as the chin-up, involve movement of one's own body weight, they are relative rather than gross measures. As Montoye et al. have noted gross strength performance for girls increases with age, while relative strength does not. That muscular endurance for girls, as measured by the sit-up, does not increase with age is probably best accounted for by the fact that muscle mass in girls increases only moderately with age, while body weight increases at a more rapid rate than during earlier years.

Pull-ups and Similar Measures

Pull-ups (palms away) and chin-ups (palms forward) are commonly included in motor fitness batteries. The AAHPERD battery includes pull-ups for boys, as do the Oregon and California tests for children. Interestingly, none of these tests recommend the pull-up test for girls. Commonly administered as substitute tests for girls are the modified pull-up and the bent arm hang. Comments relative to the administration of the pull-up for testing the muscular endurance of girls are included in Chapter 18.

There is virtually no difference in the ability of boys to perform chins between the ages of seven and twelve (Cureton 1964). Mean scores for all age groups is between one and three (Cureton 1964; Hunsicker and Reiff 1965). After age twelve pull-up performance increases proportionately with age. Like gross and relative strength measures, muscular endurance, as measured by pull-up performance, increases dramatically after puberty.

Push-ups and Other Measures

Performance on push-ups, bar dips, and other similar measures is almost identical to performance on other muscular endurance measures. Generally performance is poorer on these measures than for the chin-up or

pull-up, perhaps because the measures are not as commonly used in the public schools. Because these measures are not frequently given to girls, comprehensive data are not available.

Performances of girls on the flexed arm hang, which measures the time that the chin can be held above a bar with the elbow flexed, show relatively constant average performances for each age, ten through seventeen (Hunsicker et al. 1975). Similarly performances of the modified pull-up reflect no significant increase in performance with age. It is known, as can be attested by anyone who has administered the modified pull-up, that girls who have some muscular endurance can reach "ceiling" levels on the test. That is, these girls can perform in excess of a number of modified pull-ups which can be administered in a reasonable testing period. Girls who perform 50 or more of the pull-ups are stopped, and, therefore, the test has no discrimination power for those who exceed that level of performance. The modified pull-up was dropped from the AAHPERD test battery. There is some indication that the bent arm hang and the pull-up measures will be deleted from the AAHPERD Test Battery in the future. For those who are interested in testing the arm strength of both boys and girls of all levels of strength and muscular endurance Baumgartner (1978) has reported a test which accommodates those of lesser ability while still discriminating between those with higher arm strength and muscular endurance. The interested reader is referred to the reference at the end of the chapter for more information.

FLEXIBILITY

Flexibility can be simply defined as the length of muscle, or the ability of a joint to move through its possible movement range.

While it is generally acknowledged (Fleischman 1964) that flexibility exists in at least two separate factors, static and dynamic, this discussion will be limited to static flexibility. Corbin et al. (1978), summarize the research on flexibility as follows:

1. Flexibility is specific to each joint.
2. Strength development need not limit flexibility development, though it may if exercises are not properly conducted.
3. Length of body parts does not significantly affect body flexibility.

A study of girls age six to eighteen (Hupprich and Segerseth 1950) showed increases in flexibility on most of 12 measures prior to age twelve, with decreases in flexibility each year thereafter. However, more recent research by Milne et al. (1976) showed decreases in flexibility among children from kindergarten to grade 2. Clarke (1975) in his review of the flexibility research suggests that the decline in flexibility begins at about 10 years of age for boys and 12 for girls. The findings of Krahenbuhl and Martin (1977) are in general agreement reporting that between ages 10 and 14 flexibility decreases as body surface area increases.

Although research within sex groups indicates that length of body parts does not affect flexibility scores, it is generally accepted that girls have greater potential for flexibility after puberty on such measures as trunk flexion because of their lower center of gravity and shorter leg length. There is, however, no comprehensive comparative study of flexibility scores for boys compared to girls reported in the literature. Results of the flexibility tests included in the Kraus-Weber battery were discussed in Chapter 14.

References

Baumgartner, T. A. "Modified Pull Up Test." *Research Quarterly* 49(1978):80.

Clarke, H. Harrison. *Application of Measurement to Health and Physical Education*, 4th ed. Englewood Cliffs, N.J.: Prentice-Hall, Inc., 1967.

———. *Physical and Motor Tests in the Medford Growth Study*. Englewood Cliffs, N.J.: Prentice-Hall, Inc., 1971.

———. "Joint and Body Range of Movement." *Physical Fitness Research Digest* 5(1975): 16.

Corbin, Charles B.; Dowell, Linus J.; Lindsey, Ruth; and Tolson, Homer. *Concepts in Physical Education*, 3rd ed. Dubuque, Iowa: Wm. C. Brown Company Publishers, 1978.

Cureton, Thomas K. *Improving the Physical Fitness of Youth*. (A monograph of the Society for Research in Child Development.) Yellow Springs, Ohio: The Antioch Press, 1964.

Fleischman, Edwin A. *The Structure and Measurement of Physical Fitness*. Englewood Cliffs, N.J.: Prentice-Hall, Inc., 1964.

Hunsicker, Paul A. and Reiff, Guy G. "Youth Fitness Report: 1958-1965-1975." *Journal of Physical Education and Recreation* 48 (1977):33.

Hupprich, Florence L. and Segerseth, Peter. "Specificity of Flexibility in Girls." *Research Quarterly* 21(1950):25.

Jones, Harold E. *Motor Performance and Growth*. Berkeley: University of California Press, 1949.

Krahenbuhl, G. S. and Martin, S. C. "Adolescent Body Size and Flexibility." *Research Quarterly* 48(1977):797.

Metheny, Elanor. "Breathing Capacity and Grip Strength of Preschool Children." *University of Iowa Studies in Child Welfare* 18(1941): 1.

Milne, C. et al. "Relationship Between Grade, Sex, Race, and Motor Performance of Children." *Research Quarterly* 47(1976):726.

Montoye, Henry I. *An Introduction to Measurement in Physical Education*. Indianapolis: Phi Epsilon Kappa Fraternity, 1970.

Montoye, H. J. and Lamphier, D. E. "Grip and Arm Strength in Males and Females." *Research Quarterly* 48(1977):109.

Montpetit, Richard R.; Laeding, Lawrence, and Montoye, Henry J. "Grip Strength of School Children, Saginaw, Michigan: 1899 and 1964." *Research Quarterly* 38(1967):231.

Childhood Obesity 17

Charles B. Corbin
Kansas State University

THE BABY FAT MYTH

Obesity in adults has long been a concern of laymen, educators, physicians, and scientists. That too many adults are "too fat" is well documented (Keys and Brozek 1953). Until recently, obesity has been considered a malady prevalent only in adults — the idea that there should be a concern for the too fat child having been rejected by many. In fact, many have taken a position that "baby fat is a sign of good health." The "Baby Fat Myth" has led many a parent to resist help for an obese child on the assumption that children will "grow out" of their obese condition.

There is convincing evidence that "juvenile obesity persists into adult life" (Heald 1966). Those who were too fat as children were too fat as adults (Stunkard and Burt 1966).

A study in a selected school system indicated a 20 percent increase in the prevalence of childhood obesity in the last decade (Johnson et al. 1956a). Studies by Tanner and Whitehouse (1962) and Corbin (1969) also attest to the high incidence of obesity among children. Contrary to the thesis that children get leaner as they grow older, the typical child increases in adipose tissue with age.

It appears, therefore, that obesity is a problem which plagues children as well as adults and is a problem which should be given attention early in childhood. The Experiments of Knittle and Hirsch (1968) and Hirsch and Knittle (1970) show that both the size and the number of fat cells increases in early childhood. They present convincing evidence indicating the importance of controlling weight early in life. In all likelyhood children who are too fat develop "extra" fat cells, thus increasing the chances of becoming too fat adults. Further, Oscai (1974) has shown that exercise early in life may help limit the growth of fat cells and therefore reduce the chances of adult obesity. Clearly "baby fat" is not necessarily a sign of good health. It is important that body fatness problems be dealt with early in life.

CRITERIA FOR ASSESSING FATNESS OF CHILDREN

Commonly, the criterion for assessing obesity or overweight among children is the height-weight chart. This procedure has several limitations. Tanner and Whitehouse (1962) make the following comment on the subject:

Though standards for height and weight are certainly useful in following the growth process of individual children and in assessing the health and nutrition of different populations and social groups, they are not sufficient by themselves to answer many important questions. They do not tell us with any degree of assurance, for example, how fat or thin a child is relative to his fellows or relative to his state at a previous age. A child who is above average weight for his height may be a fat child, or he may be a muscular child, or he may even be a child with heavy bones. Conversely, a child who is underweight for his height may be simply lean or may be lacking in muscle or in bone mineralization. Even a gain in weight, in children, cannot be taken as evidence that fat has been put on, as it usually can in adults. (Tanner and Whitehouse 1962, p. 446.)

The fact that height-weight ratios may not reflect overweight or obese conditions is illustrated by the fact that professional football players were "overweight" in terms of height-weight measures but were actually "thin" in terms of body fat content (Welham and Behnke 1942).

The Wetzel Grid (Wetzel 1941) was developed to evaluate "physical fitness in terms of physique (Body Build), developmental level, and basil metabolism." The grid which has proven to be very useful in recognizing abnormal changes in height-weight relationships, uses three basic components: physique channels, developmental levels, and developmental ratios. While extremely useful as a tool for studying child growth and development, it is essentially a sophisticated longitudinal height-weight chart and is limited as a tool for assessing fatness of children at any given point in time. The reader is referred to the grid instruction manual for further details (Wetzel 1941).

The X-ray procedure for assessing distribution of subcutaneous fat levels of children has been used extensively by Reynolds (1951) at the Fels Research Institute for the Study of Human Development. A summary of his research is included in a later section of this chapter.

The underwater weighing procedure is probably the most valid method of assessing body fatness but because of the lack of a comprehensive study using children as subjects, this technique will not be discussed at length in this chapter. There have been sev-

eral procedures which have been widely used to measure fatness among children which correlate reasonably well to body fatness as determined by the underwater weighing procedure. Perhaps one of the most frequently used methods of assessing fatness of children is the skinfold procedure. The tricep and subscapular skinfold are good simple criteria for assessing body fatness (Seltzer and Mayer 1965). These measurements, "obtained by using a suitable caliper on selected sites, have been shown by comparison with results of other methods to give good indications not only of subcutaneous fat (about 50 —of the total fat) but also of total body fat" (Seltzer and Mayer 1965, p. 104). More recently, Katch and McArdle (1973) have reported good correlations between body circumferences and body fatness. To date the procedure has not been perfected for use with children.

SKINFOLD MEASUREMENTS IN CHILDREN

As noted in an earlier chapter there is an increased interest in health related physical fitness in the schools. One of the important components of health related fitness is body composition. The AAHPERD Taskforce charged with the revision of the Youth Fitness Test has noted the importance of screening children for body fatness as a part of fitness testing. The taskforce has plans to include a skinfold test in future revisions of the test (Falls, 1978).

Of all skinfold measures the tricep is the easiest to measure and is felt to be the most representative of total body fatness. Seltzer and Mayer (1965) suggest that there is no special advantage to using skinfold measures in addition to the tricep when screening children for obesity. While this may be true for "screening", which implies the identification of children with special problems, the tricep alone may not be as good a discriminator among non obese children as some have thought. Zuti and Corbin (1978) have shown that this measure is good for some ages but not necessarily for others. Likewise, the measure does not predict body fatness equally well for both sexes. If skinfold measures are to be used for more than simple screening it appears that specific prediction formulas will have to be developed for each sex and age group. Youngberg (1978) has reported a formula for use with fifth grade girls, and several formulas have been developed for use with adults of either sex and of different ages. General standards for screening obesity using the tricep skinfold are presented in Table 17.1.

The standards plotted in Table 17.1 are statistically based. Using one standard deviation above the mean as the cutoff point, the standards were established. Accordingly, by definition 16 percent of the original sample were obese. The fact that children acquire fat with age presents a problem. This arbitrary standard implies that children are "allowed" to acquire more fat as they grow older. If the tricep measure is truly an indicator of body fatness, increases in fatness with age should not be considered a "desirable" phenomenon. Rather fat accumulation should be relatively constant with age. Of course, increases in amounts of fat deposits during adolescence for girls are expected, as are the decreases in fatness at puberty for boys. It is, however, hard to accept a standard which "allows" increases in body fatness with age after physical maturity. While it is easy to understand how children and adults get fatter as they get older, it is hard to justify the standards in as

TABLE 17.1
Obesity Standards for Caucasian Americans.*

Age (Years)	Minimum Triceps Skin-fold Thickness Indicating Obesity (Millimeters)	
	Males	Females
5	12	14
6	12	15
7	13	16
8	14	17
9	15	18
10	16	20
11	17	21
12	18	22
13	18	23
14	17	23
15	16	24
16	15	25
17	14	26
18	15	27
19	15	27
20	16	28
21	17	28
22	18	28
23	18	28
24	19	28
25	20	29
26	20	29
27	21	29
28	22	29
29	22	29
30-50	23	30

*From Carl C. Seltzer, and Jean Mayer. "A Simple Criterion of Obesity." *Post Graduate Medicine* 38 (1965): 101. (Copyright by McGraw-Hill, Inc., used by permission.)

much as statistics show that both children and adult may accumulate too much fat as they grow older.

Results of studies designed to establish skinfold standards for Canadian (Pett and Ogilvie 1956), British (Tanner and Whitehouse 1962), and American children (Corbin 1969) are summarized in Figure 17.1.

Regardless of any international comparisons that could be made, it can be seen that children need not get fatter as they get older. British children do not increase in tricep skinfold with age. Further, it can be seen

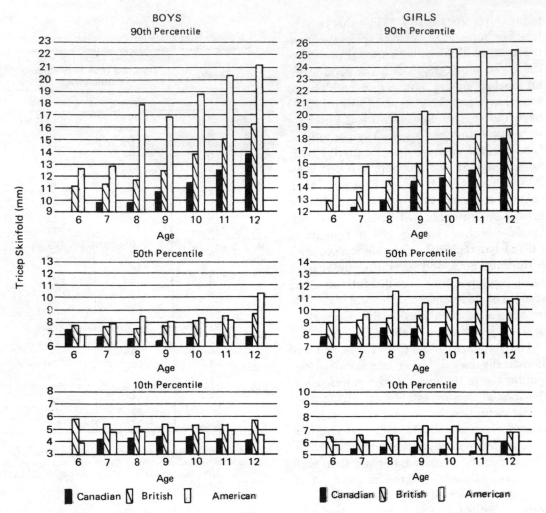

Figure 17.1. A Comparison of Tricep Skinfold Thicknesses of American, Canadian, and British Children. (From Charles B. Corbin, "The Fatness of Our Youth." *TAHPER Journal* 37 (1969):5, used by permission.)

that too many American children exceeded the generally accepted, though arbitrary, obesity standards presented by Seltzer and Mayer.

Skinfold data for children are also presented by Montoye (1965) as part of the Tecumseh Study, Clarke (1971) as part of the Medford Study, and Cureton (1964)

as part of the Illinois Sports Fitness Study. These studies, though providing additional and valuable information, did not present information which would modify the facts as previously presented in this chapter. The interested reader is referred to these sources as a basis for additional and a more indepth study of skinfold thicknesses of children.

X-RAY ASSESSMENTS OF CHILDHOOD FATNESS

Reynolds (1951) has reported results of a thirteen year study designed to assess subcutaneous fat levels throughout youth. Using X-ray procedures, children were followed over a period of years and growth curves were plotted. Over 300 children were studied and some 8500 X-ray pictures provided data for analysis. Measurements were made on as many as fourteen different body areas. Like the results of the skinfold studies, Reynolds' study revealed that girls had greater distribution of fat than boys with the mean fat concentration increasing at a more rapid rate for girls than for boys after puberty. The greater amounts of fat for girls as compared to boys is reflected at all ages in measurements except the neck at age 10.5. Reynolds found greater fat thicknesses in early maturing children (chronologically and maturationally) than among late maturing children. He also pointed to the strong relationship between hereditary factors and fatness. Like others, Reynolds pointed out that weight and height alone are not necessarily valid criteria for the diagnosis of obesity.

MAINTENANCE OF "DESIRABLE" FAT LEVELS IN CHILDREN

Although the hereditary predisposition to obesity is a significant factor to consider in determining reasons for obesity in early life, children are not different than adults in that a balance between caloric intake and expenditure is necessary for control of body fat. However, the idea that caloric restriction is the most important factor in the onset of childhood obesity has been challenged (Johnson et al. 1956b; Corbin and Pletcher 1968).

Studies have shown that inactivity is a more relevant factor than is overeating for the development and maintenance of childhood and adolescent obesity (Johnson et al. 1956b). Bullen et al. (1964) took movies of obese and non-obese girls while engaged in sports activities. The obese girls were extremely inactive but when askd to judge their activity levels, felt that they were quite active.

Corbin and Pletcher (1968) did a study similar to those presented in the preceding paragraph. They tested the diet and physical activity patterns of obese and non-obese elementary school boys and girls. Dietary recall procedures and cinematographic analysis yielded results similar to those of Johnson et al. which support the contention that . . . "inactivity may be as important or more important than excessive caloric intake in the development and maintenance of childhood obesity" (Corbin and Pletcher 1968, p. 922). Some suggestions for treating the obese child in the public school setting have been offered by Pangrazzi (1978). The interested reader is referred to this source.

The discussion presented in the preceding pages of this chapter is not intended to imply that caloric restriction is unimportant in controlling childhood obesity. Rather, the discussion is meant to relate the importance of activity to maintenance of normal body fat levels as well as the prevention of childhood obesity.

BODY COMPOSITION AND MOTOR PERFORMANCE

For most types of motor activities body fatness limits the ability to perform. Excess body fatness requires extra work to perform a specific task, thus results in relatively inefficient performance. There are exceptions such as long distance swimming, but in general motor performance is effected by body fatness. Cureton (1975) has shown that body composition effects AAHPERD test results and Gutin, et al. (1978) has shown a relationship between body composition and Maximum VO_2. It should also be noted that being "too fat" is not the only body composition problem which may effect motor performance. Ribisl (1974) is only one of many who warn of the dangers of excessive weight loss for sporting events such as wrestling. Excessive weight loss without proper medical attention can result in poor performance as well as poor health. The problems of excessive weight loss are magnified for young children who are still growing and developing.

References

Brozek, J. and Keys, Ancel. "The Evaluation of Leanness-Fatness in Man: Norms and Interrelationships." *British Journal of Nutrition* 5(1951):194.

Bullen, Beverly A.; Reed, Robert B., and Mayer, Jean. "Physical Activity of Obese and Non Obese Adolescent Girls Appraised by Motion Picture Sampling." *American Journal of Clinical Nutrition* 14(1964):211.

Clarke, H. Harrison. *Physical and Motor Tests in the Medford Boys' Growth Study*. Englewood Cliffs, N.J.: Prentice-Hall, 1971.

Corbin, Charles B. and Pletcher, Philip. "Diet and Physical Activity Patterns of Obese and Non Obese Elementary School Children." *Research Quarterly* 39(1968):922.

Corbin, Charles B. "Standards of Subcutaneous Fat Applied to Percentile Norms for Elementary School Children." *American Journal of Clinical Nutrition* 22(1969):836.

Cureton, K. J. et al. "Relationship between Body Composition Measures and AAHPER Test Performance of Young Boys." *Research Quarterly* 46(1975):218.

Cureton, Thomas K. *Improving the Physical Fitness of Youth*. (A monograph of the Society for Research in Child Development). Yellow Springs, Ohio: The Antioch Press, 1964.

Falls, H. "Revision of the AAHPER Youth Fitness Test Battery." A paper presented to the National Conference on Aerobic Exercise, Tulsa, Oklahoma, October, 1978.

Gutin, B. et al. "Morphological and Physiological Factors Relating to Endurance Performances of 11- and 12-Year-Old Girls." *Research Quarterly* 49(1978):44.

Heald, F. P. "Natural History and Physiological Basis of Adolescent Obesity." *Federation Proceedings* 25(1966):4.

Hirsch, J. and Knittle, J. L. "Cellularity of Obese and Nonobese Adipose Tissue." *Federation Proceedings* 29(1970):1518.

Johnson, Mary Louise; Burke, Bertha S., and Mayer, Jean. "The Prevalence and Incidence of Obesity in a Cross Section of Elementary and Secondary School Children." *American Journal of Clinical Nutrition* 4(1956b):231.

Katch, F. and McArdle, W. D. "Prediction of Body Density from Simple Anthropometric Measures in College Age Men and Women." *Human Biology* 45(1973):445-54.

Keys, Ancel and Brozek, J. "Body Fat in Adult Man." *Physiological Review* 33(1953):245.

Knittle, Jerome L. and Hirsch, Jules. "Effect of Early Nutrition on the Development of Fat Epididymal Fat Pads: Cellularity and Metabolism." *Journal of Clinical Investigation* 47 (1968):2091.

Montoye, Henry J.; Eptein, F. H., and Kjelsberg, M. O. "The Measurement of Body Fatness: A Study in a Total Community." *American Journal of Clinical Nutrition* 16(1965): 417.

Oscai, L. "Exercise or Food Restriction: Effect on Adipose Tissue Celluarity." *American Journal of Physiology* 27(1974):902.

Pangrazzi, R. "Treating the Obese Child in the Public School Setting." *AAHPER Research Consortium Symposium Papers* 1(1978):58.

Pett, L. B. and Ogilvie, G. F. "The Canadian Weight-Height Survey." *Human Biology* 28(1956):177.

Reynolds, Earle L. *The Distribution of Subcutaneous Fat in Childhood and Adolescence.* Evanston: Child Development Publications, 1951.

Ribisl, P. "When Wrestlers Shed Pounds Quickly." *The Physician and Sports Medicine* 2(1974):30.

Seltzer, Carl C. and Mayer, Jean. "A Simple Criterion of Obesity." *Post Graduate Medicine* 38(1965):101.

Sloan, A. W.; Burt, John J., and Blyth, Carl. "Estimation of Body Fat in Young Women." *Journal of Applied Physiology* 17(1962): 967.

Stunkard, Albert J. and Burt, Victor. *A Report Given to the Sixth Multidiscipline Research Forum of the American Medical Association, 1960.*

Tanner, J. M. and Whitehouse, R. H. "Standards for Subcutaneous Fat in British Children." *British Medical Journal* 155(1962): 446.

Welham, W. C. and Behnke, Albert R. "Specific Gravity of Healthy Men: Body Weight — Volume and Other Physical Characteristics of Exceptional Athletes and Naval Personal." *Journal of the American Medical Association* 118(1942):498.

Wetzel, Norman C. *Instructional Manual in Use of the Grid.* New York: NEA Service Inc., 1941.

Youngberg, L. "Prediction of Body Density in Pre-Adolescent Girls." Masters Thesis, Oklahoma State University, 1978.

Zuti, W. B. and Corbin, C. B. "Modified Procedure for Underwater Weighing Children." A paper presented to the American College of Sports Medicine, Washington, May, 1978.

The Physical Fitness of Children: A Discussion and Point of View

18

Charles B. Corbin
Kansas State University

In studying the motor development of the human, in this case the physical fitness of children, we are forced because of the nature of our data, to look at performance levels for "normal" children. As discussed in Chapter 1 of this text, the study of "typical" children is not a bad approach to studying human behavior. However, if we truly are to discover the human's potential for performance we must project beyond the actual performance of children to speculate about what performance would be like given ideal developmental circumstances.

PHYSICAL FITNESS DIFFERENCES BETWEEN BOYS AND GIRLS

Though the preceding chapters have shown that there are differences in health related fitness performance of boys and girls, the most dramatic differences do *not* occur in childhood. In fact what differences do occur prior to age 11 of 12 are quite small. The average boy and girl are quite similar in Maximal O_2 per Kg. of Body Weight, strength as measured by dynamometers, and muscular endurance. Girls are slightly fatter and perhaps a bit more flexible prior to age 11 or 12. However, in field tests or non lab performance tests such as the items of the AAHPERD test, girls have slightly lower scores than boys even before age 12.

Possible reasons for the differences which do exist between boys and girls in childhood are listed below:

1. Many of the differences in health related fitness are most noticeable in the years 10, 11, 12. This may reflect the earlier maturation of girls and could easily explain the fat differences. The fat differences might also contribute to lesser performances in field tests of fitness.

2. The fact that what differences do exist are most dramatic in field tests may suggest a lesser motivation among girls to do well on such tests.

Whatever the reasons, for differences between the sexes, it is clear that girls are capable of all kinds of physical performance. Rarick et al. (1975) after studying many children of both sexes emphasize the capability of girls noting, "It is clear from the foregoing that while the motor performance levels of boys and girls in the range 6 to 9.9 years may in the average differ considerably, the basic components which underly a major part of the motor domain for the two sexes are highly similar (p. 110). The sex differences in performance are much more dramatic after age 11 or 12. These differences are discussed more thoroughly in Chapter 30.

SKILL VS. HEALTH-RELATED PHYSICAL FITNESS

For operational purposes, physical fitness factors have been grouped in two general categories, skill-related and health-related physical fitness. While the differences between the two fitness types are affected by many factors, it does appear that performance patterns for the two differ. The health-related factors, which involve physiological-muscular changes, require rather intensive work to reflect performance changes for pre-adolescent children. On the other hand, performances on the perceptual motor skill-related fitness factors are plotted graphically as a straight line. Beginning in early childhood and continuing into adulthood, these performances improve with age. Figure 18.1 depicts the "typical" performance curves for health and skill-related physical fitness.

The reason for the differences in the curves may be related to physiological potential for performance (especially for health-related fitness prior to age twelve), the greater "social" value for success in skill performance as opposed to health-related fitness, or the lack of any planned effort to improve health fitness, which requires a more intensive daily effort than does skill-related fitness.

GROSS VS. RELATIVE PHYSICAL FITNESS

Physical fitness can be measured in terms of gross or relative performance. For example, strength can be measured in terms of the total number of pounds of total strength (gross), or the total strength score can be corrected for body weight by dividing one's body weight into the total strength score (relative). Some fitness tests, such as pull-ups, are by their very nature relative (the

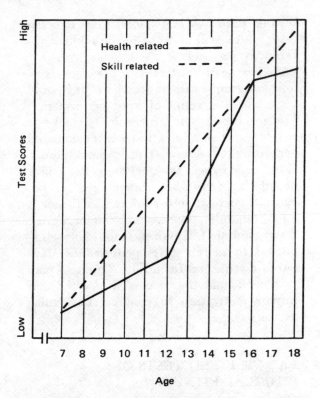

Figure 18.1. Differences in performance between health and skill related fitness.

performer is lifting his or her own body weight), while others, like grip strength, are gross; some are a combination of the two.

First, it must be said that performance curves can reflect one picture for gross performance and a completely different one when relative performance is considered. When comparisons are to be made, the differences between gross and relative performance should be specified. Often differences between two groups, such as children and adults, are less pronounced when compared using relative performance rather than gross performance. In fact, gross measures can discriminate against smaller performers. Ricci (1970) has gone so far as to suggest a moratorium on physical fitness testing until we can successfully develop tests which will account for individual differences.

As has been illustrated in previous chapters, children cannot compare favorably with adults in terms of gross performance. For example, their Maximal O_2 Intake is much less than adults, but when calculated according to body size equals that of adults. If children expect to equal the performance of adults in distance running merely because their relative cardiovascular fitness is equal to adults, they would be in for a great disappointment. Children should not be expected to match gross performance standards established for adults. To do so may very well limit the success of children and impair motivation to continue in regular exercise.

LAB VS. FIELD TESTS OF PHYSICAL FITNESS

Field tests of physical fitness serve a very legitimate educational purpose because they are easy to administer and great numbers of subjects can be tested. The weakness of the field test is that social, motivational, and other factors can easily contaminate the test results. Laboratory tests, when administered on a one-on-one basis, convey to a subject a seriousness of purpose which often is reflected in a more nearly maximal performance. Also, the fact that tests like the bicycle test for PWC use heart rate or O_2 uptake as the criterion makes them less likely to be affected by motivation than a test where time for distance is the criterion. Both field and lab tests should be considered in assessing the physical fitness of children, but basing the performance capability of children on field tests alone is to grossly underestimate their fitness levels.

CRITICAL DEVELOPMENT STAGES

Critical developmental stages refer to the time in the life of an individual when changes in behavior are most likely to occur at rapid or optimal rates. It is true that physical fitness, for example, can be developed at any age given appropriate overload, nutrition, etc. However, the rate of improvement of physical fitness will not be the same at every age, nor will the potential for improvement be the same at every age. Since every child cannot work to accomplish every aspect of fitness every year of life, it would seem desirable to determine the "critical development stages" for each separate aspect of fitness. The child could then concentrate on different aspects of fitness development at specific ages, when improved fitness would be most likely to occur. Instead of each child trying to achieve all aspects of fitness at one time (and risk achieving none), the child could accomplish each as he or she concentrates on that aspect during periods of optimal development. For example, prepubescent children can perform significant feats of health-related fitness (see next section on trainability), but would be better to concentrate on these areas later when gains are easier to see and motivation to continue exercise is great. Skill-related fitness has a potential for much earlier development; thus it seems that these aspects should be emphasized early in the child's life when graded success is not only possible, but likely.

This writer does not want to imply that children should not be exposed to all aspects of fitness development at all age levels. Rather it is suggested that specific aspects of fitness be emphasized at ages when development is most likely. Motivation to achieve full potential for physical fitness is a serious concern for those interested in developing physical fitness. Perhaps we would be better to teach for a "desire to exercise" early in life by emphasizing fitness development when improvements are most likely to occur.

THE TRAINABILITY OF CHILDREN

In the previous section it was noted that the child's potential for developing health related fitness development is less than that of the adolescent. This does *not* mean that children cannot train or be trained to do significant performances involving health related fitness. There are too many examples of outstanding running, swimming and other performance feats to deny that children can be trained. However, there is evidence that training for exceptionally high levels of health related fitness may be quite inefficient in childhood (prior to age 11 or 12).

It has already been noted that Astrand found motivational problems with obtaining maximal performances of very young children. Chourbagi (1973), on the basis of his research with olympic athletes, suggests that children below 10 "cannot stand the rigorous training necessary" for high level feats of health related fitness. This is not to suggest that the performance of such training will physiologically harm the child but rather to suggest that the benefits of such training may not equal the effort required to get them. Massicotte and McNab (1974) and Ekblom (1969) have indicated that the threshold of training for children is higher for children than for adults for cardiovascular fitness. This may in part explain why many studies (Cummings et al., 1969; Daniels and Oldridge, 1971; and Stewart and Gutin, 1976) have failed to find improvements in cardiovascular fitness among children after lengthy training programs.

The previously presented information and a knowledge of the normative data for all aspects of health related fitness, leads to the conclusion that the development of health related fitness is relatively inefficient in childhood. Children can be trained but the effort-benefit ratio is not good. In adolescence, because of accompanying changes in muscle mass, body size, etc. the benefits will increase for a given expenditure of effort.

If children are training for absolute performance accomplishments such as running against adults or lifting against adults, the effort necessary for a given benefit is even greater. The child would have to train especially hard to offset the developmental differences which exist. It is not hard to see why this would lead to problems in becoming motivated to train. If the performance is limited to persons of similar developmental level the problems would be lessened. Likewise, in activities which require relative rather than gross performance components, the advantage in some cases may actually go to the child because of the lesser body weight and size (gymnastics for example). However, even in these cases the person must have exceptional levels of health related fitness which do not come easy for children.

To summarize, children can train or be trained to achieve high levels of health related fitness, but the cost in effort is high. Unless the child is extremely motivated to train or unless there is some compelling reason for the training, it appears that most children would be best encouraged to maintain reasonable levels of health related fitness in childhood but to save efforts at intense training for a time when the effort-benefit ratio is more efficient.

INAPPROPRIATE EXERCISES

The purpose of this text is not to expound on exercise techniques. However, since optimal development of physical fitness is the concern of this section of the text, a few comments concerning inappropriate exercises seem in order.

Several recent reports (Flint 1964; Soderberg 1966) have drawn attention to the possible dangers of the leg-lift, the straight leg sit-up, the push-up, and other exercises. In spite of these warnings, these tests and exercises are still widely used without precaution. Even if there is no danger to the physically fit, results of the preceding chapters show that many children are not fit enough to use some of the exercises commonly administered in school. The fit may not experience problems associated with inappropriate exercise, but exposure to inappropriate exercises in childhood may result in injury when these exercises are used later in life by the unfit adult.

Further, it is hard to understand why boys, regardless of fitness potential, are required to perform pull-ups (many cannot do one), while stronger girls are not given this test. It would seem that better testing procedures would be to test weak children, regardless of sex, with one test and stronger children with another. Finally, this writer is concerned about testing procedures which require, or at least allow, children to perform extreme numbers of test item repetitions. The wisdom of performing 100 sit-ups is questionable. With no regular exercise as a prelude, children perform high repetitions as mentioned above. It would seem that one could tell what he wants to know about the child without the need for excessive repetitions of a test item, such as the sit-up.

SUMMARY

On the basis of the preceding four chapters, some general statements concerning the physical fitness of children seem appropriate:

1. Children have great potential for physical fitness performance. While their gross performances rarely equal those of adults, within their own size limitations, children are virtually unlimited in their performance potential.

2. American children have not nearly achieved their physical fitness potential. Evidence indicates that they may be fatter and less fit than would be desirable.

3. In childhood girls can achieve health related fitness similar to boys. The factors which contribute to successful accomplishment is similar for both sexes. Differences in health related fitness between the sexes are more dramatic in adolescence (see Chapter 30).

References

Chourbagi, Z. Y. "The Age Factor in Competitive Sports." In *Sport in the Modern World*, edited by O. Grupe et al. Heidelberg: Springer-Verlag Berlin, 1973.

Cummings, G. R. et al. "Failure of School Children to Improve in Cardiovascular Fitness." *Canadian Medical Association Journal* 101 (1969):69.

Daniels, J. and Oldridge, N. "Changes in O_2 Consumption of Young Boys During Growth and Training." *Medicine and Science in Sports* 3(1971):161.

Eklom, B. "Effects of Physical Training in Adolescent Boys." *Journal of Applied Physiology* 27(1969):350.

Flint, M. M. "Selecting Exercises." *Journal of Health, Physical Education and Recreation* 35(1964):19.

Massicotte, D. R. and MacNab, R. "Cardiorespiratory Adaptations to Training at Specified Intensities in Children." *Medicine and Science in Sports* 6(1974):242.

Rarick, G. L. and Dobbins, D. A. "Basic Components in the Motor Performance of Children 6 to 9 Years of Age." *Medicine and Science in Sports* 7(1975):105.

Ricci, Benjamin. "For a Moratorium of Physical Fitness Testing." *Journal of Health, Physical Education and Recreation* 41(1970):28.

Soderberg, G. L. "Exercises for the Abdominal Muscles." *Journal of Health, Physical Education and Recreation* 37(1966):67.

Stewart, K. J. and Gutin, B. "Effects of Physical Training on Cardiorespiratory Fitness in Children." *Research Quarterly* 47(1976):110.

Section 7

Perceptual-Motor Development

Perceptual-Motor Development: A Theoretical Overview

19

Harriet Williams
University of Toledo
Karen DeOreo
Kent State University

Over a century ago, Sechenov, a Russian physiologist, suggested that all human behavior could be thought of as a product of three very closely interrelated processes: (1) a sensory or afferent input; (2) a cortical or central process; and (3) an efferent or motor output. He further hypothesized that the motor or efferent process followed after and was based upon the outcome or effectiveness of the first two processes (Williams 1964, 1968). If for the sake of clarity and simplicity, we were to lump the first two processes together and call them "perception" and label the latter efferent process "movement" or overt behavior, we find that what Sechenov was suggesting was that all of man's behavior could be thought of as a series of perceptual events followed by a series of motor or behavioral acts. In other words, this formulation suggests that the processing of specific sensori-perceptual or afferent information is both prerequisite to and necessary for adequate execution of overt motor acts. The implication is, of course, that if the processing of such afferent information is slow or inaccurate, the probability of the subsequent motor or behavioral act being unskillful and/or maladaptive is considerably greater than if the processing of such afferent information is rapid, precise, and efficient. Thus according to Sechenov, most of man's behavioral or motor acts (whether as an adult or as a child) are, in large part, a product of the efficiency of the perceptual or afferent processes which precede them and upon which they are based.

It is because there is this very strong and identifiable link between overt motor behavior and sensori-perceptual or afferent processes that the term perceptual-motor has been coined and used so widely. It is this writer's belief that the use of this term is an attempt to draw attention to the importance of afferent or perceptual processes in human behavior. Thus motor learning is not just motor learning but perceptual-motor learning and motor development is not simply motor development but perceptual-motor development. In other words, learning and/or development are inherently linked to sensori-perceptual processes — processes which in essence provide the foundation upon which all such behaviors are built.

SENSORI-PERCEPTUAL PROCESSES AND MOTOR BEHAVIOR

What exactly are we talking about when we speak of sensori-perceptual or afferent processes? Sensori-perceptual processes, regardless of the kind of behavior ultimately involved, initially involve "sensory input." That is, sensori-perceptual processes have to do with the picking-up or taking-in of infor-

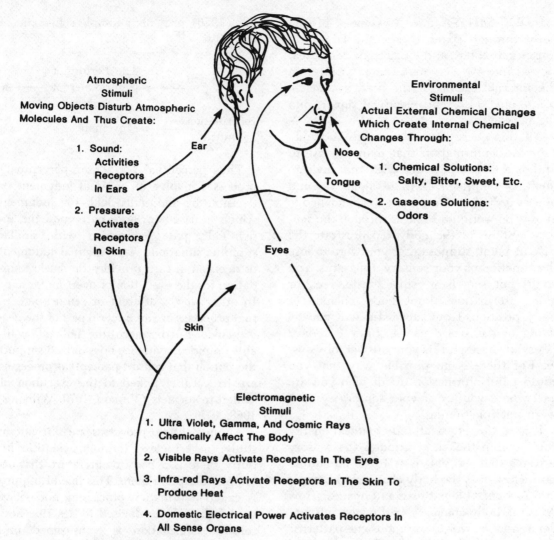

Atmospheric Stimuli
Moving Objects Disturb Atmospheric Molecules And Thus Create:

1. Sound:
   Activities
   Receptors
   In Ears

2. Pressure:
   Activates
   Receptors
   In Skin

Ear

Nose

Tongue

Eyes

Skin

Environmental Stimuli
Actual External Chemical Changes Which Create Internal Chemical Changes Through:

1. Chemical Solutions:
   Salty, Bitter, Sweet, Etc.

2. Gaseous Solutions:
   Odors

Electromagnetic Stimuli

1. Ultra Violet, Gamma, And Cosmic Rays Chemically Affect The Body

2. Visible Rays Activate Receptors In The Eyes

3. Infra-red Rays Activate Receptors In The Skin To Produce Heat

4. Domestic Electrical Power Activates Receptors In All Sense Organs

Figure 19.1. Sensory information pickup.

mation from the external (and/or internal) environment of the individual.

Let's take a look at these sensori-perceptual processes in an attempt to more accurately define and understand what they are. Man's body is constantly being bombarded by physical and chemical energy from our environment. This energy is picked up by our exteroceptors and takes the form of mechanical vibrations; chemical changes in the environment, and electromagnetic waves. These energy forms are illustrated in Figure 19.1.

In addition to the physical and chemical energy from our external environment, man's body is also stimulated by energy from within the body itself. This energy comes from two sources; the proprioceptors and the interoceptors. Movement of the body through space causes the labyrinth, muscles, tendons, and joints to fire electrical signals into the nervous system. Changes in the internal organs of the body (stomach, colon, etc.) also send electrical signals into the nervous system.

All this energy forms the one and only source of information that man can use to understand and interact with the environment. In simple terms, there is one way and one way only that man gains knowledge about the world and that is through the sensory systems of the body. To illustrate the case at point, suppose that you were to lose the function of your sensory apparatus. You could not see, hear, smell, taste, feel, or gain information about body balance or body position. How successful will you be living in our world as we know it today? "Very unsuccessful" is your answer, obviously. For there is no possible way that you could gain information about who you are and where you are if your sensory systems were not functioning.

It is to this physical and chemical energy coming into the body through the sensory systems that we will now focus our attention. How does the body change light waves into recognizable patterns and images? How does the body change sound waves into understandable words and musical patterns? This process of change, called perceptual process, has been studied by many scientists. The typical method of study deals with the observation of information going into the body through the senses (input). This is followed by observation of the resultant motor behavior (output). Based upon the type of input and consequent output, inferences are then made about the perceptual processes occurring in between. Marten-

iuk (1976) presents a simple schematic of this flow.

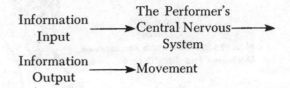

Thus perceptual (or sensori-perceptual) processes involve an internal judgment or decision by the individual — a judgment which is based in large part upon the individual's past experience with similar stimulus situations. This internal judgment or decision in turn provides the basic foundation for the execution of overt motor acts. In other words, afferent or sensori-perceptual processes are an integral part of the performance. Furthermore, the bulk of available empirical evidence does indeed support the notion that sensori-perceptual processes are irrevocably linked to the execution of skilled motor acts (Vernon, 1970; Williams, 1968, 1970).

Although these processes are difficult to study; nevertheless, through scientific inquiry there is a body of literature that attempts to explain them. This line of inquiry is called information processing and many models have been devised to describe how sensory information is transformed into meaning.

INFORMATION PROCESSING AND MOTOR BEHAVIOR

Massaro (1975) conceptualized information processing as a psychological phenomenon which has as its goal the understanding of the stimulus-response relationship. Stimulus being the physical and chemical energy entering the body through the sensory system and response being the observable behavior resulting thereafter. Important to this understanding of stimulus-response is the basic assumption that there are a number of processing stages which occur between the initiation of the stimulus and the observable motor response. As the information enters the human body through the sensory system, it encounters the first processing stage where it is acted upon and sent on to the second processing stage. The actions of each processing stage take time due to the particular transcription characteristics performed in that stage. Each stage is assumed to be successive.

Although the names of the various processing stages vary depending upon which information processing model you are following, the general overall theme is very similar among others. Figure 19.2 represents, in schematic form, the basic aspects of the processing stages (Williams, 1968). An explanation of each stage follows:

Phase I. Information Pick Up

The primary purpose of this stage is to receive information from the environment through the senses and to provide the following stage with an accurate description of the environment. Incoming information is identified and classified (Marteniuk, 1976). Through a process called feature detection, the incoming physical signal is changed into a neurological code which is held in preperceptual storage for a very short time (250 m seconds). The purpose here is to determine whether or not a particular feature is present. During preperceptual storage a readout of features is generated (Massaro, 1975).

An example of the operation of Phase I can be seen through a child's attempt to catch a ball. The ball is seen in the air as it is moving toward the child. Information about the flight of the ball, its speed and direction, is picked up by the visual receptors. The position of the catcher to the body in space is picked up by the proprioceptive system. Extraneous elements in the visual and proprioceptive fields are blocked out and the process of selection and/or attention are operating within the child. This allows the child to block out irrelevant cues and to concentrate upon the pertinent elements in the visual and proprioceptive field that deal with the motor act of catching. Thus the initial step in the sensory integration process is the picking up or providing the system with certain relevant sources of sensory information (Lappin, 1971; Williams, 1968, 1973; Wing, 1972).

Phase II. Interaction of Stimulus Information

Now that the information is in the system, what happens next? It is sent immediately to the main analytic unit of the system for further processing and analysis. However, only a small percentage of information originally entering the system is retained long enough to reach the main analytic unit. At this point in the sensory integration process, a great deal of the original sensory information picked up is lost before it can be sent to the main analytic unit. At this time the short term memory processes assume an important role (Biederman, Checkosky, 1970; Henderson, 1972; Druker and Hagen, 1969). If short term memory is adequate, a larger percentage of the information is retained within the system. Thus, there is more data

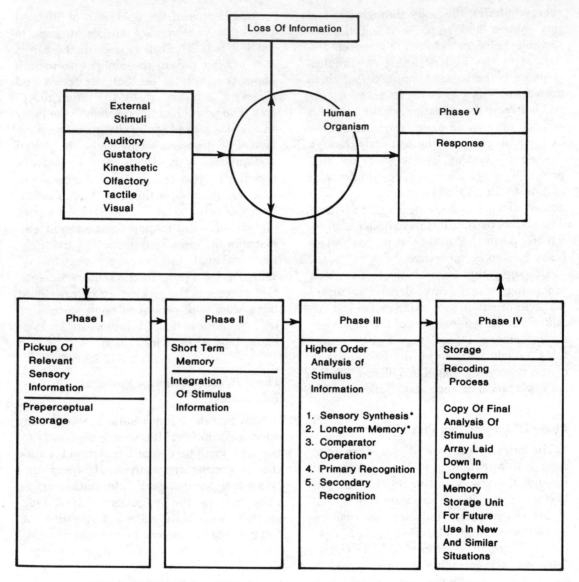

Figure 19.2. Sensory integration process.

for processing and use in the decision making process leading to the motor act, which in the case above is catching. Therefore it can be seen that the short term memory processes allows for more precise analysis of present stimulus conditions.

Phase III. Higher Order Analysis of Stimulus Information

The purpose of this phase is to analyze the information received from Phase II in such a manner that a plan of action in relation to the current task objectives can be determined (Marteniuk, 1976). The readout of features generated from preperceptual storage is matched with the features in long term memory that have corresponding descriptions. Current contextual information is also included. In this manner the information is transcribed into synthesized memory through the primary recognition process (Massaro, 1975).

Specifically, three main operations are to be considered here. The first of these is sensory synthesis. This is where both present and past sensory information are compared, analyzed, and synthesized. The final interpretation of sensory input occurs here. The second operation is long term memory storage. This is where the information from, for example, the child's past experience with similar ball catching situation is stored. This information is used as a frame of reference against which new data are organized and categorized. The third operation is the comparator (Williams, 1968). This is a monitering activity which continues to provide information about ongoing changes in the visual and proprioceptive fields, such as that of the catcher in our example. This keeps the system up to date about external and internal environments so that final decision can be precise and relevant to the situation at hand.

During the secondary recognition process, synthesized memory is transformed into units compatable with generated abstract memory. The role of this process is to achieve a match between the synthesized precept and information held in long term memory so that choices and alternatives can be made. This match can be referred to as conception since it involves analysis of synthesized memory for meaning (Massaro, 1975).

Phase IV. Storage

As in our example above, once the motor act of catching is completed the copy of the final analysis of the sensory data is preserved in the comparator until the act of catching is complete. Some time later the final copy of the stimulus array is laid down in more permanent form in the long term memory storage unit where it can be called upon for future use in new but similar ball catching situations.

Also operating in this phase is a recording process. This process attempts to further extract meaning from the information of an abstract and generalized nature. The higher order rules and strategies come into effect here; the resultant analysis is recirculated back through generated abstract memory (Massaro, 1975).

Phase V. Response

The end result of the first four stages of processing occurs here, in stage five, through the observable behaviors that follow specific sensory information pick up. Most responses involve some type of motoric response-be it running, writing, talking, or eye blinking. Seldom does the intake of sensory information result in inaction. Except, in extreme cases, where one is "frozen" with fear.

And so it is, that the sensory information process can be viewed from beginning to end as a perceptual-motor process . . . information pick up — perceptual interpretation — motor response.

 ## PERCEPTUAL-MOTOR DEVELOPMENT: A DEFINITION

In light of the foregoing theoretical formulation, it seems reasonable to suggest that the concept of perceptual-motor development is one which deals with changes or improvements in the child's afferent or sensori-perceptual capacities. These are changes grounded in a steady and continuous improvement in the child's capacity to perceive (to pick up and evaluate internally) increasingly more complex kinds and quantities of sensory information. Thus as perceptual-motor development proceeds, there is an accompanying increase in the refinement of the sensori-perceptual capacities of the child. This of course allows for greater control of overt motor acts. Behaviorally, this means that the child runs more efficiently, throws more skillfully, draws pictures with greater accuracy, and more detail, and so on ad infinitum. The concept of perceptual-motor development then is one which deals with age-related changes in the child's capacity for exerting more and more refined afferent control over overt motor behavior.

INFORMATION PROCESSING: ADULT VS. CHILD

It is clear to the observer that young children and adults do not function similarly in the task of information processing. Adults are highly efficient information processors who quickly take in only cues that are relevant to the task at hand. There is seldom wasted energy. Processing is rapid and the response is quite accurate. By comparison, the young child is slower and frequently irrelevant cues are picked up. Depending on the difficulty of the task, the response is likely to range all the way from totally wrong to highly accurate. What causes this sharp contrast between the abilities of children and adults on information processing tasks? A look at some of the fundamental processes may shed some light on this question.

The first process to consider is information pick up. Can the child pick up as much sensory information from the environment as the adult? The answer to this question is yes. The child can pick up as much information and even, up to a point, more information than the adult. Essentially, the child is equipped with the same sensory apparatus as the adult. For example, the visual receptors transduce light energy into the same neural code for the child as for the adult. The same is true for the auditory system and for all the other sensory systems. Research has shown that children pick up as much stimulus information from the environment as the adult (Haith et al., 1970a; 1970b; Haith, 1971; Sheingold, 1971). If this is true, then, how is it that adults are better than children? The difference must exist later in the stages of the information process.

Let's consider next the short term memory processes and how children and adults differ on this function. Children tend to lose information from the system at a much more rapid rate than adults do. Within one to five seconds after the stimulus information has been presented the child will lose 60% or more of the information (Haith, 1971; Haith et al., 1970a, 1970b; Liss and Haith, 1970). Since adults do not lose information as rapidly they have more information available upon which to make decisions. Two factors which effect the efficiency of the short term memory process are attention and rehearsal strategies. Attention is getting the right information into the system to begin with. Young children don't engage in planful scanning (Vurpillot, 1968). They do not know how to search the visual spectrum to pick up task relevant information for decision making. On the other hand, adults are quite skillful in picking out relevant information. Studies have shown that older individuals tend to block out incidental or irrelevant information almost entirely (Druker and Hagen, 1969). Adults take in less information than the child, but the information that is taken in is almost totally task relevant. The young child tends to overcrowd the system with both relevant and irrelevant information. Therefore the system must process large quantities of information if even a modest amount of task relevant information is to be retained. This process makes retention of information much more difficult for the child.

Another factor to consider in short term memory is the use of rehearsal. Rehearsal strategies, also called encoding strategies, have to do with the retention of information within the system beyond a very short time. Rehearsal strategies allow the system to retain information for an extended period of time. Encoding is the capacity of the system to chunk incoming information into large, meaningful units and to place these chunks into a "frame of reference". Studies have shown that both less intelligent individuals and children do not use the chunking operation in dealing with complex sensory input (Hagen, 1971).

How are these "frames of reference" developed and what is their importance to optimal functioning? This is where the long term memory must be considered. Long term memory is concerned with the development and use of multidimensional frames of reference and their retention in the system. The development of frames of reference is dependent upon the increased capacity of the system for processing multiple sources of sensory information. Behavioral data point out that a major characteristic of growth and development in children is a decrease in the separate use of individual sensory systems and an increase in use of multimodal or intersensory information (Aiken, 1972; Aiken and Griffin, 1972; Balter and Fogarty, 1971; Bartholomeus and Doehring, 1972; Birch and Lefford, 1967; Blank and Bridges, 1964; Daehler, 1971; Gaines and Raskin, 1970; Goodnow, 1971; McGrady and Olson, 1970; Wohlwill, 1971). The child, as he grows and develops, demonstrates an increasing ability to use information from a single sensory system to assist in the processing of information obtained from another sensory system. Consequently the key to efficient operation in terms of long term memory processes is the increased capacity for intersensory integration (Birch and Lefford, 1967). Since adults have already perfected the simultaneous and integrative processing of multiple sources of sensory information they are far more efficient in terms of the long term memory process than children.

DEVELOPMENTAL CHANGES IN SENSORI-PERCEPTUAL PROCESSES

If perceptual-motor development is directly linked to efficient sensori-perceptual or afferent processes, then we need to be concerned with such processes and to know something about the nature of the changes that take place in them during the child's growth and development. Although such changes are described in slightly different language by different authorities (Birch and Lefford 1967; Braine 1965; Nash 1970), there is at least some general agreement that these developmental changes in sensori-perceptual processes tend to manifest themselves in three major forms: (1) a shift in the hierarchy of the dominant sensory systems; (2) an increase in intersensory communication; and (3) an accompanying improvement in intrasensory discrimination.

The Shift in Dominance of the Sensory Systems

The first of the developmental changes in sensori-perceptual processes is seen in the consistently and universally observed shift from the dominance or pre-eminence of the use of sensory input from tactile-kinesthetic or proximo receptors to the use of input from teloreceptors, mainly the eyes, for the control and/or modification of behavior. Perceptual-motor development in the child thus is characterized by a shift in the reliance on tactile-kinesthetic or somato-sensory information to a primary reliance on information from the visual system as a basis for regulating or modifying motor acts. This move to dominance by the visual system represents a shift from the use of input from sensory systems with relatively elementary or crude information processing capacities to the use of input from a sensory system which has much more highly refined information processing capacities. The visual system is, of course, the most advanced of all the sensory systems with regard to the speed and precision with which it can supply information to the individual about the surrounding environment.

A good example of this change in the pre-eminence of the sensory systems is seen in the young child's attempts to jump rope while two adults turn it. If one observes a four-year-old under such circumstances, it becomes obvious immediately that the child simply cannot coordinate bodily movements to the movement of the rope. In other words, this child is not able to use, in any precise way, the visual information derived from the swinging of the rope to initiate and/or carry on a successful jumping response. To perform successfully in this situation, the child has first to establish his/her own rhythm or pattern of jumping. Once this rhythm or pattern of movement is established, the rope can be added, but the movement of the rope must always be coordinated by the rope turners to coincide with the pattern of movement already established by the child. This suggests of course that the four-year-old child is still quite dependent on tactile-kinesthetic (bodily) cues in performing motor acts and cannot as yet effectively use specific visual cues to successfully initiate or regulate motor behavior.

In contrast to this, the child of seven or eight years, when faced with a similar situation, does not have to be led into the skill of rope jumping by first establishing his or her own pattern of bodily movement. The child has little or no difficulty in coordinating rope jumping behavior with visual cues derived from the movement of the swinging rope. This suggests that there has been or that there is in progress a shift from the reliance on tactile-kinesthetic cues to the use of visual information for the regulation of motor acts. Reliance on visual cues of course, allows the child to make more rapid and precise judgments about the environment to which he/she must adjust. This in turn means that the child is capable of more refined, better coordinated motor acts—partly because the child *can* make better use of sensory information available in the environment.

Improved Intersensory Communication

The second clearly observable change in sensori-perceptual processes in the young child is that of improved intersensory functioning or intersensory communication. This simply means that as the child grows and develops he/she is increasingly better able to interrelate or match up information from several sensory systems simultaneously. As increased intersensory functioning occurs, the child matches up what is heard with what is seen; he/she evaluates what is seen against what is felt; and compares what is felt with both what is seen and what is heard and so on. Thus as the child grows and develops, he/she becomes more and more skilled in using multiple sensory inputs in directing motor behavior. The child can use visual cues and sound cues as well as tactile-kinesthetic cues to help adapt behavioral responses to the precise environmental conditions in which he/she finds himself/herself.

To illustrate, in the case of the rope jumping behavior, we saw that the older child was able to use visual input in initiating the rope jumping response more effectively than the younger child. In the case of improved intersensory communication, the maturing child develops an ever increasing capacity for interrelating the visual cues derived from the movement of the swinging rope to the sounds produced by the rope as it comes in contact with the surface of the ground and to rely on a combination of these two sources of sensory input as a basis for initiating and carrying-out

the rope jumping response. A part of the outcome of improved intersensory functioning then is a more efficient rope jumping performance because the child can pick-up and use more information from the environment.

Perhaps one of *the* most important characteristics of perceptual-motor development is this very definite and identifiable trend toward multisensory (multimodal) functioning and away from unimodal or isolated functioning of the sensory systems. This move toward multisensory functioning is important because it is believed to be a reflection of the growing integrative powers of the brain — powers which allow the child to match up or evaluate input from a variety of sources before a given movement or motor response is decided upon. That this process of intersensory communication is neither fixed nor fully functioning at birth is clearly supported by the numerous descriptions of the early sensori-motor stages of the child's development. Such periods of development are universally described as stages during which the various sensory systems function independently of one another. Perceptual-motor development in the young child then is characterized by a definite and identifiable trend away from a reliance on single sources of sensory information and toward the use of multiple inputs.

Improved Intrasensory Discrimination

The third major change which occurs in sensori-perceptual processes of the child (and which seems to occur simultaneously with the appearance of improved intersensory communication) is an increase in the discriminatory powers of the individual sensory systems themselves. In other words, each individual sensory system develops a more and more refined capacity for differentiation and/or discrimination. This improved intrasensory functioning is clearly reflected in the child's increasing ability to see more and more detail in the visual surroundings and to detect even small differences or similarities in various visual stimuli experienced in the environment. For example, with improved intrasensory discrimination the child is able to make finer and finer discriminations about the speed, direction and pattern of movement of the swinging rope. As a consequence of this increased discriminatory power, the child is better able to coordinate the movement of the body to the movement of the rope and thus rope jumping behavior improves.

In general, all three of these basic changes in sensori-perceptual processes play a vital role in the child's total perceptual-motor development and are the means by which the child gains greater and greater afferent control over motor responses. As a result of such changes, the child perceives more about the spatial environment and thus becomes more effective in adapting behavior to whatever specific environmental circumstances he/she may be faced with.

If perceptual-motor development is viewed, as it should be, as the product of the increasing refinement and differentiation of sensori-perceptual processes, then discussions of perceptual-motor development in children must necessarily look not only at changes in the motor characteristics of the growing, developing child but also at modifications in the perceptual makeup of the child which occurs during these same developmental years. The following chapters present a brief description of the perceptual *and* motor behaviors which characterize the early years of perceptual-motor development in the child.

Perceptual-Motor Systems

Though there are many sensory systems which contribute significantly to the Perceptual-Motor Development process, only three, the visual, auditory and kinesthetic systems are of major concern. For most gross motor skills the visual and kinesthetic systems are most important. Thus only these two systems will be in depth in this text. Chapter 20 will concentrate on the visual system while Chapter 21 will focus on the kinesthetic system.

References

Aiken, L. S. "Intermodal Consistency in Visual and Auditory Pattern Perception." Unpublished paper presented at the thirteenth annual meeting of the Psychonomic Society, St. Louis, Missouri, 1972.

Aiken, L. S. and Griffin, L. R. "Visual and Auditory Processing of Common Pattern Class Structure." *Perception and Psychophysics* 12(1972):492.

Balter, L. and Fogarty, J. "Intra- and Intersensory Matching by Nursery School Children." *Perceptual and Motor Skills* 33(1971):467.

Bartholomeus, B. N. and Doehring, D. G. "Acquisition of Visual-Auditory Associations by Good and Excellent Readers." *Perceptual and Motor Skills* 35(1972):847.

Biederman, I. and Checkosky, S. F. "Processing Redundant Information." *Journal of Experimental Psychology* 83(1970):486.

Birch, H. G. and Lefford, A. "Visual Differentiation, Intersensory Integration and Voluntary Motor Control." *Monograph of the Society for Research in Child Development* 32(Serial No. 110), 1967.

Blank, M. and Bridger, W. H. "Cross-Modal Transfer in Nursery School Children." *Journal of Comparative and Physiological Psychology* 58(1964):277.

Braine, L. G. "Age Changes in the Mode of Perceiving Geometric Forms." *Psychonomic Science* 2(1965):155.

Daehler, M. W. "Children's Visual Regard and Manual Activity in Retention of Information about Spatial Position." *Perceptual and Motor Skills* 33(1971):71.

Druker, J. F. and Hagen, J. W. "Developmental Trends in the Processing of Task-Relevant Information." *Child Development* 40(1969): 371.

Gaines, B. J. and Raskin, L. M. "Comparison of Cross-Modal and Intra-Modal Form Recognition in Children with Learning Disabilities." *Journal of Learning Disabilities* 3(1970):243.

Goodnow, J. J. "Matching Auditory and Visual Series: Modality Problem or Translation Problem?" *Child Development* 42(1971): 1187.

Hagen, J. W. "Some Thoughts on How Children Learn to Remember." *Human Development* 14(1971):262.

Haith, M. M. "Developmental Changes in Visual Information Processing and Short-Term Visual Memory." *Human Development* 14 (1971):249.

Haith, M. M.; Morrison, F.; and Sheingold, K. "Tachistopic Recognition of Geometric Forms by Children and Adults." *Psychonomic Science* 19(1970):345.

Haith, M. M.; Morrison, F.; Sheingold, K.; and Mindes, P. "Short-Term Memory for Visual Information in Children and Adults." *Journal of Experimental Child Psychology* 9(1970): 454.

Henderson, L. "Spatial and Verbal Codes and the Capacity of STM." *Quarterly Journal of Experimental Psychology* 24(1972):485.

Lappin, J. S.; Snyder, C. R.; and Blackburn, C. "The Encoding of Perceptual Information in the Organization of Individual Stimulus Patterns." *Perception and Psychophysics* 10 (1971):123.

Liss, P. and Haith, M. M. "The Speed of Visual Processing in Children and Adults: Effects of Backward and Forward Masking." *Perception and Psychophysics* 8(1970):396.

Martenuik, R. G. *Information Processing in Motor Skills.* New York: Holt, Rinehart and Winston, 1976.

Massaro, D. W. *Experimental Psychology and Information Processing.* Chicago: Rand McNally, 1975.

McGrady, H. J., Jr. and Olson, D. A. "Visual and Auditory Learning Processes in Normal Children and Children with Specific Learning Disabilities." *Exceptional Child* 36 (1970):581.

Nash, John. *Developmental Psychology: A Psychobiological Approach.* Englewood Cliffs, N. J.: Prentice-Hall, Inc., 1970.

Sheingold, K. "A Developmental Study of Short-Term Visual Storage." Unpublished Doctoral Dissertation, Harvard University, Cambridge, Mass., 1971.

Vernon, M. D. *Perception through Experience.* New York: Barnes and Noble, 1970.

Vurpillot, E. "The Development of Scanning Strategies and Their Relation to Visual Differentiation." *Journal of Experimental Child Psychology* 6(1968):632.

Williams, Harriet G. "The Development of Selected Aspects of Visual Perception in Infancy and Childhood." Unpublished Seminar Paper, University of Wisconsin, Madison, Summer 1964.

————. "A Neuro-Psychological Approach to Perceptual-Motor Functioning." Paper presented at MAPECW, Zion, Illinois, 1968.

————. "Visual Perception: A Review." Unpublished Paper, University of Toledo, 1970.

Wing, A. and Allport, D. A. "Multidimensional Encoding of Visual Form." *Perception and Psychophysics* 12(1972):474.

Wohlwill, J. R. "Effect of Correlated Visual and Tactful Feedback on Auditory Pattern Learning at Different Age Levels." *Journal of Experimental Child Psychology* 11(1971):213.

Characteristics of Visual Perception 20

Karen DeOreo
Kent State University
Harriet Williams
University of Toledo

Human visual perception ranks in complexity with speech and passes through comparable developmental phases (Gesell et al. 1949). The development of such capacities in infancy and childhood is so subtle, swift and esoteric that it does not always declare itself in conspicuous stages. Thus it becomes more than a difficult task to observe and accurately describe the nature and course of such development in the young child. Still during every stage of physical growth during infancy and childhood, the visual mechanism seems to undergo rather specific changes—changes which are then manifested in identifiable changes in the visual behavior patterns of the growing, developing child.

The instances of cooperative interplay between the visual system and the kinesthetic system are innumerable. The visual system is a critical source of information to the kinesthetic system. Frequently a motor task is attempted by an individual after first watching someone else perform. This observation of performance is recorded visually and processed in such a manner that the repetition of the observed movement is quite accurate. In fine motor movements it is seldom, if ever, that movements are made without the use of vision. The "eye guides the hand" so to speak. It is most difficult, for example, to write legibly with the eyes closed. Vision also supplies information about the results of a movement pattern so that we can see what we've done. If the movement in which we are engaged is slow enough, vision can be used to monitor the movement so that, if warrented, errors can be corrected.

In keeping with our theoretical overview presented in Chapter 19 the characteristics of visual perception will be presented in light of Visual Sensory Input — Visual Perceptual Processing — Visual Motor Response. Thus the reader will be able to trace the visual experience from sensory information transduction through perceptual interpretation to the ultimate and final visual-motor response.

VISUAL SENSORY INPUT

Envision it is the electromagnetic waves that pass through the eyeball which stimulate the receptor cells of the retina. These receptor cells contain pigments which break down chemically in the presence of specific wavelengths of light. It is this chemical breakdown which ultimately triggers the nerve impulse which is sent via the optic nerve to the primary visual cortex in the occipital lobe of the brain.

The specific path of light as it passes through the eyeball is as follows: cornea, pupil, lens, and retina. Once the light reaches the retina it is absorbed by the primary visual receptors — the rods and cones. These receptors differ in shape, location and function. The shape of the rods are long and narrow whereas the shape of the cones is short and bulb-like. In terms of location, there is a very high concentration of cones in the midsection of the retina around the fovea centralis. Moving away from the fovea there are gradually more and more rods until at the retinal periphery there is a high concentration of these receptors. Functional differences between these two receptors hinge on their degree of light sensitivity. Rods are extremely sensitive to light and are essentially receptors for night vision. As illumination increases these receptors gradually cease to function and the receptors for day vision, the cones, take over.

The actual firing of the nerve impulses along the optic nerve occurs as a result of a chemical reaction in the rods and cones. This chemical reaction is unique in each of the receptors. For the rods the photosensitive pigment is rhodopsin or "visual purple." When light reaches the rods it is absorbed by rhodopsin and bleaching occurs. At this point rhodopsin undergoes a chemical change which in turn generates the nerve impulse in the connecting neuron. For the cones the photosensitive pigments are three kinds of iodopsin each housed in separate "special" cones. Each pigment is sensitive to different wavelengths which in turn give rise to sensations of three separate colors; red, blue, and green. Therefore color vision is mediated by the cones whereas the rods respond only in black and white vision. Chemical changes which occur in the cones are similar to the chemical changes of the rods except for the different photosensitive pigments.

VISUAL PERCEPTUAL PROCESSING

The area of visual perceptual processing has received extensive study by experimental psychologists and is very complex in nature. Much information is known about visual perceptual experiences but specifically how these are mediated in the brain still eludes the scientist.

Forgus and Melamed (1976) have proposed that visual perception can be broken down into levels which can be arranged in a hierarchical fashion. They have identified five levels which range from level one, and simplest form of the visual perceptual experience, to level five, the most complex. It is their premise that what differentiates each stage of the hierarchy is the extraction of more and more information from the visual stimulus energy. The five hierarchical levels, in order from simples to most complex, are as follows:

I. The *detection* of the stimulus *energy* (light) and a discrimination of change in the stimulus energy.
II. The *discrimination of a unified brightness, figural unity,* and *orientation* as separate from the background.
III. The *resolution* of finer details which give rise to a more *differentiated figure.*
IV. The *identification* and *recognition* of a *form* or *pattern.*
V. The *manipulation* of the identified form; this happens for example, in *problem solving,* social *perception,* and where perception is related to value and motivation (Forgus and Melamed, 1976, pp. 16-17).

The preceding sections of this chapter have dealt with the first two phases of the total visual perceptual process. First visual sensory input was discussed followed by general information concerning visual perceptual processing. While it is beyond the scope of this book to do a complete treastise on the subject of visual perception, the following pages include a discussion of topics representative of the general scope of visual perception, especially the first two phases. The third phases, Visual Motor Response or output will be discussed later in this chapter.

CHARACTERISTICS OF VISUAL PERCEPTION

Visual Acuity

In order to see more clearly we turn our head and eyes toward the object of interest. This common and unconscious procedure occurs for a very logical physiological reason. Turning our eyes toward the object permits the visual image to pass through the eyeball and to fall on the retina at the fovea centralis. This is the area of highest "acuity"; or in other words the area that permits us to see sharply and clearly the fine details of the object. When visual acuity is poor, as in the peripheral areas of the retina, only gross outlines can be seen and the fine features, outlines and contours are blurred.

The sharpness and clarity of visual acuity is affected by several factors. The first of these is illumination or the amount of light available. Acuity is poor in dim light and gradually improved as illumination increases. The second factor involves contrast. Acuity improves as the contrast between an object and its background becomes sharper. The third factor deals with light of high intensity. When this intense light shines near the line of vision acuity is poor. The fourth factor was touched upon in the discussion above. When an object is sighted in such a way that the visual image falls on the fovea, acuity is sharper than when the visual image falls on the retinal periphery. Other factors that would affect visual acuity would be malfunctions of the lens and the cornea causing farsightedness (hypermetropia), nearsightedness (myopia), and astigmatism.

Visual acuity is poor in infants and continues to gradually improve up to the age of eight or nine years. Visual acuity can be categorized into two types: static and dynamic. Static visual acuity (SVA) refers to viewing a stationary object. This is also referred to as staticifixation. Neither the observer nor the object are moving. Most testing of acuity occurs in the static condition. When viewing a stationary object one might think that during the steady gaze the eye also remains steady. As it turns out this is not true for the eye actually dances about shifting the line of vision slightly. Ratliff and Riggs (1950) carefully measured fixational movements of the eye and found that there were four different kinds of movement occurring when the eye was being held steady. Description of these movements are: 1) a series of very fast tiny movements occurring at the rate of 30-70 per second, 2) slower movements somewhat larger in scope occurring at the rate of 2-5 per second, 3) very slow movements drifting from side to side, and 4) irregular jerks which may be compensating for the slow drifts. It appears that the eye is never really steady but in a state of constant motion.

The second type of visual acuity is referred to as dynamic visual acuity (DVA). This acuity deals with gazing at a moving object while the observer is either stationary or moving. This is also called ocular pursuit. When tracking a moving object the extraocular muscles come into play and work with a high degree of precision. There are three sets of these muscles around each eyeball and their primary purpose is to help the eye keep the visual image on the retina.

Fixation and pursuit movements of the eyes are also important in the development of depth perception and follow an interesting developmental trend (see Tables 20.1 and 20.2). These visual powers, which at the outset are simple and primitive, attain a high level of functional complexity by the age of six. Such development contributes in no small way to the everchanging motor skill capacities of the child. By age eight or nine years of age, children are able to track moving objects and make very precise judgments about their movement patterns (Williams, 1967).

Visual Discrimination

The ability of the visual system to perceive more and more detail of the visual world is labeled visual discrimination. This infers that we are able to make such judgments as: look alike, different from, same as, larger, smaller, rounder, taller, shorter and many others. Not only are we able to categorize, as just illustrated, but we are able to tell exactly what it is that differentiates and helps us to make the requested judgments, i.e., this circle is different from that circle because it has a line through it.

Two factors that play a strong role in visual discrimination are stimulus energy and time of viewing. The stimulus energy refers to the amount of light available. It is well known that at the two ends of visual illumination; darkness and intense light, visual discrimination is seriously impaired. However, once illumination reaches the level where we can see an object or pattern clearly our ability to discriminate detail does not necessarily get better if the light becomes brighter. The intensity of the light can be increased many times and we will still see, for example, a circle with a line through it. Conversely the light may be dimmed many times without impairing the ability to resolve the details of the object or pattern. However, there is some interplay between stimulus energy and complexity. Therefore the role of stimulus energy in enhancing visual discrimination is strong, gross and more powerful during high and low levels of illumination.

Time of viewing plays an unique and powerful role in visual discrimination. It takes more time for a complex pattern or figure to be visually perceived than for a simple figure ground experience to occur. Why is this so and what contributes to this phenomena? Werner (1935) in his classic study on contour development found that the more contours in a form the longer it will take it to be visually processed. His hypothesis was supported by Bitterman, Krauskopf, and Hochberg (1954) who presented geometric forms for .5 second to dark adapted subjects. The mistakes made in identification of the forms were related to their angles (contours). In general, the subjects tended to simplify the forms. Typical mistakes were: a square was called a circle, a triangle a circle, a cross a diamond, an X a square, etc. Circles were identified correctly most of the time. Additional studies in the area of contour development have concluded that in visually processing a form the higher the ratio of perimeter to area the more time will be required for processing (Hochberg, Gleitman, and MacBride, 1948; Krauskopf, Duryea, and Bitterman, 1954).

In reality, then, it is not the length of viewing time that is the critical element in visual perception but it is the amount of *processing time* needed to visually inspect the contours and to correctly identify the form. Stated another way, it is the length of time needed by the visual system to extract and process visual information. The more information included in the visual array the more processing time is needed. The reader is reminded of the earlier discussion of the hierarchy of visual perception proposed by Forgus & Melamed (1976) and their premise that each stage of the hierarchy involved extraction of more and more information from the visual stimulus. Thus, the processing time for level I tasks will be a great deal less than the processing time required for level V tasks. Forgus & Melamed also point out that as the levels of the hierarchy increase so does the role of experience and memory. In complex tasks the length of processing time is related to previous experience with similar tasks and memory functions.

Visual Constancy

The term visual constancy refers to the fact the certain aspects of the visual perceptual experience remain unchanged even though the physical dimensions (color, brightness, size, shape) are varied. Even though we live in a constantly changing environment there are certain visual experiences which are relatively constant. For example, a square box is perceived square whether its dimensions are 2 inches by 2 inches or 2 ft. by 2 ft. If we stand 6 ft. away from each box the size of the retinal image for each box will differ greatly — yet we still perceive squareness. The spatial orientation of each box could be varied, one tipped on its corner and the other tilted 30 degrees right, and we would still recognize the shape of each one as a square. One box could be painted blue and the other box painted green but the perception of square would not be altered. Constancies help to give our world order and stability. If we responded to *all* the changes in our physical environment our life would be one of considerable instability. Colors would change simply because we turned on the lights; sizes and shapes would change because their distance or spatial orientations were altered. Visual constancies help us order our world so that our responses can be made on predictable and reliable information.

In general, the visual constancies consist of brightness constancy, color constancy, size constancy, and shape constancy. Brightness constancy occurs as the result of light being reflected from the surface of an object. White, gray, or black objects are perceived the same regardless of whether they are viewed in shadows, cloudy conditions, twilight, or bright sunlight. Brightness constancy refers to the perceived whiteness of an object while color constancy refers to the specific wavelengths of light which are reflected giving rise to color sensations. Excluding the extreme ends of illumination, red is perceived the same in either a well lighted or dimly lighted room. Actually, color constancy includes both brightness and hue.

There are several factors that affect brightness and color constancy. The first of these is the amount of light reflected from the object itself. This is called *albedo* and is typically stated by a proportion between amount of light received and amount of light reflected back. An object that looks white may be reflecting back 85% of the received light and thus would have an albedo of .85. Objects perceived as black have an albedo of .14. Therefore, the more light reflected back by an object the more is its perceived brightness. However, perceived brightness also depends on the amount of light reflected from the background. Brightness constancy occurs as the result of innate responses to the difference between the intensity of reflected light of the object and the intensity of light coming from its background. Contrast between the object and its background also has an affect on perceived brightness. When the background is darker the object appears brighter (Wallach, 1948; Wallach & Galloway, 1946). Contrast also affects perceived color. When a ring of light surrounding an orange disk was made brighter the orange disk looked brownish (Wallach 1948). Brightness constancy and color constancy perceptions are innate and basically not learned. The observer automatically responds to the difference between the reflected light of the object and the reflected light of the surroundings. However, the accuracy of the judgments made is due to experience in the real world and attitudinal set (Forgus & Melamed, 1976).

Size constancy refers to the fact that perceived size does not change as distance from the object (decreasing retinal image) changes but remains constant. Thus the size of a cup is perceived the same when you are holding it as if you are across the room from it. At short distances, size constancy judgments are triggered by several innate processes. The first one is accommodation. This is brought about by the ciliary muscles as they contract to make the lens of the eye convex so that near objects can be brought into focus. The proprioceptive sensation of these muscles are believed to be one of the cues innately used by the organism to judge size. Convergence is a second process which provides clues for estimating size. This is brought about by the movement of the extraocular muscles of the two eyes as they attempt to bring the focused image onto the retina. The manner in which these muscles contract due to the variation in size of the object of sight provides innate cues for size approximations. Another process which assists in providing innate cues for judgments of size is retinal disparity. This is the slight difference in the visual image caused because we have two eyes that are an inch or so apart. Each eye receives a similar but slightly different picture of the world. The differences in these visual images provide information about size estimations.

For determining size estimations at longer distances cues for both size and distance are used. The innate processes mentioned above are no longer effective and cues which have been learned from experience are now brought into operation. The first clue is known size. If you know the real size of an object then its distance is more easily estimated. If two objects are placed at a distance the nearer one is perceived larger. Shadows cast by one object upon another provide information about size and distance. An object which is partially hidden by another object is perceived farther away. Linear perspective is another clue which provides the observer with size and distance information. Gradients of texture-density provide information about the size and distance of objects standing on the surface (Kling & Riggs, 1971).

Shape constancy refers to the fact that judgments of perceived shape do not change even though the spatial orientation of the object is changed. This means that even though a rectangular box is turned on its side, end, or edge, it will still be perceived as a rectangular box. Shapes are areas of the visual field that are set off by their visible contours. They have identity and position in relation to the remaining portions of the visual field. Brightness plays a role in defining shape. If the two portions of the visual field differ in luminance a brightness contour appears to separate the field into different shapes. However, if the two portions appear equal in brightness then clear cut shape perceptions are not made. If luminance of one visual region shades off gradually into another region, the shapes of both are indefinite. The perception of shape, then, requires a sharp contour between regions that differ in brightness (Kling & Riggs, 1971).

Visual Figure-Ground

Our visual world is more than a series of unrelated pieces of visual information floating into and out of our visual consciousness. Instead it has an order which consists of perceiving figures as separated from their backgrounds. This is called figure-ground perception which is a phenomenon basic to the understanding of shape and form perception. Rubin (1915, 1921, 1958) has described the differences between figure and ground as follows:

1. The figure appears to have a shape while the background is shapeless.
2. The ground appears to be behind the figure's edge.
3. The figure gives the observer the impression of a "thing"; the ground has no shape.
4. The figure appears brighter and more solid than that of the ground.
5. The figure appears to be in front of the ground.
6. The figure is more easily remembered because it is more meaningful than the ground.

What determines which of two observed areas will be the figure and which will be the ground? Wertheimer (1923) used simple line drawings and dot patterns to study these factors and his findings are listed below:

1. Proximity — when dots are placed near each other, they easily form a group with contours.
2. Area — when the boundaries of an area are made smaller, it is more strongly perceived as a figure.
3. Orientation — patterns that are aligned with the vertical and horizontal axes of space are more likely to be perceived as a figure than those aligned with oblique axes of space.
4. Closedness — areas that are bounded by closed contours form stronger figures than areas with open or incomplete contours.
5. Symmetry — areas that are symmetrical in shape are perceived as figures more frequently than those of asymmetrical shape.
6. Similarity — similar shapes tend to be grouped together as well as dots with similar brightnesses.
7. Common Fate — patterns of dots that appear to move together in the same direction are perceived as a group.
8. Good Continuation — patterns of dots grouped in such a way as to follow a uniform direction are perceived together in a straight or smoothly curving line.
9. Homogeneity or Simplicity — the visual organization of figural contours (edges and boundaries) that presents the figure in the most homogeneous or uniform way.
10. Observer's Set — When the observer is set to perceive a certain figure he/she will do so even though the laws of organization are opposed. Also, the observer may continue to perceive a figural organization even though conditions no longer favor it (figure perseveration).
11. Past Experience — a figure can be perceived even though the spacing or configuration is changed due to past experiences in perceiving the figure.

Now that the basic explanation of the figure-ground experience has been presented, let's turn our attention to the development of figure-ground abilities in children. It appears that there is some elementary form of figure-ground ability in newborn infants (Fantz, 1961). In young children visual attention is most often directed toward the ground rather than toward the figure (field dependence). This is true up to the age of 10 to 13 when there is a change toward observing the figure (field independence) (Witkin, 1954).

The ability of a child to extract relevant detail from contexts containing extraneous elements has most frequently been measured by embedded figures or figure-ground tests. In such studies objects or figures known to the child are embedded in a larger more complex pattern. When five- and six-year-olds are shown these figures, only the more advanced children are able to find the simple figure in the more complex one. Less advanced children frequently cannot pick them out at all unless the figures are very simple ones. Although there seems to be a marked improvement in performance on such tests between the ages of 8 and 13, this general perceptual capacity seems to continue to improve until 17 or 18 years of age (Ayers 1969; Mussen 1965).

Gibson (1966) also has found a significant difference between the performances of second, fourth, and sixth graders in picking out a specific form (a letter) from a context of other extraneous items. Younger children (second graders) in general required a significantly longer time to pick out the correct letter than did the older children. In a slightly different but related experiment, five- and six-year-olds were asked to judge the "lightness" of target objects when more than one object was presented at a time (Beck 1966). These children showed great difficulty in making this perceptual judgment accurately. When targets were presented singly, however, the children performed at the same level as adults. All of this seems to indicate that as the child matures, the ability to differentiate and to use perceptual detail increases. The capacity for not only seeing but also for extracting detail from extraneous contexts requires a number of years to become fully developed. Development of figure-ground processes must involve an increased capacity for handling large quantities of visual information and for differentiating that information which is relevant or useful from that which is not. It has been estimated that development of whole-part perception may not be fully complete until late adolescence (Vernon 1970).

Visual Localization

Knowing the location and orientation of objects and people in space, their direction and distance from the observer and from each other, is a function of visual localization. Coding of object direction by the eye is accomplished fairly easily since the image of objects is located in different areas of the retina. This differential location of the images on the retina results in perceived direction. However, the determination of distance and depth, a three dimensional task, from an optical image which falls on the two dimensional surface of the retina is a more complicated feat. How does the visual system code distance and depth? What clues are used and how do they develop in children? Table 20.1 summarizes the development of visual localization for children from birth to 7 years of age. This section will attempt to answer these questions through discussions of perception of depth and distance, perception of spatial orientation, and perception of movement.

TABLE 20.1
Development of Visual Localization

AGE 0-16 Weeks	16-28 Weeks	28-40 Weeks
	Recognizes depth; reaches out to grasp near objects but not distant ones. Judges distance more accurately in near space than in far. Shows preference for solid as opposed to flat objects. Avoids deep end of visual cliff.	Heightened but still undifferentiated awareness of spatial intervals separating two objects or an object and his person. Ability to manipulate closely juxtaposed. Spatial relationships increasing: takes one cube and pushes another one with it. Depth perception still meager but growing: often peers into cavity of a cup.

AGE 40-52 Weeks	One Year	Two Years
Increased awareness of depth. Three-Dimensional space world now consists of near distances and far reaches. Manifests an awareness of container and contained; solid and hollow; top and bottom, etc. Vertical surfaces have a new appeal. Builds up sense of depth through probing of index finger and prying with the eyes. Extends ocular experiences through creeping.	Becoming aware of spatial enclosure-insidedness. Continuous investigation of essential characteristics of objects-attracted by hollow objects especially. Aware that things can be either stable or mobile. Classifies all moving things into one category. Vertical sectors of space are being mastered. Identifies objects by position in space.	Increased awareness of new areas in space through climbing behaviors. Now separates near, far, and intermediate space sectors. Far space still unorganized; near space well organized. Near space-more binocularity present. Intermediate space-prevailingly monocular but some binocularity present. Far space-beginning to respond monocularly. Becoming aware of dualism in space-up-down, in-out, top-bottom. Increased visual discrimination shown in preoccuation with small objects. Likely to get things wrong-side up and reversed. Notices shapes but not directionality. Alarmed by on-coming movement: is making an important distinction between incoming and out-going spatial dimensions.

Table 20.1 (Continued)

AGE Three Years	Four Years	Five to Seven Years
More comprehensively oriented in space.	Combines spatial meridians into wholes and subunits without sacrificing continuity of space and interrelationships between components.	Space is now self-oriented: notices more and more detail in environment; notices irregularities in size and outline of objects.
Does not react diffusely to content of space world-perceives specific objects within a given area.	Can integrate more elements into perception of a situation.	Likes specific orientations in space: has definite preference for vertical sectors.
Whole is losing its wholeness: perceives more and more detail.	Demands that an object be right-side-up—increasing aware-ness of relation between own person and experimental object.	Can look out into space while maintaining specific fixation in near space.
Sees more clearly the rela-tionships between objects.	Cannot as yet handle oblique strokes.	Increased awareness of relativities of space and of orientations in space.
Interest in minute facets of space leads to enrichment of near space sector.		Has gained mastery of the oblique direction.
Perceives objects very effectively in near and distant space but may lose them visually in intermediate sectors.		
Has an increasing propensity toward horizontal sectors of space.		
Is aware of both stable and changing relationships.		

Perception of Depth and Distance. Although the terms depth and distance are very similar and are frequently used interchangeably, there is a slight difference in their meaning. Depth refers to the space between two objects in space whereby distance refers to the space between the observer and the object. Considerable capacity for depth perception appears early in infancy. At six weeks the infant is able to make some gross differentiation between objects that are nearer versus those that are farther away from him (Bower 1966). Gesell (1949) reports that binocular convergence (the ability to focus both eyes accurately on an object and thus a forerunner of true depth perception) appears, on the average, at the end of the second month. Gibson and Walk (1960) in their visual cliff experiment showed that human infants can discriminate depth as soon as they can crawl. At any rate, it appears that some primitive type of depth perception, geared to perceiving features of the environment which are ultimately essential for adaptation to and survival in the three dimensional space world of the adult, are functional in the infant even as early as one-and-one half to two months.

If the infant and/or young child perceives depth, by what means is it done? Two of the primary cues involved in adult

TABLE 20.2
Development of Dynamic and Static Fixation

AGE Neonate	4-16 Weeks	16-28 Weeks
Aware of movement of objects in first day of life.	Increasingly aware of movement in the environment but does not perceive casuality.	More facile patterns of fixation and pursuit evident.
Fixates accurately when object is only few inches away from eyes.	Shows increasingly prolonged visual activity.	Shifts gaze more freely in supine position than in sitting position.
Gives only brief, feeble glances when it is farther away.	Sustained fixation at peak of efficiency.	Fixation is most effective in near space.
Pursues moving object before accurate fixation is possible.	Scope of fixations and eye movements increased.	Visual regard of an object is more inspectional: notices details.
	Easily fixates object 1-3 feet away.	
	Can reverse pursuit movements.	
	Often overshoots in pursuit movements of the eyes.	
	Follows a dangling ring through an arc of 90-180 degrees easily.	

AGE 28-40 Weeks	40-52 Weeks	One Year
Notices movement and gestures of near-by persons.	Increased mobility in fixation and pursuit movements.	Capable of versatile head and eye movements in sitting position.
Beginning to localize positions in space.	Freely sweeps eyes across arcs of 180 degrees.	Easily follows moving objects when seated.
Eyes fixate on general target area but not with complete precision.	Fixates specific object in room: then spreads gaze to rest of room.	Tilts head backward and sideward in pursuit.
Watches intently the movements of hand in the mirror.	Increase in perceived detail: distinguishes readily ring from the string to which it is attached.	Lifts ball, releases it, intently watches it after release.
Increased ability to shift from one fixation to another.	Beginning to distinguish movements of objects from movements of own body.	Casts object from high chair-pursues it visually, fixates on object after it lands.
Fixation and attention extend farther out into space: fixates objects at greater distances more easily.	Intensely interested in movements reflected in a mirror.	
At 36 weeks: intently watches ball moving toward or across field of vision.	Aware of small movements and small changes or displacements in spatial relationships.	
	Likes to watch motion of cars, animals, and other objects.	

Table 20.2 (Continued)

AGE	Three Years	Five to Seven Years
Moves visual fixation easily from one focus to another.		Follows complicated excursions of moving objects for brief periods of time.
Releases readily at far sector, picks up at near sector-reverse also true.		Pursues easily targets moving at faster speeds.
Eyes now able to move precisely on or around a specific object.		May lose fixation but readily picks it up again.

depth perception are binocular parallax (a consequence of the fact that the eyes are set structurally, some distance apart in the head and thus each eye receives a slightly different picture of the object being viewed) and motion parallax (which derives from the movement of the head from side to side as one looks at a number of objects located at different distances). These two processes require an integration of two or more visual images derived from the object or scene being observed, and thus involve a high degree of coordination or teaming of the two eyes-binocularity. There are, however, single image, monocular cues that also function in adult depth perception. These include such things as real (distal) size, relative size, familiar size, shadows, aerial perspective, interposition, linear perspective, and gradients. The question then is, is the visual system of the young child capable of the integration necessary for the use of binocular and motion parallax cues in depth perception or does the infant rely instead on single image cues; that is, on monocular cues which do not require such integration?

In the newborn infant (2-3 days old), neither true monocularity nor binocularity as such seem to be present. Within the first week, however, monocularity begins to dominate the child's visual processes and he/she seems to be more adept at using a single eye than in using the two eyes together (Gesell et al. 1949). With continuing growth, a transitional period occurs — a period which is clearly marked by the alternating use of monocularity and binocularity in viewing the environment of objects in the environment (one to two months). Binocularity, however, becomes the primary force in vision at about two months and much advancement can be noted in the coordinated use of the two eyes in the weeks and months that follow (Fantz 1961b; Gesell et al. 1949). Parallel with this development, there is, in terms of depth perception, an identifiable transition from a kind of primitive, innate sense of stereopsis to a more refined perception of depth which seems to be well on its way to maturity by the end of the fifth year.

Experiments by Bower (1966) have also indicated that even at the early age of six to eight weeks, binocular parallax and motion parallax (both of which are dependent on binocularity) are the most important cues in the infant's perception of depth. At this age when monocular cues alone were available, the infant could not discriminate depth as readily as when binocular cues were present. It is conceivable that monocular cues are not useful to the infant simply because they do not provide enough information about depth in a situation. In other words, it may be that the visual system of the young infant is such that specific kinds of visual information are required for the child to be able to judge depth and if such sources of information (which are apparently binocular in nature) are not available the infant cannot perceive or judge depth accurately.

As growth continues, binocular and monocular cues become better integrated and ultimately the older child (6-7 years) or the adult can judge depth as accurately with monocular (reduced cues) as with binocular cues (Johnson and Beck 1941; Vernon 1970).

Perception of Spatial Orientation. Perception of spatial orientation as it is defined here refers to those perceptual behaviors in which the child shows a recognition or awareness of the orientation or position of objects in three-dimensional space. The normal human adult can readily see the difference between these two figures: N and Z. This visual difference is so striking that we are likely to think of these two forms as two completely distinct shapes rather than as different spatial orientation of the same shape (Z=N rotated 90°) (Watson 1966). The mature skills of visual perception permit the adult, in most cases, to readily resolve differences in object orientation and to either regard or disregard such differences, depending upon their relevancy to the situation.

The child's visual organization of space follows, in general, a near to far sequence. The child first organizes near space, perceives details and builds up complex spatial relationships and orientations there, and then gradually extends this organization farther and farther out into space. Visual organization of these spatial sectors, however, often overlaps for the child begins to visually define and organize in far space before completely mastering of the near space sector. Thus a child may be oriented in near space but not nearly so well organized or oriented with respect to more distant sectors of space (Gesell et al. 1949).

The human infant, at a very early age, is capable of perceiving both the shape and the orientation of external objects, but when both sources of information are available, the primary response of the visual mechanism is to shape. In other words, the perception of shape appears to be more basic than the perception of orientation or direction. As the visuo-perceptual mechanism matures, the simultaneous processing of multiple visual inputs is possible and the child can thus respond to either or both perceptual qualities of shape and spatial orientation (2-4 years).

It is of interest to note that children seem to master spatial directions and thus orientation of objects in a fairly orderly sequence (Gesell et al. 1949; Jeffrey 1966; Katsui 1962; Rudel and Teuber 1963). First, the verticals are mastered; this is followed by mastery of the horizontal, and last by control over the apparently more complex oblique or diagonal spatial directions. A child of two or two and one-half years of age is as likely to get things upside down as right-side up (Gesell et al. 1949; Vernon 1970). That is, the child is as content to look at a picture book upside down or in a tilted position as in its normal orientation. This would suggest that the child has not yet completely outlined the vertical or up-down sector of space. Children of three and four years of age, however, can distinguish a vertical line from a horizontal one, and thus the four-year-old demands that the picture book be right-side up. Mirror images or right-left reversals are still very difficult for these

children and they often fail to distinguish between two oblqiue lines which are oriented differently in space (Rudel and Teuber 1963). This perceptual inadequacy is evidenced in the fact that when asked to copy a shape which is tilted obliquely in one direction or another, the three-year-old may copy the shape in an upright position. Either the child perceives only the shape and not the tilt or is unable to regulate movements so as to be able to reproduce it in the tilted position.

Children of this age are still greatly influenced in their recognition of certain forms by the orientation of that form. Preschool children, for example, are more frequently correct in their identification of geometric forms when they are viewed in an upright position than when viewed in an inverted one (Ghent and Bernstein 1961).

Within the next few years, considerable advancement occurs in the visual-perceptual skills for six-seven-, and eight-year-old children. They show little or no difficulty with discriminations involving vertical and horizontal lines or with upright and inverted figures and most of them can learn rather easily to tell the difference between a horizontal and oblique line (Rudel and Teuber 1963). Thus by six the child readily notices the orientation of plane figures on a page (Rice 1930-32). Discriminations involving vertical and oblique lines however, are a little more difficult as are discriminations involving two oblique lines, and even seven- and eight-year-olds may have difficulty with these (Rudel and Teuber 1963). Katsui (1962) has noted that in a number of eight-year-olds, there is still a high frequency of right-left or mirror reversals. Thus even at eight, perception of spatial orientation may still be far from complete, and adaptive motor patterns are still in the making.

Perception of Movement. How can an observer tell that an object is moving, is stationary, or vice versa? The retinal image is ambiguous to the locations and motions of objects in space. For example, the tilted image of an object on the retina may be caused by the object being tilted in space or by the observer being tilted in space. In one case, the object is tilted while in the other, the object is upright. For the perception of movement the retinal image is in motion. This can be caused by the object itself moving or by the object remaining stationary and the observer moving. Correct perceptions of movement not only take into account the retinal image but also include the knowledge of body position and movement. The visual system actually perceives movement in two major ways. The first is when the image of an object remains stationary on the retina while the eye pursues the object. This suggests that the sensation of movement arises from the eye movements used to track the object. The second is when the eye is stationary and the image of the object moves across the retina. In this case, the sensation of movement would arise from the differential excitation of the visual receptors. An exception to this occurance is saccadic eye movements which cause the retinal image to move but produce no sensation of movement to the observer. Although the perception of movement is presented as being composed of two major functions, there are other less understood factors which lead the observer to experience the perception of movement.

The two functions described above involve primarily the way the neural units (rods and cones) respond to specific displacement in the retinal image. Other factors may involve the way an observer remembers a sequence of events. Movements take time to run their course yet the observer can recognize and compare movement sequences to each other. There must be some mechanism whereby the observer can remember an entire change of temporal events. Movement is not a simple sensory experience, but composed of several different processes which contribute to a complex perceptual experience.

In the study of movement experiences, of interest to the experimenter is the minimum amount of distance over which a movement must occur in order to be detected. Also of interest is the amount of time needed by the observer to detect the movement. This is called a velocity (distance/time) threshold. It has been found that the velocity threshold when fixating a moving object while some parts of the visual field are stationary, is 1 to 2 minute/seconds. However, when only a moving object is fixated, the velocity threshold changes to 20 minute/seconds (Kling and Riggs, 1972). The fact that the velocity threshold increases greatly when there is no stationary background for the moving object suggests that spatial references play an important role in the perception of movement.

Since information from the visual system by itself presents a rather uncertain picture of movement events and the location of objects, the observer must use information from the proprioceptive system for assistance. Knowledge of the position of the eyes, head, and body helps in locating objects and in executing successful actions toward them. Movements that are aimed towards objects in space must carefully combine the information which comes from the retinal image with information which comes from the eyes, head, and body. Proprioceptive information which responds to the internal state of our muscles and joints, as well as to the constant pull of gravity, is essential for the refined perception of movement in space.

It was mentioned above that saccadic eye movements do not produce a sensation of movement to the observer. Saccadic movements are tiny movements of the eyeball which occur several times a second. Even through the observer feels that the eyes are being held steady, as in staring at an object, in reality the eyeballs are literally dancing around in their sockets. Yet, the world appears to remain fixed in space and we continue to function totally unaware of these tiny continuous eye movements. One explanation for this phenomenon is that as the eye moves the entire retinal image moves maintaining a constant relationship between its segments, and thus no movement is perceived. Another explanation is that voluntary eye movements have occurred then no movement is perceived. Complete understanding of the role of saccadic eye movements and their contribution, or lack of it, to the perception of movement is not clear.

VISUAL-MOTOR OUTPUT

The output which occurs as a result of visual-perceptual processing is chiefly comprised of two components which operate in close cooperation with each other. The first component results from the action of the eyes as they explore the world; the second component occurs from the action of the hands and body. Thus the term visual-motor is most commonly used in referring to both components. It is seldom that the intake of visual information is not followed by the performance of a motor act. In this section the two components will be discussed as they occur in fine visual motor acts and gross visual motor acts.

Fine Visual-Motor Skills

The major period of growth for fine visual-motor coordination skills takes place during the first year of life. During this time, the basic operation involved in eye-hand coordination appear, and development in the years that follow consists largely of the refinement, extension and/or use of these basic operations in an ever expanding manipulation and exploration of the spatial environment of the child.

The visual component of eye-hand coordination behaviors appears to involve four major stages (Gibson 1966; Harris 1966; Williams 1964). Each of these stages clearly involves changes in the basic sensori-perceptual makeup of the child; changes which are reflected in the ever-improving and constantly expanding repertoire of eye-hand coordination skills which the child displays. The initial stage of development of eye-hand coordination includes the period from birth to sixteen weeks and is best described as a stage of static visual exploration. The infant, during this stage of development, seems to have a genuine visual predilection for the hands and spends a large percentage of waking time fixating intently on the hands while lying in the crib.

The second stage of eye-hand coordination development, which covers the seventeenth to the twenty-eighth week, is one which is characterized by active and repeated visual exploration of objects in the child's environment. This active visual manipulation of objects seems to be a kind of ocular grasping and is probably a forerunner of actual manual prehension and manipulation. Thus at about twenty weeks, the infant seems to literally "pickup" an object with the eyes, drop it and then pick it up again visually.

The third stage of eye-hand coordination development (28-40 weeks) is one in which the visual mechanism of the child seems to prompt or take the lead in initiating specific grasping and/or manipulative responses. (It should be noted, however, that although such movements are more selective and better controlled than before, they are still frequently inaccurate and misdirected). Perhaps the most important characteristic of this stage of eye-hand coordination development is the newly acquired ability of the child to correct reaching, grasping movements through intensified activity of the visual mechanism. For example, during this stage the child seems first to locate an object or toy with the eyes, then initiates a movement toward the toy. As the child reaches for the object, visual fixation relaxes. Frequently this initial movement is in error and when it is, the child's visual fixation of the object intensifies and the child adjusts or corrects the reaching response. Focus on the toy is maintained throughout this time and when the hand finally comes into contact with the toy, visual fixation becomes even more intensified. Then as the object is grasped and manipulated, the eyes continue to explore it visually. This sequence of behavior suggests that the child is going through a step-by-step process of interrelating what is seen with what is felt and vice versa. In so doing, the child may be building up a more refined capacity for using what he/she sees (vision) to guide or direct what he/she does (manipulation), an important step in the total cycle of eye-hand coordination development.

The final stage of eye-hand coordination development begins at approximately 40 weeks and continues throughout the years of middle childhood. This period of development consists mainly of acquiring a more refined control of eye-hand coordination behaviors and of extending them to the performance of a wide variety of tasks.

From birth, arms and hands are in constant motion. The movements consist of awkward jerks, random hittings, and opening and closing of the fingers. The child in exploring the world and makes much use of the hands. Manipulation in combination with the senses enables the child to understand size, distance, and textures, and orientation to directions. Not until about the second month, when the eyes are coordinated and able to focus, can progress be made in the development of prehension. Even then, eyes and hands remain uncoordinated.

The development of the motor component of fine visual-motor coordination begins with movements not under voluntary control by the infant, in other words, the reflexes. These reflexes play an important part in the development of eye-hand coordination for fine-motor skills. The grasp reflex is present at birth and is integrated/inhibited around 2 months of age. The grasp reflex is primarily accomplished with the first two fingers and the heel of the hand. The thumb is curled into the palm and not utilized in grasping. The tonic neck reflexes are the dominating force for head and arm position.

By the end of the first month the infant is beginning to lift the chin and gain momentary head control. This is followed by development of the shoulders which help to raise the chest while in the prone position. As the infant lies supine in the ATNR position one eye is observing the hand on the face side. This is considered to be the first in the development of eye-hand association, and is followed by hand reaching responses for the first time. Although the hand reaching responses are being developed, the infant cannot consciously direct the hand and grasp a perceived object.

By four months of age the infant has gained stability in the trunk for support sitting, and holding the head erect in the midline position. The infant can now begin to shift visual attention to objects at different distances and tracks moving objects quite well. At this point the grasp reflex is beginning to be integrated into a conscious grasp known as the palmer grasp. The thumb is now adducted to the side but still not utilized to help in the grasping of objects.

Around 6 months of age the tonic neck reflexes are integrated. Maintenance of an erect position and free rotation of the head is seen. The arms can be used asymmetrically when the head is held at the midline position, and the eyes begin to direct the hand in goal oriented tasks.

At 9 months of age the pincer grasp is developing, thus aiding the infant in picking up objects with the index finger and thumb. The ability to consciously release objects is also being developed, however, not fully demonstrated until about the age of 11 months (Strauss and DeOreo 1979).

During the second year of life, the visual and motor components continue to develop in close cooperation with one another. Manipulation and exploration of objects occupy a large portion of the child's time. The visual motor activity of this period serves as the precursor to self-help skills and later writing skills.

In Table 20.3 a brief summary of the development of fine visual motor coordination from birth to 8 years is given. At one year a child will reproduce a few imitative scribblings. At 2 years, refinement of the scribbling are noted with the child reproducing perseverated (multiple line drawing) patterns of vertical and horizontal lines. At

TABLE 20.3
Development of Fine Visual-Motor Coordination

AGE Neonate	4-16 Weeks	16-28 Weeks
Visual activity affects action patterns but the two are not well coordinated. Fixation on an external object brings about complete cessation of bodily activity.	Age of prehension approaching. Looks at object, then at hands; immobilizes eyes, and legs then activates.	Picks up object with eyes; makes feeble attempts at contact or prehension of it. Preparation for prehension continues: often looks at object, then at hand, then back to the object and back to hand. Integration of visual-tactile-kinesthetic impressions seen in the greatly increased eye-hand-mouth activity. Grasps objects only if placed in hand. Retains object in hand briefly. Holds toys actively. Reaches for toys suspended above head.
AGE 28-40 Weeks	**40-52 Weeks**	**One Year**
Eye-hand activity shows endless variations. Fixates object: reaches for object and fixation relaxes: grasps object and fixation intensifies. Fixates target: overreaches it manually; intensifies fixation and adjusts reach. Reaches for ball with two hands; eyes and hands work in unison.	Grasping is facile and smoothly coordinated. Organizes space world by manipulating toys in limitless ways. Objects begin to acquire fixed dimensions and permanency. Pushes ball a short distance, pursues it with eyes, then creeps to it; repeats whole cycle. Picks up objects. Recovers objects dropped. Reaches persistently. Reaches purposefully. Transfers objects from hand to hand.	Prehension becoming refined. Eyes no longer riveted to manipulations. Eyes are more facile when sitting than when standing or walking. Keeps eyes on container when placing object in it. Eyes follow rather than direct activity. Visual and manual releases expulsive; not under control. Picks up objects and throws them on the floor or out of the playpen. Holds pencil with fist and scribbles imitatively. Makes vertical strokes with pencil (18 months) Drinks fom cup and can self-feed, but is awkward.

Table 20.3 (Continued)

AGE 28-40 Weeks	40-52 Weeks	One Year
		Pounds easily with small wooden mallet.
		Stacks blocks 3 high.
		Places 1″ pegs in holes.
		Turns two or three pages at a time.
		Spontaneous scribbling.
		Imitates vertical and horizontal strokes.
		Extended reach and grasp.
		Pincer grasp-thumb and index finger.
		Voluntary release of objects.
		Puts object into containers.

AGE Two Years	Three Years	Four Years
Eyes assume a more directive role in guiding motor activities but are slower in shifting visual focus.	Hands used constructively to direct and confirm visual responses.	Eye-hand relationships not tightly bound: leads to multiplicity of visual and motor responses.
Eyes shift smoothly from near to intermediate sectors of space.	Deploys hands without direct supervision of eyes.	Eyes enjoy a certain autonomy: hands not needed to support visual manipulations.
Visual perception locates and prompts manipulation of objects.	Hands are used more selectively in visual exploitation of objects.	Depth perception reaching new horizons.
Eyes direct when child shifts object from one location to another.	Manipulates more discriminatingly and skillfully.	Tends to orient movement from center of periphery.
Looks and then acts.	Drawings better defined; lines made with more control.	Puts some detail in drawing.
Looks at container, at object, and back to container, then places object in container.	Copies circle.	Copies circle and square but not triangle.
Can interrupt activity, look away and then give full visual attention to previous activity.	Copies cross.	Oblique lines.
Still dependent on manual contact, cannot readily identify or locate object in space by voluntary visual and adjustment alone.	Handles crayon in adult manner.	Oblique cross.
	Cuts with scissors.	Draws a recognizable face.
	Picks up small objects.	

TABLE 20.3 (Continued)

AGE Two Years	Three Years	Four Years
Tendency to overhold and over-release in manipulations.		
Feeds self without too many spills or accidents.		
Makes horizontal strokes with pencil.		
Stacks blocks six high.		
Turns one page at a time.		
Strings beads.		
Holds crayon with fingers.		
Copies vertical stroke.		
Copies horizontal stroke.		
Imitates circular strokes.		
AGE Five Years	**Six Years**	**Seven Years**
Uses knife for cutting and spreading.	Copying tasks become less laborious.	Demonstrates preference for pencils instead of crayons.
Horizontal and vertical strokes mastered; obliques still a problem.	Demonstrates fair ability to block print letters.	Demonstrates ability to make uniform size in letters, numbers, etc.
Can copy square and triangle but not a diamond.		Comparative size of human figure is more accurate.
Displays increased fine finger control (such as involved in playing musical instruments).		
Can color within lines.		
Cuts fairly accurately.		
Begins to draw combination of two forms.		
Draws recognizable man, body, and extremities.		
AGE Eight Years		
Can copy a diamond.		
Begins cursive writing.		
Letters are more uniform in alignment.		

three years of age the child can copy visually presented figures of a circle and cross. The four-year-old can copy a square, oblique lines, and oblique cross. Five-year-olds begin to color within the lines, cut and paste simple things. They can draw triangles, and begin to draw combinations of two or more forms. At six years the child demonstrates fair control for block printing, however, some letters may be reversed. It is not uncommon for some children to reverse their letters occasionally until around 8 years of age. The seven-year-old's ability to reproduce geometric figures matures. The oblique lines have been sufficiently mastered, thus enabling the child to reproduce a fair drawing of a diamond. It is not until the eighth year that reproduction of a diamond with acute angles 60 degrees or less is accomplished. Usually between the seventh and eighth years, the child is confronted with the task of developing cursive writing skills. This does not suggest that their skills might not be developed at an earlier age. (Berry 1967, Cratty and Martin 1969, and Gessell 1946).

Gross Visual-Motor Skills

Although all movements that are made use visual information in one way or another, some more commonly accepted gross visual-motor skills are throwing, catching, kicking, striking, and ball bouncing. The successful performance of these skills requires the visual system to work in close cooperation with the motor system. In throwing, the visual system must relay information about the location of the target to the motor system. The motor system in turn, programs a movement series that will enable the ball to be thrown to the target area. In catching, kicking, and striking, the eyes are required to track the oncoming ball so that the motor act can be carried out at exactly the right time. In ball bouncing, the eyes monitor the movement of the ball as it rebounds from the floor so the hands can be commanded by the motor system to be in the appropriate position to maintain the bouncing action.

The development of these gross motor visual skills in young children depends upon the gradual maturing of both the motor and visual systems. Basically, gross motor visual skills are those activities that require movement of the large muscle of the body in coordination with visual tracking. The success of the movement depends on the accuracy of the visual system. These skills involve an object or implement which is usually a ball, bat, or racket.

The environment must include these objects or, for example, no throwing and catching will develop. Also, the addition of another person is instrumental in developing these skills. Throwing and catching are best performed with two or more people and the same is true of striking and kicking.

Below, these gross motor skills are discussed; highlighting developmental progression. Since throwing and kicking are covered in Chapter 9, only catching, striking, and ball bouncing will be discussed.

Catching. The use of the hands to stop and control a moving ball, whether it is bouncing, rolling, or in the air is generally considered catching. In attempting to catch a ball, the methods used appear in definite stages (See Figure 20.1). The beginning attempts are characterized by the use of the whole body to clasp the ball. These attempts are followed by the use of two arms and less general movement. Gradually the movement to catch the ball with one or two hands is practiced and per-

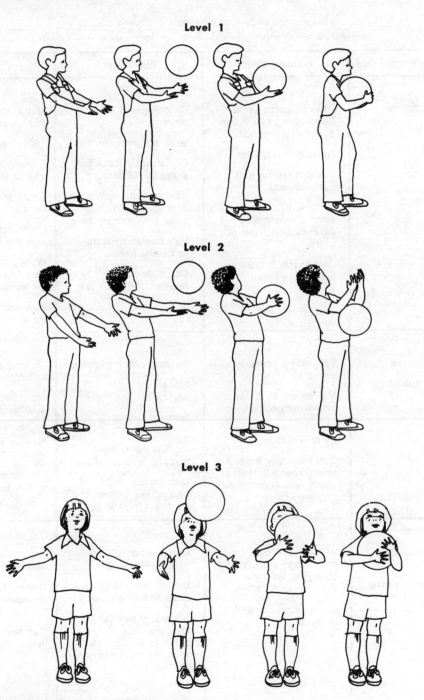

Figure 20.1. The develomental sequence of catching. (Wickstrom, R. L., *Fundamental Motor Patterns,* 2nd ed., 1977. Philadelphia: Lea & Febiger Redrawn from Wild, N., Research Q., Am. Assoc. Health, Phys. Ed., 1938.)

TABLE 20.4
Development of Gross Visual Motor Skills in Younger Children

AGE Two Years	Three Years	Four Years	Five Years
CATCHING Not able to catch. Unable to visually track ball.	Able to catch some balls using the 2-arm-body trap method. None are proficient. Turns head as ball approaches. Catches with both arms straight and extended in front of body. Can catch 9 1/2" ball two out of three trials.	Catching skill improving. 29% are proficient. Can visually track ball some of the time. Catches with both arms extended in front of body with elbows bent. Ball contacts mostly arms and hands. Can catch 9 1/2" ball two out of three trials.	Catching skill continues to improve. 56% are proficient. Can visually track the ball all the time. Catch with elbows bent and at body sides. Catches mainly with the hands. Weight transferred to rear foot as ball is received. Can catch 9 1/2" ball three out of three trials.
STRIKING Not able to strike. Unable to visually track ball.	Can strike some objects. Movement in anterior-posterior plane. Movement entirely by arm action. Can hit softly tossed ball three out of five times with hand or fist.	Striking skill improving. Movement more horizontal. Some trunk rotation apparent. Occasional weight transfer to forward foot. Can hit ball from batting tee five out of six trials (plastic bat.)	Striking skill continues to improve. More definite trunk and hip rotation. Weight shift to forward foot. Can hit ball from batting tee five out of five trials (plastic bat).
BALL BOUNCE Not able to bounce ball. Unable to exert visual motor control.	Attempts at ball bouncing: includes swinging wildly at the dropped ball. Little or no contact is made.	Can perform a drop catch sequence. Use of two hands to drop and catch ball. Control of ball is fair. Can continue drop-catch pattern for 15 seconds continuously.	Actual rhythmic ball bouncing is achieved. Ball contact tends to be a slapping motion with an open hand. Can bounce with both hands 15 seconds. Can bounce with right hand 15 seconds. Can bounce with left hand 15 seconds.

TABLE 20.5
Development of Gross Visual Motor Skills in Older Children

AGE Six-to-Seven Years	Eight-to-Nine Years	Ten-to Twelve Years
CATCHING Refinement of catching pattern. Skill gradually improves. Absorbing force begins to be evident. Weight transfer used effectively.	Good catching pattern evident. Use of mechanical principles apparent and improving. Can catch fly balls of moderate distance and height. Can catch ground balls of moderate distance and speed.	Mature, mechanically correct catching pattern used. Can catch fly balls of greater distances and heights. Can catch ground balls of greater distance and speed.
STRIKING Refinement of striking pattern. Skill gradually improves. Greater range in the backswing. Can hit softly tossed ball six out of seven trials (plastic bat).	Good striking pattern evident. Use of mechanical principles apparent and improving. Can hit softly pitched softball with regulation bat.	Mature, mechanically correct striking pattern used. Can hit softball pitched with greater force using regulation bat.
BALL BOUNCING Refinement of ball bouncing pattern. Skill gradually improves. Greater control exhibited. Can ball bounce using alternating hands 15 seconds.	Good ball bouncing pattern evident. Greater control exhibited. Can ball bounce using uneven rhythmic patterns for 15 seconds.	Continued refinement and improvement of skill. Good control of rhythmic elements evident. Can vary sequential and temporal elements of bounce pattern at will.

fected. The size of ball effects the child's ability to catch. A large percentage of 5-year-olds who can catch well, can catch a 5″ ball easily (Gutteridge, 1939).

During the transition from the beginning catching attempts to mature form, there are maked arm positions. These are: 1) the ball is addressed with the arms straight, 2) then with the arms slightly bent in front of the body, and 3) with the arms bent considerably with the elbows more at the side of the body (Wickstrom, 1970).

Striking. Striking is hitting an object with some part of the body or with an implement which is under control by the hand. Information concerning the performance of striking skills in preschool children is extremely sparce.

Early forms of striking can be described as an overarm motion occurring in the anterior-posterior plane. As striking skills develop, the child seems to progress from striking in the vertical plane downward through a series of oblique planes to the horizontal plane. Early attempts to strike in the sidearm pattern can be described as follows: 1) the movement is initiated by arm action which is followed by limited pelvic rotation, 2) pelvic and trunk rotation appear as the result of the swing rather than a contributing force, and 3) progression in the development of the sidearm striking pattern is indicated by more forward weight shift, a greater range of joint actions, and more separation of rotatory elements in the patterns (Halverson, Robertson, 1966). In children less than 30 months old, the striking pattern persistently used was the overarm striking pattern which was adjusted to lowered heights of the ball by bending forward at the waist.

Progress in the development of an effective striking pattern is indicated by the following changes: 1) more freedom in the swing with increased range of motion at the various joints, 2) more use of the forward step or a forward weight shift to initiate the pattern, 3) more definite hip and trunk rotation preceding the action of the arms in the swing, 4) more uncocking of the wrists.

Ball Bouncing. Ball bouncing is not usually considered a fundamental motor skill, but it is included here because of the variety of ball bouncing games traditionally found among children today. Also, visual-motor control of balls is found in several of the most popular sports in our culture. Without this important coordination, performance in these sports would be greatly impaired.

Early attempts at ball bouncing by the two- and three-year-old child are crude at best. The ball is dropped and then hit at wildly. Contact is seldom achieved and the ball rolls away. The four-year-old can learn to carry out a drop catch sequence after a little practice. The ball is not always under control. The drop catch is performed with a two-hand drop and a two-hand catch. By age five, the child is able to consecutively bounce the ball using both hands or one hand alone for at least fifteen seconds. Ball contact tends to be with a slapping motion with an open hand. Mastery of even rhythmic bounce patterns, using alternating hands, is achieved at seven to eight years of age. Uneven rhythmic bounce patterns are mastered around the age of nine to ten years.

References

Ayers, J. *Southern California Perceptual Motor Tests.* Los Angeles: Western Psychological Corporation, 1969.

Beck, J. "Age Differences in Lightness Perception." *Psychonomic Science* 4(1966):201.

Berry, K. E. *Developmental Test of Visual Motor Integration: Administration and Scoring Manual.* Chicago: Follett Publishing Company, 1967.

Bitterman, M. E.; Krauskopf, J.; and Hochberg, J. E. "Threshold for Visual Form: A Diffusion Model." *American Journal of Psychology* 67(1964):205-19.

Bower, T. G. "The Visual World of Infants." *Scientific American* 215(1966):80.

Cratty, B. M. and Martin, S. M. *Perceptual-Motor Efficiency in Children.* Philadelphia: Lea & Febiger, 1967.

Fantz, R. L. "The Origin of Form Perception." *Scientific American* 204(May 1962a):66-72.

Fantz, R. L. "A Method for Studying Depth Perception in Infants." *Psychological Record* 11(1961b):27.

Forgus, R. H. and Melamed, L. E. *Perception: A Cognitive-Stage Approach.* New York: McGraw-Hill, 1976.

Gesell, A. and Ilg, F. L. *The Child from Five to Ten.* New York: Harper and Row, 1946.

Gesell, A.; Ilg, F. L.; and Bullis, G. E. *Vision: Its Development in Infant and Child.* New York: Paul B. Heober, Inc., 1949.

Ghent, L. and Bernstein, L. "Influence of the Orientation of Geometric Forms on Their Recognition by Children." *Perceptual-Motor Skills* 12(1961):95.

Gibson, E. J. "Developmental Study of Visual Search Behavior." *Perception and Psychophysics* 1(6) (1966):169.

Gibson, E. J. and Walk, R. D. "The Visual Cliff." *Scientific American* 202 (4)(1960): 67.

Gutteridge, M. V. "A Study of Motor Achievements of Young Children." *Archives of Psychology* 244(1939):1-78.

Halverson, L. E. and Roberon, M. A. "A Study of Motor Pattern Development in Young Children." Report to National Convention of AAHPER, 1966.

Harris, J. C. "Development of Hand-Eye Coordination in Infants and Children." Unpublished Seminar Paper, University of California, Berkley, December 1966.

Helson, H. and Feher, E. V. "The Role of Form in Perception." *American Journal of Psychology* 44(1932):79-102.

Hochberg, J. E.; Gleitman, H.; and MacBride, P. D. "Visual Thresholds as a Function of Simplicity of Form." *American Journal of Psychology* 60(1948):341-42.

Jeffrey, W. E. "Discrimination of Oblique Lines by Children." *Journal of Comparative Physiological Psychology* 62(1966):154.

Johnson, B. and Beck, L. F. "The Development of Space Perception: I. Stereo-scopic Vision in Preschool Children." *Journal of Genetic Psychology* 58(1941):247.

Katsui, A. "A Developmental Study on the Perception of Direction in Two Dimensional Space." *Japanese Journal of Psychology* 33 (2)(1962):63.

Kling, J. W. and Riggs, L. A. *Sensation and Perception. Experimental Psychology*, edited by Woodworth and Schlosberg, vol. 1. New York: Holt, Rinehart, and Winston, Inc., 1972.

Krauskopf, J.; Duryea, R. A.; and Bitterman, M. E. "Threshold for Visual Form: Further Experiments." *American Journal of Psychology* 67(1954):427-40.

Mussen, P. H. *The Psychological Development of the Child.* Foundations of Modern Psychology Series. Englewood Cliffs, N. J.: Prentice-Hall, 1965.

Ratliff, F. and Riggs, L. A. "Involuntary Motions of the Eye During Monocular Fixation." *Journal of Experimental Psychology* 40 (1950):687-701.

Rice, C. "The Orientation of Plane Figures as a Factor in Their Perception by Children." *Child Development* 1-2 (1930-31):111.

Rubin, E. *Synoplevede Figurer.* Copenhagen: Gyldendalke, 1915, pp. 432, 438.

Rubin, E. *Visuell Wahrgenommene Figurer.* Copenhagen: Glydendalske, 1921, pp. 432, 438.

Rubin, E. *Figure and Ground.* In *Readings in Perception,* edited by D. C. Beardslee and M. Wertheimer. Princeton: Van Nostrand, 1958, pp. 194-203.

Strauss, R. and DeOreo, K. L., *Assessment of Individualized Motor Skills,* Region XXIII, Austin, Texas: Texas Education Agency, 1979.

Vernon, M. D. *Perception through Experience.* New York: Barnes and Noble, 1970.

Wallach, H. and Galloway, A. "The Constancy of Colored Objects in Colored Illumination." *Journal of Experimental Psychology* 366 (1946):119-26.

Wallach, H. "Brightness Constancy and the Nature of Achromatic Colors." *Journal of Experimental Psychology* 38(1948):310-24.

Watson, J. S. "Perception of Object Orientation in Infants." *Merrill-Palmer Quarterly* 12 (1966):7.

Werner, H. "Studies on Contour." *American Journal of Psychology* 47(1935):40-64.

Wertheimer, M. Untersuchungen zur Lehre von der Gestalt: II. *Psychologische Forschung,* 1923, 4, 301-350. Abridged translation by M. Wertheimer: *Principles of Perceptual Organization.* In Readings in Perception, edited by D. C. Beardslee and M. Wertheimer. Princeton, N.J.: Van Nostrand, 1958, p. 433.

Wickstrom, R. L. *Fundamental Motor Patterns.* Philadelphia: Lea & Febiger, 1970.

Williams, H. G. "The Development of Selected Aspects of Visual Perception in Infancy and Childhood." Unpublished Seminar Paper, University of Wisconsin, Madison, Summer 1964.

Witkin, H. A.; Lewis, H. B.; Hertzman, M.; Mackover, K.; Meissner, P. B.; and Wapner, S. *Personality through Perception.* New York: Harper, 1954.

Characteristics of Kinesthetic Perception

21

Karen DeOreo
Kent State University
Harriet G. Williams
University of Toledo

The visual system allows us to see where we are going and to locate objects in our environment. The auditory system permits us to hear sound and to obtain meaning from it. But, there is another sensory system which receives its information not from mechanical energy outside of the body, but from the actions of the body itself. This is the kinesthetic system and it is supplied with information from the muscles, tendons, joints, and vestibular system. Basically, kinesthesis can be defined as the sensations and perceptions which occur as the result of bodily movement. Thus, every time we move sensory information is being sent to the cerebral cortex keeping it informed about the positions of body parts and their rate and extent of movement. The cortex in turn uses this information to decide what new movement should be initiated and consequently issues the neural command to move.

The kinesthetic system, like all the sensory systems, does not operate in isolation. Information from the cutaneous receptors, visual receptors, and auditory receptors is integrated with kinesthetic information to provide the cortex with a complete picture of our external and internal environment. As was pointed out in the preceding chapter, the visual system is a critical source of information to the kinesthetic system. In order to function effectively, we must perceive objects in our external environment so that our movements can be adjusted accordingly. This cooperative interplay is what keeps us from running into doors, tripping over chairs, and from being run over by cars, trains, etc.

Organization of this chapter is similar to that of the chapter on vision. The characteristics of kinesthetic perception will be presented in keeping with the theoretical overview presented in Chapter 19 — Kinesthetic Sensory Input — Kinesthetic Perceptual Processing — Kinesthetic Motor Response.

KINESTHETIC SENSORY INPUT

Essentially, kinesthetic sensory input is provided by receptors located in the muscles, tendons, joints, and the vestibular apparatus. There is some disagreement in the literature concerning kinesthetic receptors. Some authors include the cutaneous receptors since they do provide information during movement, but since this information provided by these receptors is minimal they will not be included in this discussion.

Located within the skeletal muscle fibers (also called extrafusal fibers) are muscle spindles which are small organs containing two types of sensory receptors. Spindles, which are actually composed of specialized muscle fibers called intrafusal fibers, are found in all muscles of the body and have a higher density in muscles that control fine and precise movement. The spindles lie in parallel with the muscle fibers and are sensitive to muscle stretch. The two receptors located within the spindle are the annulospiral endings and the flower-spray endings. The annulospiral endings are located centrally and spiral around the intrafusal muscle fibers. These afferent neurons are large, low threshold, and fast conducting neurons. During rest they emit a low frequency discharge. However, during linear stretch these receptors increase their firing greatly and when the muscle is actively contracted cease firing altogether. Located on either side of the annulospiral endings and attached to the intrafusal fibers are the flower-spray endings. These afferent neurons are small, high-threshold, and slow conducting neurons. Stretching of the muscle causes these receptors to fire. When active contraction occurs and stretch is released, the flower-spray endings become quiet, emitting only a small low level discharge.

What role spindle receptors play in kinesthetic perception? Basically, it is believed that they are used in the control of movement and posture without giving rise to conscious sensation. They provide a sense of active movement. Postural adjustments which are reflexive in nature are mediated by the spindle afferents. Movements of the body through space and in relations to gravity cause the spindles to fire thus maintaining a constant array of changing postural reflexes which enable us to perform effectively in our environment. It is also believed that spindle afferents play a role in providing feedback to the cerebral cortex about voluntary movement (Eccles, 1973). Thus, every time we move, the central nervous system is being provided with information concerning the rate and extent of the intended movement. This information can then be used to adjust the next intended movement if needed.

Another kinesthetic receptor is located in the tendon which attaches the muscle to the bones of the body. This receptor is commonly called the Golgi tendon organ and works in close cooperation with the muscle spindles. Although it functions similarly to the spindles, it is uniquely different in that it is stimulated by *both* stretch and active contraction of the muscle (Geldard, 1972). Thus it appears to be a general muscular tension recorder with a higher threshold than that of the spindles. The Golgi tendon organs show no resting discharge and seem to adapt less rapidly than the spindles. It appears then, that the muscle spindles discharge rapidly at low levels of stretch and the Golgi tendon organs begin firing rapidly at higher levels of tension (Dickinson, 1974).

Like the spindles, it is believed that the Golgi tendon organs have no role in conscious kinesthetic perceptions. Their role appears to be two-fold: a) to initiate the clasp knife reflex and b) to supply the higher brain centers with information about the degree of active muscle contraction. The clasp knife reflex occurs when the degree of tension that is put on a muscle becomes so great that it threatens to tear the muscle loose from the bone. The tendon receptors send impulses into the spinal cord which in turn sends inhibitory impulses to the muscles to cease contraction. This removes the tension from the tendon receptors and thus protects the muscle and tendons from damage. Also, like the spindles, it is probable that the tendon organs play an important role in providing feedback about the degree of contraction existing in the muscle. This information is used to monitor and regulate the strength of muscular contraction. Impulses from the Golgi tendon organs enter the spinal cord and ascend to the cerebellum. There are no afferents that reach the cortex by any direct route.

A third set of kinesthetic receptors is actually a combination of three receptors which are located in the joints of the body. These receptors have been recognized as contributing to discrimination of movement in the joints. This discrimination is quite precise with the movements at the hip and shoulder being detected more readily than movements at the fingers and toes (Laidlaw & Hamilton, 1937). It appears that the joint receptors are more sensitive to movement itself than to the actual direction of movement. As each joint moves through its range of motion the patterns of receptor firing vary. As the joint angle changes, different receptors become more sensitive and increase their firing for the next 10-15 degrees. As movement continues, these receptors reduce their rate of firing and gradually cease as their angle of sensitivity is passed. This pattern of increasing-decreasing neural discharge is repeated throughout the entire range of motion without reference to the direction of movement. The specific receptors responsible for recording the various positions of the joint are the spray-type endings and the Golgi-type endings which are located within the ligaments and joint capsule respectively. The third receptor, the pacinian corpuscle, is responsible for reporting information concerning the movement itself. These receptors are located within the joint capsule and are stimulated by velocity. Impulses from the joint receptors project into the spinal cord and ascend to the cerebellum, thalamus, and on into the somatic cortex.

The final set of kinesthetic receptors is located in the vestibular system which is situated in the inner ear. This system is composed of five parts; the superior, posterior, and horizontal semicircular canals and the utricle and saccule. The actual receptor organs are embedded inside these structural parts. For the canals the receptor organ is the crista ampullaris and for the utricle and saccule the receptor organ is the macula.

The overall functions of the vestibular system of the inner ear are summarized as follows:

1. Maintenance of upright posture and equilibrium using the antigravity muscles of the trunk and body for control of postural reflexes.
2. During bodily movement to help the muscles of the eyes maintain visual fixation.
3. Mediation of the body righting reflexes using muscles of the head, neck, and shoulders. When the body is off balance in relation to gravity, the head is immediately righted followed by the neck, shoulders, and body.
4. To merge with receptors from the muscles, joints, and tendons to apprise the central nervous system of the body's orientation in space.
5. To contribute to the overall perception of bodily movement in a manner similar to the other kinesthetic receptors.

KINESTHETIC PERCEPTUAL PROCESSING

There does not seem to be a clear-cut body of literature concerning kinesthetic perceptual processes. Kinesthetics is the commonly accepted term used to describe the perceptual experiences which occur as a result of afferent input from the muscles, tendons, joints and vestibular system. However, exact descriptions of the perceptual events which comprise kinesthesis are either unclear or nonexistant. The reason for this state of affairs is probably due to the uniqueness of function and structure of the kinesthetic system. In vision and audition, the individual receptor organs are similar in structure, function, and location. Their source of stimulation comes from the external environment. In the study of these receptor systems, researchers have been able to manipulate the input of sensory information and observe the effects of this manipulation. On this basis, assumptions have been made about the perceptual events unique to these sensory systems. For the kinesthetic system experimental manipulation is not so easy. First of all, the receptor organs are uniquely different and located far away from each other. Each receptor organ is stimulated in a different manner. This stimulation comes from internal sources and there is such an interweaving of afferent and efferent messages that it is difficult to carry out research similar to that done with other sensory systems. And so, one of the basic problems is how to measure kinesthetic perceptions. The past literature includes studies which have measured thresholds of movement at the joints; accuracy of movement reproduction, discrimination of force and extent, after-effects of kinesthetic distortion, and various balance and body orientations in space. Useful information has come from these studies, but we are a long way from understanding kinesthetic perceptions in the same manner as visual and auditory perceptions.

Currently, investigators are attempting to bridge this gap of understanding kinesthetic perception by equating kinesthesis to other sensory systems. Marteniuk, Shields, and Campbell (1972) used a lever positioning task to determine kinesthetic sensitivity in a way that could be compared to that of other sensory systems. They found kinesthesis to be as sensitive as other sensory systems.

In the following sections, the theme of equating kinesthesis with other sensory systems is used. This is an exploratory and conceptual approach at best and is an attempt to consider aspects of kinesthesis in a manner similar to that of other sensory systems. On the surface, this approach sounds feasible, but its soundness is still to be tested. Hopefully, work such as the Marteniuk, Shields, and Campbell (1972) study will continue and the near future will yield information about questions yet unanswered. The following sections of this chapter relate to some of the phenomena involving kinesthetic sensory input and kinesthetic perceptual processing. Kinesthetic motor response will be discussed later in the chapter.

Kinesthetic Acuity

The acuity of the kinesthetic system refers to the ability of the kinesthetic receptors to transmit accurate and precise information about the body's position in space to the central nervous system. The central nervous system in turn processes this accurate information and issues the necessary commands which enable us to maintain our postural orientation and to perform the necessary and desired movements for successful interaction with our environment. As long as the receptor systems and the central nervous system are functioning normally, kinesthetic acuity should be excellent. Several investigators have been interested in determining how sensitive the joints of the body are to movement. One of the early studies by Goldschneider (1889) used passive movement in exploring the sensitivity of nine joints of the body. He found that discrimination of movement at joints was quite good with the shoulder joint being the most sensitive and the ankle joint the least sensitive. He also noted that the position of the joint did not have any relationship to its sensitivity. That is, no matter in what direction the joint was moved, sensitivity to movement was the same. Ladlow and Hamilton (1937) following the same line of investigation found that the hip joint was even more sensitive than the shoulder joint. Basically, both studies revealed that the human being is capable of detecting motion in the joints after as little as .2 of a degree of movement. For the more insensitive joints, movement up to 1.3 of a degree may be necessary before detection is made. The larger joints seem to be more sensitive than the smaller joints. In a later investigation of joint sensibility, evidence was obtained that indicated for the elbow joint that sensitivity was greatest during flexion as opposed to extension. (Cleghorn & Darcus, 1952).

Although the above data indicate that the individual is extremely sensitive to movements in the joints of the body, it must be remembered that these investigations used passive movement. Would joint sensitivity be the same for active movement? Not as much information is available for active movement, but in an investigation of active and passive movements of the lower leg Lloyd and Caldwell (1965) found greater accuracy positioning for active movement. This accuracy occurred in the middle ranges of movement similar to the range employed during the normal walking cycle.

The ability of the vestibular system to detect movement has been investigated by several researchers. The vestibular system is sensitive to two kinds of movement — rotary and linear. Baically the studies have reported sensitivity ranging from .12 degrees per second (Graybiel, Kerr, Bartley, 1948) to 2.0 degrees per second (Dodge, 1923).

For linear acceleration Armstrong (1943) reported a range of 4-12 centimeters per second for vertical movement. For horizontal acceleration a range of 2 to 20 centimeters per second was reported by Clark and Graybiel (1949).

As mentioned earlier, if the kinesthetic receptor system and the central nervous system are functioning normally, kinesthetic acuity should be excellent. However, there are occasions when due to damage, disease, or misalignment, kinesthetic acuity is impaired. For example, accidental damage to an arm or leg which causes amputation of that limb will eliminate all sensory information that would normally be processed by that extremity. In this case the amount of sensory information is reduced as compared to that of the intact body. Diseases which effect the functioning of the motor system, such as cerebral palsy, muscular dystrophy, multiple sclerosis and others, result in a pattern of sensori-motor input that is different from the healthy body. Misalignment of body segments through weak postural muscles and improper gait can also result in faulty and inaccurate kinesthetic information. Lesions or malfunctions in the cortical motor area, basal ganglia, cerebellum, and brain stem reduce the efficiency of the processing of kinesthetic information and resultant motor performance is impaired.

Kinesthetic Discrimination

In this section movement will be considered in terms of the individual's ability to discriminate differences. These differences may be in movement extent, velocity or force. Marteniuk, Shields, and Campbell (1972) studied the sensitivity of the kinesthetic system in an effort to compare it to other sensory systems. Using active movement, their subjects were asked to reproduce movement lengths of 45 degrees, 90 degrees, and 125 degrees by moving a lever which was mounted on ball bearings. One hundred trials were given for each movement length. These investigators determined that subjects were able to reproduce movement lengths with a high degree of precision demonstrating sensitivity similar to that of the visual and auditory system.

The ability to recognize various movement lengths was studied by Marteniuk (1971). His subjects learned four different lengths by moving a level until it hit a block. Subjects were permitted as much practice as they wished prior to the test session. When each subject felt that the four movements had been learned the test phase began. At this point the subject moved the lever until it was stopped by the block and then identified the movement length. In the next four experiments the subjects learned 6, 8, 10, and 16 different movements. Results indicated that the maximum number of correct responses was six, occurring when fifteen different movements were used. It was concluded that the kinesthetic sense was capable of fairly precise recognition of movement.

The accuracy and recognition of varying degrees of movement force was studied by Russell and Marteniuk (1974). The procedures were identical to the above study except the subjects learned different force levels. The maximum number of correct responses was 3½ force levels. It was demonstrated that the kinesthetic system could accurately identify differences in movement force.

Kinesthetic Figure-Ground

Basically, the figure-ground experience is one in which the individual "tunes in" one set of stimuli while ignoring another competing set of stimuli. In visual figure-ground, the observer sees the figure while ignoring all the lines and drawings of the background. The phenomena of visual figure-ground experience is well documented. But is there a figure-ground experience in the kinesthetic system and if so how does it operate?

The answers to these questions are exploratory at best, but the best available source of information appears that kinesthetic selective attention may be similar (Marteniuk, 1976). It is pointed out that the individual selects out of the environmen information that is relative to the task at hand. This information is then processed in lieu of other available information. The purpose for this selection process is due to the fact that the central nervous system has limited processing capacity and is incapable of dealing with all incoming information. So in order to perform the task successfully and efficiently, the performer must choose the most relevant information for processing. This selection of relevant stimuli is one of the factors which differentiates the performance of children and unskilled adults from those of the skilled performer. The unskilled individual is unable to sample from the many sources of available information and thus attends (pays attention) to either too much information or selects inappropriate information for the task at hand. Therefore, errors occur in his performance which are not observed in the performance of the skilled individual.

In considering the kinesthetic figure-ground question, our attention must shift from information coming from the external environment to information coming from the internal environment — specifically from the kinesthetic receptors. The question of interest is whether the individual can selectively attend to kinesthetic messages while ignoring others? The answer to this question would appear, on the surface at least, to be yes. Let us examine this position by first considering the organization of a kinetic melody (Sage, 1977; Luria, 1966). A kinetic melody refers to the sequential chain of movement segments which combine together to form a movement pattern or skill. These movement segments must occur in the right order and must flow one into another with precise timing. In order for this flow to be accomplished, the pattern of motor impulses must be varied first to one segment, then to the second segment, and so on until the movement sequence is completed. As these motor impulses command the movement of each segment, the kinesthetic receptors are concurrently sending feedback information into the central nervous system. The individual can then choose to attend to the entire flow of the movement pattern or isolate a segmental portion of the pattern and attend to is kinesthetic feedback only. For example, while performing the golf swing, the individual notices that the flow of the downswing is faulty. On the next swing he/she decides to monitor the movements of the hip while ignoring the feedback from all other portions of the swing. This monitoring is indeed possible for the individual to accomplish and provides a basis for possible error correction. Performers can selectively attend to individual movement segments, and based on the kinesthetic feedback vary the force, velocity, direction, or extent of movement. This ability would seem, then, to be similar to a figure-ground experience and would be more highly developed in individuals of greater skill. As mentioned earlier, the novice would be unable to select appropriate segments of the movement pattern initially and therefore would be unable to identify specific segments in need of monitoring for correction.

Kinesthetic Memory

Memory functions play a vital role in all learning experiences including those dealing with acquisition of motor skills. In an earlier chapter, discussion involved the role of short-term memory (STM) and long-term memory (LTM) in information processing. In this section we will be concerned with the function of short-term memory in the learning of physical skills. Basically, STM is information that is remembered for short periods of time — up to approximately 60 seconds without rehearsal. It has limited capacity in terms of amount of information remembered and looses information rapidly. In motor skills, STM functions in two ways. The first way involves remembering the feedback from a prior performance long enough to analyze it and to modify the next attempt. The second way occurs in a teacher-learning situation and involves the remembering of the teacher's instructions and/or demonstration long enough to perform the motor act.

What types of information concerning the movement pattern would be found in STM? Information concerning the direction and extent of the movement, its speed, the sequential timing of the movement segments, muscular effort, neural pattern of motor impulses, and actual location of body segments would be essential for efficient motor evaluation to occur (Marteniuk, 1976). This is quite an expansive list of information and how each of these elements function in movement reproduction is not clearly understood. Marteniuk and Roy (1972) studied the use of distance and location cues in movement reproduction. They found that subjects who used only distance cues could not reproduce movements as accurately as subjects using location cues. Laobs (1973) in a study of retention of distance and location cues used rest and counting backwards as two conditions during 12 second retention intervals. He found that with location cues there were no differences in subjects' reproduction accuracy between immediate reproduction and delayed reproduction with a rest interval. However, when the delayed reproduction subjects counted backwards during the retention interval they became less accurate than the immediate reproduction group. For distance cues, regardless of rest or counting in the interval, the delayed production subjects always performed more poorly than the immediate production subjects. It appears that locations cues are retained longer than distance cues.

The capacity of the STM can be increased. For non-motor (verbal, visual and auditory) information it would appear that the STM capacity is 7 items for letters and 5 items for words (Fitts and Posner, 1967). However, individuals tend to remember chunks of information rather than isolated details. This means that incoming information is grouped together in a meaningful way. Miller (1956) holds that most individuals can hold 7 + 2 chunks of information in STM. The amount of information held in a chunk can vary from small to large. The teacher can help the learner to create chunks of meaningful information, thereby, increasing STM capacity. Rehearsal of information in STM can also increase retention. When pertinent movement information is the center of the individuals attention and focus, its retention is strengthened. On the other hand, when impertinent movement information is the focus of attention prior to

movement the retention of the movement is less accurate (Stelmach, 1974).

Kinesthetic Localization (Body Awareness)

This section will deal with the body's ability to localize its position in space. To accomplish this effectively requires the intricate coordination of all the kinesthetic receptor systems as well as the cooperation of the other sensory systems. Another term more commonly used in the literature to refer to the body's ability to move efficiently in space is BODY AWARENESS. Body awareness as it will be used throughout this discussion refers to the multi-dimensional image which the individual possesses as a "physical entity" (Fisher and Cleveland 1958; Kugel 1969; Schilder 1950; Schontz 1969). More specifically, it refers to the awareness, identification and/or evaluation of the proportions, dimensions, positions and movements of the individual's body, and/or body parts.

The concept of body awareness seems to be an important one in perceptual-motor development primarily because recently many child development experts (Kephart 1964a, 1964b; Nash 1970) have suggested (often without any clearcut scientific support) that it is only as the child begins to define the dimensions of the body and body parts and to identify the various positions and/or movements which they may take in space, that he/she is able to differentiate easily and accurately among the corresponding sectors of the external space world. Since the body is, in fact, a three-dimensional object immersed in space, it is conceivable that the young child might rely heavily on bodily identifications and dimensions as reference points for initial judgments and/or perceptions about dimensions of external space.

Thus, in general it is hypothesized that the young child comes to know the body and ultimately external space world through appropriate changes in sensori-perceptual apparatus; changes which are the direct result of the motor experiences which the child has during the early development years. According to this point of view, difficulties associated with body awareness development (and thus with spatial awareness in general) would be mainly the result of some deficit or lack in appropriate sensori-motor experiences afforded the child during this time. (It should be pointed out that at present there is little if any empirical evidence to support or negate this line of reasoning.)

More specifically, body awareness is believed to be made up of four basic components: (1) body schema, (2) body image, (3) body insight, and (4) body concept. It is postulated that these components may align themselves hierarchically. Thus body image could not develop without information from body schema; body insight could not evolve without information from body image; and body concept could not develop without information from body insights. There is obviously much overlapping in the development of these components and the exact time of their evolution in a child's life is speculative. It is also important to note that once these four components develop in a child that they do not remain static but are constantly changing to reflect the child's environmental influences. Each of these four components are discussed below with emphasis on their definition and role in the development in the young child.

Body Schema. The first component of body awareness development can be referred to as the "sensori-motor" component largely because it is believed that, in the beginning, basic body awareness character-

istics of the child are derived from information provided to the child through sensori-motor mechanism, that is, from the sensori-perceptual feedback resulting from the activity of the body itself (Kugel 1969; Schontz 1969). For example, at birth, the infant seems to be essentially unaware of what is and what is not his/her body . . . of where the body ends and where the external space world begins. The infant uses then, so to speak, the afferent feedback from the bodily actions to establish a crude awareness of the dimensions and limitations of the physical being and thus begins to establish the separateness of body from that of external surroundings. This sensori-motor component, it is believed, is the nucleus around which all other elements of body awareness develop or resolve. Needless to say, this component of body awareness is always present and plays an important part in the development of body awareness characteristics throughout the life of the child but particularly so in the early years (0-5 years).

More specifically this component of body awareness if formed from motor activity that is primarily designed to maintain posture, position, attitude, and equilibrium as these elements come into play through static and dynamic movement (deQuiros and Schrager, 1978). At this level, posture is viewed as the reflex activity of the body characterized primarily by flexion and extension in relation to space. Position is defined as the species specific postures such as sitting, standing, etc. Attitude includes all of the reflex actions that return the body to characteristic human postures. Equilibrium (balance) comes into play as the human moves in relation to gravity and space and is responsible for the reciprocal innervation of the skeletal muscles as they are pulled upon by gravity. Equilibrium allows the body to adopt and control postures, positions, and attitudes. As the child is forming body schema through these elements, there is a constant modification coming from the interaction with the environment.

It would appear that body schema is the foundation or framework upon which the rest of the body awareness components are built. Specific contributors to body schema would be postural reflexes, righting reactions, protective reactions, developmental events of the first year of life, equilibrium reactions, and low-level balance activities.

Body Image. This component of body awareness is formed from the information we gather about ourselves. It is associated with the feelings and/or opinions which the child develops about the body — particularly with respect to its structural (appearance, height, weight, size, etc.) and functional (performance) characteristics. It is the direct result of our biological and environmental feedback systems which combine to form a pictorial representation of our body in the mind. In other words, how the body appears to oneself. The biological feedback system is one that is governed by the laws of growth and development. For example, the eight-month-old infant who is crawling will be forming quite a different pictorial representation than the child who has begun to walk. The child is also learning that the body has two sides — two arms, two legs. Both sides of the body can be asked to move simultaneously or one side can be called on to move alone. The environmental feedback system is one that provides a continuous flow of new experiences which constantly modify the body image. Also, within the environment the actions of others will contribute to the body image formulation. Thus there is a social component which contributes to the feelings and emotions about oneself.

Since very little scientific investigation has been devoted to this topic at all, one can at best only speculate about this so-called "feeling" component. Since the scene is ripe for speculation, let us speculate.

As body awareness develops in the young child, feelings and opinions about "self" as a physical reality grow based primarily on what the child knows of his/her own physical capacities and/or bodily characteristics. These opinions are the beginnings of the infinitely more complex self-perception process which ultimately forms the basic nucleus of personality development. This suggests of course that the young child needs to have as many positive (personally involving and rewarding) experiences in the "physical" realm as possible. In other words, the child needs to have the opportunity to learn about "self" as a physical being. To do so, a child must actively use the body and experience its many capabilities and assets, its limitations, and liabilities. Thus, the opinions that the young child develops about "self" as a physical being are inextricably interrelated with overall personality development and these opinions begin to develop and function early in the life of the child. It need not be stated of course that a great deal of very sophisticated research will be required before the relative amount of fact and fiction inherent in such a postulation is clearly established. Fundamentally, the body image should be considered as the sum total of all the influences mentioned above into a single mental picture of the physical body accompanied by a set of emotional feelings about its effectiveness in the environment.

An important contributing element to the development of body image is the child's emerging LATERALITY. This is seen in the appearance of a conscious internal awareness of the two sides of the body (Alexander and Money 1967; Kephart 1964b; Swanson 1955). The young child, largely through motor experiences, becomes increasingly more aware that the body has two distinct sides — a right and a left side. Again the child may not, at this stage of development, know the verbal labels of right and left but does know that he/she has two hands, two feet, two eyes — in effect two sides to the body — two sides which although similar in size and shape are distinctly different in that they occupy decidedly different positions in space.

It has been asserted by some that the development of the awareness of the spatial dimensions of the body is the foundation upon which the child begins to outline similar dimensions in external space (Douglass 1965; Kephart 1964b). Although such an assumption seems to be theoretically plausible, there has in fact been little if any direct experimental evaluation or observation of such a phenomenon in the growing, developing child.

In the establishment of laterality a SENSORY DOMINANCE becomes apparent. Sensory dominance refers to the preferential use of one of the eyes, hands, or feet over the other. The reason for the development of such preferential use of different body parts is not clearly understood, but it is a universally observed developmental process (Wilson and Reisen 1966). If the individual develops a preference for the use of the eye, hand and foot on the same side of the body, he/she is said to have pure dominance. If any one of the preferred body parts happens to be on the opposite side of the body, the child is said to have mixed dominance. Sensory dominance is usually assessed by observing the body part or parts used most consistently by the child in performing prescribed tasks. Flick (1967) and Belmont and Birch (1963)

provide some developmental guidelines for the ages at which sensory dominance seems to be established in young children (see Table 21.1. No data are presently available on children younger than four years of age.

With regard to HANDEDNESS, it would appear that as early as age four, the majority of children have established a definite hand preference (Belmont and Birch 1963; Flick 1967). (At this age, approximately 84 percent are right-handed; some 8 percent left-handed). Ambivalence in handedness seems to be more prevalent in children five through eight years of age than in younger children. There appears to be a return to a decided and stable hand preference in the majority of nine and ten-year-old children. In general, the data suggest that although hand preference may be established at an early age, one is likely to observe some unstable, ambivalent periods of preferential hand use during the course of its final development. In other words, hand preference may not become a fixed or permanent thing until the age of nine or ten.

Data provided by these same investigators (Belmont and Birch 1963; Flick 1967) clearly indicate that children do not exhibit, at any age, the same degree of lateralization in EYEDNESS as they do in either handedness or footedness. At any given age up to ten, as many as 20-25 percent of all children fail to show a clear-cut preferential use of one eye. Older children (9-11 years), however, do tend to show a much greater preference for the use of one eye over the other. Overall, the data again suggest that many children may never establish a definite eye preference and that those who eventually do are likely to go through a definite period of ambivalence with regard to preferential eye use. The period of ambivalence again seems to be focused on the five to nine age range.

TABLE 21.1
Percent Pure Versus Mixed Sensory Dominance by Age

	Dominance	Age			
		* 4 yrs	** 5-6 yrs	7-8 yrs	9-11 yrs
Handedness	Pure (right and left)	92%	81 %	81 %	94 %
	Mixed	8%	19 %	19 %	6 %
Eyedness	Pure	97%	73 %	68.7%	78.8%
	Mixed	3%	27 %	31.3%	21.2%
Footedness	Pure	No Data	94 %	94 %	98 %
	Mixed	No Data	6 %	6 %	2 %
Hand-eye Preference	Pure	No Data	37.5%	41.7%	63.5%
	Mixed	No Data	62.5%	49.3%	36.5%

* After Flick (1967); N = 453.
**After Belmont and Birch (1963); N = 148.

In contrast to both handedness and eyedness, FOOTEDNESS or preferential use of one foot over the other seems to be established early (by the age of five) and to remain quite stable thereafter. Very little if any tendency toward ambivalence in foot preference (according to these data) is observed at any age and its total absence from the five to nine age range, where ambivalence of eye and hand preference seems to be the general rule, is particularly striking. Much more data however need to be accumulated on these different facets of sensory dominance before any definite statements can be made.

Preferential use of a given eye with a given hand shows a definite age trend. Five and six-year-olds tend to exhibit a definite mixed EYE-HAND PREFERENCE (the preferred eye is on the side opposite the preferred hand); seven and eight-year-olds are evenly divided in this respect with approximately half of the children exhibiting mixed eye-hand preferences and the other half pure eye-hand combinations; nine-, ten-, and eleven-year-olds however, show a definite tendency toward pure eye-hand combinations (preferred eye and hand are on the same side of the body). This suggests that there is a trend toward the condition of pure-hand dominance in the majority of individuals with age but that the fixing of such sensory dominance characteristics in the individual does not occur until nine or ten years of age. This clearly suggests that important changes in eye and/or hand preferences may occur during the five to nine age range.

The basis or significance of sensory dominance in the individual is not clearly understood but several attempts have been made to link the appearance of such characteristics in the individual to the development of CEREBRAL DOMINANCE (Bauer and Wepman 1955; McFie 1961; Penfield and Roberts 1959; Zangwill 1960). Cerebral dominance refers to the fact that, physiologically, the interpretive functions of the cerebral cortex are usually highly developed in one cerebral hemisphere only. This hemisphere then is known as the "dominant" hemisphere. Although at birth the two hemispheres of the brain apparently have nearly equal potential for becoming the "dominant" hemisphere, it has been observed that in nine out of ten human beings, the left cerebral hemisphere becomes the dominant hemisphere (Wilson and Reisen 1966). In the remainder of the population, either dual dominance (both cerebral hemispheres develop equally) or right hemispheric dominance occurs. Right hemispheric dominance, however, is even more rare than dual dominance. It has been asserted that cerebral dominance is reflected in the individual in the appearance of sensory dominance (handedness, eyedness, footedness). Complete or pure dominance in the form of a right-eyed, right-handed, right footed individual would be the preferred state because it reflects total or complete left hemispheric dominance. Mixed dominance, on the other hand, would be less desirable because it indicates incomplete or inadequate cortical development. Mixed dominance has thus been linked (even causally) with a wide variety of perceptual, cognitive and motor dysfunctions observed in the growing, developing child. It should be made clear, however, that to date, there is little or no empirical evidence to support the notion that cerebral dominance is revealed in the hand, eye or foot preferences of the individual or that there is any direct relationship between mixed and/or pure domi-

nance and the perceptual, cognitive or motor capacities of the young child (Belmont and Birch 1965). The true significance and/or role of sensory dominance in the child's development has yet to be established.

As the infant begins to move around in the environment by crawling and walking, new movement experiences are available which contribute to body image development. These movement experiences can be generally classified as fundamental motor skills and include all the skills that are basic to the learning of more complicated sports, recreational, and dance skills.

Success/failure experiences play a critical role in forming the emotional aspect of body image. If the child obtains desired objects without undue frustration, a feeling of success is experienced. This applies to events such as climbing onto the chair, going down the steps, etc. The more quickly the child experiences mastery over the environment the more successful and the more positive will be the feelings about "self." Conversely, if the child is plagued with frustration and lack of successful mastery over the environment negative feelings about "self" based on this failure may develop.

The values of parents and their reinforcement system also play an important role in the development of body image. A child quickly learns what activities produce parental attention and approval. Some parents discourage movement and active exploration of the environment. They may be fearful that the child will get hurt or they may simply not want their house messed up. Children who are raised in a home that restricts movement may develop body awareness problems. The values of the parents quite likely affect the child's body image development.

Body Insight Body Insight is actually the precursor to body concept except that body concept is believed to involve verbalization whereas body insight does not. Insight involves the knowledge (concept) of one's own body and the relationship of its parts to each other. It also includes the understanding of how the body and its parts move in space. Essentially body insight is a continuation of the already on-going body schema and body image. As the child proceeds in the developmental schedule, he/she gradually becomes more aware of movement in space. This awareness is centered around the spatial needs of the child's own body and its segments.

Recognition and identification are processes that typify body insight activities. However, verbalization of these events is generally reserved for the body concept component of body awareness. A commonly used assessment strategy is the identification of body parts and the performance of children on this task varies widely.

The process of accurately naming and/or identifying the various parts of the body and their functions progresses at different rates in different children. The rate of development of such capacities seems to be most affected by the relative amount of emphasis placed upon the development of such concepts by persons with whom the child comes in contact during these early developmental years (Williams 1965). Data collected on a group of Midwest children suggest that the majority (69 percent) of children by five or six years of age can accurately identify the major body parts (eyes, ears, hands, knees, etc.) and fail only slightly more often in naming more remote body parts (elbows, wrists, heels, etc.). After the age of eight or nine, mistakes in correct identification of body parts are rare (Williams 1970). See Table 21.2.

The understanding of body space concepts has been continuously developing since the child's early months. The child is able to recognize and understand various

TABLE 21.2
Body Part Identification, Right-left Awareness, and Directionality
as a Function of Age

Age	Body Part Identification*	Right-left Discrimination**		Directionality**
		Eyes Open	Eyes Closed	
5 yrs	55%	——	——	——
6 yrs	69%	71.5%	64.2%	52%
7 yrs	88%	86.8%	88.7%	56%
8 yrs	95%	89.7%	92.5%	69%
9 yrs	94%	93.6%	95.3%	80.8%
10-12 yrs	100%	——	——	——

* After Williams (1970); N = 240.
**After Swanson and Benton (1955); N = 158.

body space concepts quite awhile before being able to verbalize them.

At 18 months of age the child can understand and say "up" and "down." At 21 months, "on-off" concepts are spoken followed by "in-out," "turn around," and other side concepts at 2 years. By age three, "over-under," "front-back," "big, high, long and tall" are added to the child's expressive vocabulary. After age four, the space words are used more exactly and in combination. The following years are characterized by use of space concepts in the child's expanding environment and continual expansion and deepening of meanings (Gesell and Ilg. 1946).

Body Concept. This component of body awareness refers to the verbalized knowledge one has about one's own body and its relationship to near and far space. With the onset of the development of speech, the child enters the world of conceptualization. Because the child can now verbalize (with varying degrees of effectiveness), he/she is capable of building a conceptual framework with regard to the spatial makeup of the body. Now, not only is the child aware of different spatial features of the body from a sensori-motor point of view, but is also able to verbalize or conceptualize about them. The mechanism of verbalization appears to be an important part of the process of abstracting or internalizing the phenomena of body awareness and may play a particularly important role during the early years of development (Kugel 1969; Piaget 1952).

The conceptual component of the development of body awareness is characterized in large part by the acquisition of the following capacities: (1) rapid and precise verbal identification of body parts and their functions (2) spontaneous right-left discrimination of body dimensions; and (3) easy discrimination of the dimensions of external space (directionality). Since, for all intents and purposes, body part identification was discussed in the previous body insight section the discussion in this section will only consider right-left discrimination and directionality

RIGHT-LEFT DISCRIMINATION is defined as the ability to spontaneously label or identify the right-left dimensions of the body (Ayres 1969). Assessment of the level of development of the right-left discrimination capacities of the child is usually determined by observing the child's behavior in responding to such statements as "Show me your right hand" or "Touch your left ear". The spontaneity and accuracy of the child's responses are taken as an indication of the degree of development of his right-left discrimination capacities. The age trends for the development of right-left discrimination capacities as reported by Swanson and Benton (1955) are shown in Table 21.2.

By five and one-half to six years of age, the majority of children (71.5 percent) are able to spontaneously distinguish between the right and left sides of the body. On the other hand, a large number of children at this age still show considerable confusion in identifying with any consistency the right-left parts of the body. Not until approximately eight to nine years of age does this conceptualization process seem to be completely stabilized in the majority of children (90-94 percent). It is also of interest that at every age except five years the child is consistently more accurate in identifying the right-left dimensions of the body if allowed to respond with the eyes closed.

Ayres (1969) reports that below the age of five most children perform at no better than chance level in the identification of right-left body parts. In other words, children younger than five, when asked right-left discrimination questions, simply guess at what is right or left but seem to have no well-established stable concept of such bodily dimensions.

DIRECTIONALITY, or the ability to identify various dimensions of external space, is speculated to be an outgrowth or extension of the development of the conceptualization of the spatial dimensions of the body. For example, right and left in external space exist only as they relate to the individual's own body and thus vary according to the position of the body at any given moment in time or space. Up-down and front-back dimensions of external space also exist (at least in the beginning) largely in reference to the body and its position in space. In the beginning, the child seems to rely upon the stable spatial referents established for his/her own body in helping to identify and understand the dimensions of the external space world. The process of the conceptualization of external space reaches its zenith then when the child develops a stable and independent conceptual framework of the external spatial environment. That is, the conceptualization of external space is complete when the child can spontaneously identify positions, dimensions and directions of objects or persons in external space without having first to consciously and deliberately refer to his/her own body.

The implication is that if the conceptualization of the body's spatial dimensions is inadequate, the child will find it difficult if not impossible to develop an adequate conceptualzation of external space. Thus a child who has difficulty in discriminating among various spatial patterns and/or positions of letters (b's=d's; p's=q's, etc.)

it exists largely because of a lack of an adequate conceptual framework of the dimensions of his/her own body (Albitreccia 1959; Kephart 1964a, 1964b). As simple and straight forward as the foregoing may seem, it should be made clear that there is little if any empirical evidence to either support or negate this point of view.

Evidence reported by Swanson and Benton (1955) gives some empirical support to the notion that the conceptualization of external space (directionality) does lag slightly behind the conceptualization of the spatial dimensions of the body (see table 21.2). These data, however, deal only with the conceptualization of right-left spatial dimensions and provide no information about any cause-effect relationships. Still it is clear from such data that at any given age, the number of children who can spontaneously identify the right-left dimensions of external space is considerably less than the number who can accurately identify the right-left dimensions of their bodies. Furthermore, it would appear that although 87 percent of all children can identify accurately the right-left dimensions of the body by the age of seven, similar ease in identifying the corresponding right-left dimensions in external space (on another object or person) does not occur until much later (approximately age nine).

KINESTHETIC-MOTOR RESPONSE

After kinesthetic information has been received and processed what types of kinesthetic motor responses can be now expected to occur? It would be nice if the answer to this question could be presented here in A, B, C terms, However, the issue is not that simple. *All* movement is actually a kinesthetic-motor response but the confounding lies in that a purposeful movement is usually based on synthesized information from all the sensory systems. As mentioned earlier, the input to response model so easily applied to the visual and auditory systems does not apply as readily to the kinesthetic system. However, there are classes of movement behaviors that most children do exhibit and these will be presented here. It is quite clear that a reciprocal relationship must exist between these movement behaviors and kinesthetic perceptual events. One could not exist without the other. Also, gradual and ever improving kinesthetic perceptions must be based on the feedback obtained from these movement behaviors.

Basically, the simplest way to address the classes of movement behaviors just mentioned is through the discussion of the developmental progression of movement from birth to maturity. In Chapter 4, Table 4.1, the movement responses of the newborn infant are given. This table shows quite clearly the amount and type of movement patterns present at birth. In Hottinger's discussion it was pointed out that early movement is reflexive in nature. In other words, not under voluntary control. As the infant matures these reflex movement patterns are gradually brought under voluntary motor control — usually by 6 to 9 months of age. Basic reflexive patterns are sometimes referred to as the building blocks of voluntary, complex movement. The continuation of the development of motor abilities is shown in Table 4.3. It can be observed that sitting alone occurs around 6 months of age whereas walking occurs around 13 months. Once the child is able to get around in the environment the child becomes obsessed with the movement of his/her own body and

is in perpetual motion all day long, except for the nap periods. The following months are characterized by movement exploration of the environment. As growth proceeds a new class of motor behaviors begin to evolve. First effective movements of the body parts are learned then fundamental gross motor skills. These motor characteristics of perceptual-motor development are important because they represent the most direct manifestation of the changes in sensori-perceptual processes taking place in the child. The period of most rapid development of motor behaviors during early perceptual-motor development is the period from the third to the sixth year, the preschool years (Williams 1965). During this span of time most of the basic locomotor, ball-handling and fine eye-hand coordination skills appear and undergo rapid development. Thus the major emphasis here will be on descriptions of motor behaviors most characteristic of perceptual-motor development during the preschool years. Descriptions of the gross motor behavior patterns of the preschool child are shown in Table 21.3.

Although the foundation for the development of gross motor behavior patterns is in fact being laid down from birth onward, the appearance of most such patterns, in any kind of finished form, does not occur until sometime during the second or third year. The span of years from three to six then seems to be a period of accelerated growth in terms of the acquisition of gross motor skills. What occurs during this period of development of course is directly related to the nature and extent of the advances made in development during the earlier years of life.

In general, the three-to-four-year-old child does not display the "whole body responses" so typical of the motor acts of the younger

TABLE 21.3
DEVELOPMENT OF LOCOMOTOR SKILLS
Ages 2 to 5 Years

LOCOMOTOR SKILL	Two-year-old	Three-year-old	Four-year-old	Five-year-old
RUNNING	Run characterized by overall stiffness (waddle). Frequent falling down and tripping. Minimal overall control of run pattern.	Run with lack of control in stops and starts. Overall pattern more fluid than 2-year-old. Run with flat foot action. Inability to turn quickly.	Run with control over starts, stops, and turns. Speed is increasing. Longer stride than 3-year-old. Non-support period lengthening. Can run 35 yards in 20-29 seconds.	Run well established and used in play activities. Control of run in distance, speed, and direction improving. Speed is increasing. Stride width increasing. Non-support period lengthening.
GALLOPING	Unable to gallop	Most children cannot gallop. Early attempts are some variation of the run pattern.	43% of children are attempting to learn to gallop. During this year most children learn to gallop. Early gallop pattern somewhat of a run and leap step.	78% can gallop. Can gallop with a right lead foot. Can gallop with a left lead foot. Can start and stop at will.
HOPPING	Unable to hop	Can hop 10 times consecutively on both feet. Can hop 1-3 times on one foot. Great difficulty experienced with hop pattern. Attempts characterized by gross overall movements and a lot of arm movement.	33% are proficient at hopping. Can hop 7-9 hops on one foot. Hop pattern somewhat stiff and not fluid.	79% become proficient during this year. Can hop 10 or more hops on one foot. Hop characterized by more spring-like action in ankles, knees, and hips. Can hop equally well on either leg.

TABLE 21.3 (continued)

LOCOMOTOR SKILL	Two-year-old	Three-year-old	Four-year-old	Five-year-old
CLIMBING	Climbing action mostly confined to climbing onto and off of low chairs, stools, bed, etc. Stair climbing is difficult and a mark time foot pattern is used.	Ascends stairs using mark time foot pattern. During this year, ascending stairs is achieved with alternate foot pattern. Descending stairs mostly with mark time foot pattern. Climbing onto and off of low items continues to improve with higher heights being conquered.	Ascends stairs using alternate foot pattern. Descends stairs with alternate foot pattern. Can climb a large ladder with alternate foot pattern. Can descend large ladder slowly with alternate foot pattern.	Climbing skill increasing. 70% can climb a rope ladder with bottom free. 37% can climb a pole. 32% can climb a rope with bottom free. 14% can climb an overhead ladder with 15 degree incline. Climbing included more challenging objects such as trees, jungle gyms, large beams, etc.
BALANCE	Walks balance beam in a sideways manner.	Balance beam walking pattern characterized by mark time sequences. Can traverse 25 ft. walking path that is one inch wide in 31.5 seconds with 18 step-offs. Can walk 3″ wide beam forward 7.4′, backward; 3.9′. 44% can touch knee down and regain standing position on 3″ wide beam.	Balance beam walking pattern characterized by alternate shuffle step. Can traverse 25 ft. walking path that is one inch wide in 27.7 seconds with 6 stepoffs. Can walk 3″ wide beam forward 8.8′, backward 5.8′. 68% can touch knee down and regain standing position on 3′ wide beam.	Balance beam walking characterized by alternate step pattern. Can traverse 25 ft. walking path that is one inch wide in 24.1 seconds with three stepoffs. Can walk 3″ wide beam forward 11′, backward 8.1′. 84% can touch knee down and regain standing position on 3′ wide beam.

TABLE 21.3 (continued)

LOCOMOTOR SKILL	Two-year-old	Three-year-old	Four-year-old	Five-year-old
SKIPPING	Unable to skip	Skip is character-ized by a shuffle step. Can skip on one foot and walk on the other. Actual true skip pattern seldom performed.	14% can skip. One footed skip still prevalent. Overall movement stiff and undiffer-entiated. Excessive arm action frequently occurring. Skip mostly flat-footed.	72% are proficient. Can skip with alter-nate foot pattern. Overall movements more smooth and fluid. More efficient use of arms. Skip mostly on balls of feet.
JUMPING	Early jumping characterized by stepping down action rather than actual jump. During this year most learn two foot jump downward.	42% are proficient. Jumping pattern lacks differentiation. Lands without knee bend to absorb force. Minimal crouch for take-off. Arms used ineffec-tively. Can jump down from 28″ height. Can hurdle jump 3 1/2″ (68%)	72% are proficient. Jumping pattern characterized by more preliminary crouch. Can do standing broad jump 8-10″. Can do running broad jump 23-33″. 90% can hurdle jump 5″. 51% can hurdle jump 9 1/2″.	81% are skillful. Overall jumping pattern more smooth and rhyth-mical. Use of arm thrust at take-off evident. More proficient landing. Can do standing broad jump 15-18″. Can do running broad jump 28-35″, vertical. Can jump and reach 2 1/2″. 90% can hurdle jump 8″. 68% can hurdle jump 21 1/2″.

child. For example, the hands, even though used awkwardly at times, can be employed adeptly and independently of other bodily movements in the performance of rather demanding visual-motor tasks. The three-to-four-year-old can place the blocks in a "tower" in the proper position with a relatively sure and steady hand; the two year old has considerably more difficulty in separating these movements from more global body responses.

The walking and running patterns of the three-year-old are quite advanced. The child walks and runs with ease and seems to have difficulty in executing these locomotor patterns only when sudden turns or quick stops are necessary. Jumping and crawling patterns are also improving and the next few years will be spent largely in refining and expanding the use of these basic locomotor skills. The three-to-four-year-old has not yet begun to master the skills of hopping, galloping or skipping (although attempts to perform are made). Ball handling skills too are just beginning to show signs of improvement. Still the three-year-old loves to play with balls and spends a great deal of time attempting to execute the crude throwing and catching patterns now possessed.

The three-to-four-year-old does seem to undergo a period of transition during which certain motor inadequacies and uncoordinations arise. Both gross and fine musculature, including the oculomotor muscles of the eyes, are involved in this developmental transition and thus the total action or motor system of the child is affected. As a result, the three-year-old often stumbles and appears awkward and uncoordinated. Overall however, the three-year-old is far advanced over the two-year-old even though he/she has yet to acquire the increased motor proficiency of the four-to-five-year-old.

Although the gross motor patterns of the four-to-five-year-old are still loosely organized, the child of this age is far better coordinated than the three-year-old. He/she runs, walks, jumps and climbs with proficiency. In addition he/she has nearly mastered the skill of hopping but has not yet put together effective skipping or galloping patterns, although these are in the making and in a few short months the child will skip and gallop in a very advanced form. Skill in catching and throwing are on the increase and as many as 20 percent to 30 percent to four-to-five-year-olds exhibit advanced throwing and catching patterns.

The four-to-five-year-old also seems to possess a high energy drive — a drive which almost always manifests itself in rather extended bursts of motor activity. These bursts of activity may have real significance for perceptual-motor development for it seems that it is during these frequent and prolonged periods of activity that the child works on the refinement of old motor patterns and adds new ones to the already rapidly expanding repertoire of motor behaviors.

The year from five-to-six seems to be a period which marks both the beginning and the end of a major growth epoch. Within limitations, this age child is something of a finished product. In general, the five-year-old is much more stable than the four-year-old, and ease and economy of movement are present in almost all ball-handling and locomotor skill patterns. The five-to-six-year-old has acquired a more refined manner of running, jumping, hopping and climbing. This age child exhibits considerable proficiency in galloping and the skipping pattern is well on its way to being mastered. Ball-handling skills are far advanced over the four-to-five-year-old.

Some 74 percent of five-to-six-year-olds have good throwing patterns and 56 percent have already developed "good" catching skills. Still further increases in proficiency in throwing and catching will take place during the sixth and seventh years. In general, although many refinements in gross motor behaviors are likely to occur in the years which follow, by the end of the fifth year, the child can perform most simple gross motor patterns.

The rapid improvement seen in gross motor skill performances during the preschool years (improvement which is ultimately seen in the proficiency displayed by the six-year-old in executing such motor patterns) is a clear behavioral indication of the important (but unseen) changes that have been taking place in the sensori-perceptual makeup of the child during these years of growth.

References

Albitreccia, S. I. "Treatment of Disorders of Body Image." *Spastics Quarterly* 8(1959): 30.

Alexander, Duane and Money, John. "Reading Disability and the Problem of Direction Sense." *The Reading Teacher* 20(1967):404.

Anderson, S. and Gernandt, B. E. "Cortical Projections of Vestibular Nerve in Cat." *Acta Oto-laryngol., Stockholm, Suppl.* 116(1954): 10-18.

Armstrong, H. G. *Principles and Practices of Aviation Medicine,* 2nd ed. Baltimore: Williams and Wilkins, 1943.

Ayers, Jean. *Southern California Perceptual-Motor Tests.* Los Angeles: Western Psychological Corporation, 1969.

Bauer, Robert W. and Wepman, Joseph M. "Lateralization of Cerebral Functions." *Journal of Speech and Hearing Disorders* 20 (1955):171.

Belmont, Lillian and Birch, H. G. "Lateral Dominance and Right-Left Awareness in Normal Children." *Child Development* 34 (1963):257.

Boring, E. G. *Sensation and Perception in the History of Experimental Psychology.* New York: Appleton-Century-Crofts, 1942.

Clark, B. and Graybiel, A. "Linear Acceleration and Deceleration as Factors Influencing Non-Visual Orientation During Flight." *Journal of Aviation Medicine* 20(1949):92-101.

Cleghorn, T. E. and Darcus, H. D. "The Sensibility to Passive Movement of the Human Elbow Joint." *Quarterly Journal of Experimental Psychology* 4(1952):66-77.

deQuiros, J. B. and Schrager, O. L. *Neuropsychological Fundamentals in Learning Disabilities.* Academic Therapy Publications, 1978.

Dickinson, J. *Proprioceptive Control of Human Movement.* Princeton Book Company, 1974.

Dodge, R. "Thresholds of Rotation." *Journal of Experimental Psychology* 6(1923):107-37.

Douglass, Malcolm P. "Laterality and Knowledge of Directions." *Elementary School Journal* 66(1965):69.

Eccles, J. C. *The Understanding of the Brain.* New York: McGraw-Hill, 1973.

Fisher, S. and Cleveland, S. *Body Image and Personality.* New York: Van Nostrand, 1958.

Fitts, P. M. and Posner, M. I. *Human Performance.* Belmont, Calif.: Brooks/Cole, 1967.

Flick, Grad L. "Sinistrality Revisited: A Perceptual-Motor Approach." *Child Development* 38(1967):415.

Geldard, F. A. *The Human Senses.* New York: John Wiley and Sons, Inc., 1972.

Gesell, A. and Ilg, F. L. *The Child from Five to Ten.* New York: Harper and Row, 1946.

Gesell, Arnold; Ilg, Frances L.; and Bullis, Glenna E. *Vision: Its Development in Infant and Child.* New York: Paul B. Heober, Inc., 1949.

Goldschneider, A. 1889. "Untersuchungen uber den Muskelsinn." Cited in *Sensation and Perception in the History of Experimental Psychology, by E. G. Boring.* New York: Appleton-Century-Crofts, 1942.

Graybiel, A.; Kerr, W. A.; and Bartley, S. H. "Stimulus Thresholds of Semicircular Canals as a Function of Angular Acceleration." *American Journal of Psychology* 61(1948): 21-36.

Kephart, N. C. "Perceptual-Motor Aspects of Learning Disabilities." *Exceptional Children* 31(1964a):201.

———. *The Slow Learner in the Classroom.* Columbus, Ohio: Chas. E. Merrill, 1964b.

Kugal, J. *Lichaamsplan, Lichaamsbesef, Lichaamsidee (Body Plan, Body Knowledge, Body Idea).* Waltersnoordhoff nv., Gronengen, 1969.

Laidlaw, R. W. and Hamilton, M. A. "A Study of Thresholds in Apperception of Passive Movement among Normal Control Subjects." *Bulletin Neurological Institute.* New York 6(1937):268-73.

Laabs, G. J. "Retention Characteristics of Different Reproduction Cues in Motor Short-Term Memory." *Journal of Experimental Psychology* 100(1973):168-77.

Lloyd, A. J. and Caldwell, L. S. "Accuracy of Active and Passive Positioning of the Leg on the Basis of Kinesthetic Cues." *Journal of Comparative and Physiological Psychology* 60(1965):102-6.

Luria, A. R. "Functional Organization of the Brain." *Scientific American* 222(March 1970):66-78.

Marteniuk, R. G., Shields, H.; and Campbell, S. "Amplitude, Position, Timing, and Velocity as Cues in Reproduction of Movement." *Perceptual and Motor Skills* 35(1972):51-58.

Marteniuk, R. G. "An Informational Analysis of Active Kinesthesis as Measured by Amplitude of Movement." *Journal of Motor Behavior* 3(1971):1.

Marteniuk, R. G. *Information Processing Motor Skills.* New York: Holt, Rinehart, and Winston, 1976.

Marteniuk, R. G. and Roy, E. A. "The Codability of Kinesthetic Location and Distance Information." *Acta Psychologica* 36(1976)471-79.

McFie, J. "The Effect of Hemispherectomy on Intellectual Function in Cases of Infantile Hemiplegia." *Journal of Neurology and Neuro-surgical Psychiatry* 24(1961):361.

Miller, G. A. "The Magical Number Seven Plus or Minus Two: Some Limits on our Capacity for Processing Information." *Psychological Review* 63(1956):81-97.

Nash, John. *Developmental Psychology: A Psychobiological Approach.* Englewood Cliffs, N. J.: Prentice-Hall, Inc., 1970.

Penfield, W. and Roberts, L. *Speech and Brain Mechanisms.* Princeton, N. J.: Princeton University Press, 1952.

Piaget, Jean. *The Origin of Intelligence in Children.* New York: International Universities Press, 1952.

Russell, D. G. and Marteniuk, R. G. "An Information Analysis of Absolute Judgments of Torque." *Perception and Psychophysics* 16 (1974):443-48.

Sage, G. H. *Introduction to Motor Behavior; A Neuropsyc Approach.* Reading, Mass.: Addison Wesley Publications, 1977.

Schilder, Paul. *The Image and Appearance of the Human Body.* New York: International Universities Press, 1950.

Schontz, F. C. *Perceptual and Cognitive Aspects of Body Experience.* New York: Academic Press, 1969.

Stelmach, G. E. "Retention of Motor Skills." In *Exercise and Sport Sciences Review,* edited by J. D. Wilmore. New York: Academic Press, 1974.

Swanson, Robert and Benton, A. L. "Some Aspects of the Genetic Development of Right-Left Discrimination." *Child Development* 26(2) (1955):123.

Williams, Harriet G. "Visuo-Perceptual and Motor Development in the Pre-School Child." Unpublished Seminar Paper, University of Wisconsin, Madison, Spring 1965.

———. "Visual-Perception: A Review." Unpublished Paper, University of Toledo, 1970.

Wilson, Paul D. and Reisen, A. H. "Visual Development in Rhesus Monkeys Neonatally Deprived of Patterned Light." *Journal of Comparative Physiological Psychology* 61 (1966):87.

Zangwill, O. L. *Cerebral Dominance and Its Relation to Psychological Function.* Edinburgh: W. R. Henderson Trust (Oliver and Boyd), 1960.

Section 8

Factors Influencing Motor Development

Factors Influencing Motor Development: Introductory Comments

22

Robert M. Malina
University of Texas

The development and refinement of skillful performance in motor activities is one of the major developmental tasks of childhood. All children, barring significant developmental retardation, have the potential to develop and learn a variety of fundamental and special motor activities. Such motor acts comprise an integral part of the developing child's behavioral repertoire. Further, it is through the medium of movement activities that many of the child's experiences with his/her environments, especially early experiences during the first decade of life, are largely mediated.

This section is organized into four chapters. The first is introductory in nature. The second chapter in the section deals with biologically related factors which influence motor development and performance. The third and fourth chapters deal with environmentally related factors. The focus of the third is on general environmental factors while the fourth focuses on social-psychological factors, or one specific type of environmental factors, which influence motor development and performance. A separate chapter on factors influencing motor development in adolescence is included in Section 10. Adolescence is treated as a separate unit since the timing of the adolescent growth spurt and its physiological and behavioral concomitants are quite variable. Nevertheless, many of the correlates of motor performance operating during childhood also operate in adolescence.

Many factors influence the motor development and activity of children during infancy and childhood. This discussion considers a number of factors which have been related to motor development and performance during this period. These factors can be viewed as correlates of motor development and performance in the sense that they might be related to and/or might condition or modify the expression of the underlying neuromotor processes. To what extent, for example, is the emergence, integration and refinement of motor responses genetically based? To what extent is the progress from immobility to a mature pattern of movement mediated by maturational processes? Or, to what extent is the development of motor responses influenced by the cultural and subcultural patterns in which the child is reared? The foregoing are general questions that must be considered in the assessment of motor development during infancy and childhood.

Though the factors which influence motor development are many and are interrelated, for the purposes of this discussion they will be divided into two categories: Biologically related factors, and environmentally related factors. Because they are so important to motor development, social-psychological factors, a subcategory of environmentally related factors, will be given a special attention.

BIOLOGICALLY RELATED FACTORS

There are many biological factors which influence motor development and motor performance. Some of these were discussed in Chapter 2. In this section such factors as general genetic endowment, body size including body size at birth, physique, and rate of maturation will be discussed.

ENVIRONMENTALLY RELATED FACTORS

Among the environmental factors discussed in this section are rearing and sex differences, birth order, ethnic considerations, and cross cultural considerations. In addition social-psychological considerations such as socialization, social reinforcement, social facilitation, and personality are discussed. All of these factors are important in the total motor development process.

BIOLOGICAL-ENVIRONMENTAL INTERACTION

In this section many different biological and environmental factors which influence motor development are discussed. As discussed in Chapter 1 these factors cannot be considered individually but must be dealt with together as we study the total person. Motor development is a gradual process of continuing modification of movement patterns based upon the individual's genetic potential, the residual effects of prior experiences, and the new movement experience per se. The developing infant and young child must also adapt to the demands and stresses imposed by his/her environments, and in turn, these environments will have an impact on the child's progress in the motor sphere. Hence, motor development is a product of an organism-environment interaction and perhaps covariation. The kinds of interactions can vary in different cultures, e.g., kinds of stimulation and expected responses. It is hoped that after reading this section, the vast array of actual and potential organism-environment interactions and covariations, and the effects of these on motor development will become apparent.

Biologically Related Correlates to Motor Development and Performance during Infancy and Childhood

23

Robert M. Malina
University of Texas

Although this chapter will consider several biologically related correlates of motor development and performance, studies of the developmental sequences and stages should not be overlooked. The fundamental motor skills of infancy and childhood develop sequentially, and the sequence is generally uniform while the rate of development varies. There are, however, possible exceptions to the sequence of early motor development which deserve consideration, as do factors related to variation in rate. Variation in the sequence of motor development might be related to a number of factors in the environments of the developing child, such as different rearing conditions, opportunity for practice, availability of toys and equipment, extent of infantile stimulation, and so on. A commonly cited example of a sequential exception in early motor development is that noted by Mead and Macgregor (1951, p. 181) in a small sample of Balinese children:

Where the American children go from frogging to creeping on all fours, then to standing and walking, with squatting coming after standing, the Balinese children, who do much less creeping . . . combine frogging, creeping, and all-fours behavior simultaneously in a flexible, interchangeable state, from which they go from sitting to squatting to standing.

Mead and Macgregor relate this sequential variation to the manner in which Balinese adults carry their children (passively, involving minimal interaction).

The motor programming of an Eskimo youth to hunt (Laughlin, 1968) also provides possibilities for sequential variation in motor development. The programming includes a series of general and specific activities beginning very early in childhood, at the age of walking. Activities include, for example, special tendon lengthening exercises and throwing exercises from a seated position designed for hunting from a kayak. The special exercises in turn are reinforced in turn by a series of games.

The range of normal variation in motor development during infancy and early childhood, though rather substantial, is perhaps extended by various cultural practices, demands, and sanctions. There is thus a need for further descriptive developmental data which incorporates significant correlates as critical variables.

The descriptions of ages and stages of motor development might also be considered in terms of the timing of entry into a specific stage of motor behavior, the rate of attaining the stage, and the duration of the stage of motor behavior. For example, are certain stages in a developmental sequence passed through more rapidly than others? How long might a stage last? Can the length of a particular stage be modified by environmental circumstances? If so, when and to what extent? What might be the ideal age to introduce attempts to enhance motor competence? What stages are more discriminating in terms of predicting subsequent motor behavior? Note, however, that motor development, like development in general, is a continuous process, upon which researchers superimpose stages or levels, which themselves may vary between investigators.

GENETIC

Twin studies have been used to estimate genetic influences on motor development and performance. Studies of twins during infancy indicate greater similarly among monozygotic (identical) than among dizygotic (fraternal) twin pairs, i.e., greater within pair differences for fraternal twins (Bouchard, 1978). Two early studies of sitting-up and walking in infant twins (Sklad, 1972) indicate greater concordance (similarity) among monozygotic twins (67% and 69%) than dizygotic twins (35% and 30%) for first efforts at walking. The timing of sitting-up behavior, however, was almost equally concordant among both identical and fraternal twins (82% and 76% respectively). Although twin data on other aspects and subsequent motor development during infancy and early childhood are not extensive, they do indicate a close correspondence in the development of motor activities among monozygotic twins early in life (see Gesell, 1954). Monozygotic and dizygotic twins,

however, do not differ significantly in levels of motor attainment from each other, nor do first-born and second-born twins differ from each other in early motor development. Twins, however, do show a consistent developmental lag in motor development compared to singletons from three months to three years of age (Dales, 1969; Witherspoon, 1965).

In an early study of motor performance in children five through nine years of age, Vickers, Poyntz and Baum (1942) noted a greater degree of similarity of gross motor performance on a modification of the Brace scale* in siblings and twins than in unrelated children. The data thus suggest a possible familial pattern for gross motor ability during middle childhood. Using gross motor skills in monozygotic and dizygotic twins 11 to 25 years of age, Kovar (1974) noted that speed (running) and explosive power (jumping, throwing) are more influenced by genetic factors than other motor tasks (e.g., errors in a coordination task, bent arm hang). Analyzing the running pattern of monozygotic and dizygotic twins 9 through 12 years of age, Sklad (1972) observed greater similarity in the kinetic structure of running performance in the monozygotic twins.

Studies utilizing such motor skills as pursuit rotor tracking, hand steadiness, card sorting, tapping speed, and two hand coordination tasks also indicated a high degree of heritability; i.e., there is closer agreement between the motor performance of identical twins as compared to fraternal twins (see Bouchard, 1978). However, results of twin studies are discordant and equivocal for nerve conduction velocity, reaction time,

*The Brace test of motor ability is a graded series of stunts on which the child must manage the movement of his/her body.

and reflex time. In a study by Komi, Klissouras and Kavvinen (1973), female dizygotic twins showed as much variability in the neuromuscular tasks as did monozygotic twins, leading the authors to conclude that such measures might be more susceptible to environmental influences in girls than in boys.

Observations derived from studies of motor development and performance of twins, though important, leave several unanswered questions. For example, are monozygotic twins more similar in motor tasks due to genetic similarity or due to environmental pressures for similarity? Or, how important is the role of mutual imitation in the motor development of twins? Similar questions can be extended to the genetic basis of the rate of learning motor skills. Sklad (1975) compared the learning curves and rate of improvement in monozygotic and dizygotic twins during the course of learning three motor tasks — ball throwing, tapping, and precision movements. Monozygotic twins were more similar in motor learning than the dizygotic twins. Further, performance levels and rate of learning appeared to be more influenced by genetic factors in boys than in girls. More recently, Marisi (1977) noted a high degree of genetic determination of initial levels of performance on a pursuit rotor apparatus. However, with practice, the strength of genetic determination diminished systematically.

The preceding indicates that genetic factors are important correlates of motor development and performance. This genetic basis can also be viewed as representing potential; whether the potential is attained or developed, is dependent upon the environments in which the child is reared. Genes need a substrate upon which to act, and the nature of the substrate can influence the course of development.

STATUS AT BIRTH

Since birth marks the transition from a uterine to an extrauterine existence, it is of interest to view the relationship between status at birth or shortly thereafter, a subsequent motor development. Rosenblith (1966), for example, reported a highly significant prognostic relationship between neonatal assessment of motor behavior and fine and gross motor development as assessed by the Bayley scales of infant development at eight months of age. The motor items tested during the neonatal period included the following: head reaction in prone position, coordinated crawling motions in the prone position, vigor of responses to cotton and cellophane, grasp or strength of pull on a four-pound spring balance, and an overall rating or muscle tonus.

In a similar approach, Edwards (1968) related condition at birth as assessed via Apgar scores to motor performance at four years of age. The Apgar rating is an assessment of viability at birth and includes assessments of heart rate, repiratory effort, muscle tone, reflex irritability, and color. Motor performance items tested at four years of age included both fine and gross motor tasks. The former included the Porteus maze III and IV, Wallin peg board B, copying forms, and stringing beads, while the latter included a line walk, hopping on the right and left foot, and a ball catch. Apgar scores taken at one and five minutes after birth were significantly related to both fine and gross motor performance levels at four years of age. Within the total Apgar series, the muscle tone rating was the single best predictor of motor performance at four years of age.

The significance of the preceding observations is indeed puzzling, and needless to say rather complex. An infant's status at birth is strongly related to maternal factors, especially as far as birth weight is concerned (Penrose, 1961; Tanner, 1974). Birth weight, excluding premature infants, is, in general, not consistently related to motor development status at four months of age (Solomons and Solomons, 1964), to the age at walking alone (Pinneau, 1961), and to gross motor coordination at four years of age (Edwards, 1968). On the other hand, fetal movements during the last trimester of pregnancy are significantly related to postnatal motor development during the first year of life (Richards and Newbery, 1938; Walters, 1965). Are fetal movements related to the maternal intra-uterine environment and those factors affecting pregnant women, for example, emotional stress, smoking, maternal age, nutritional status, etc., or do they reflect inherent motor capacities of the developing fetus? To this we can add the infant's physical condition at birth (Apgar scores), which is perhaps related to the birth process and delivery room procedures (for example, anesthesia). It is apparent, therefore, that a variety of factors, many of which are maternal, are already operating at this early stage of life, and perhaps may have a relationship to motor development. Specific operation of these influences and undoubtedly others in mediating and modifying early and subsequent motor development are not clear.

LOW BIRTH WEIGHT AND PREMATURITY

Individuals vary in size at birth and also in gestational age. There is much concern for the growth of low birth weight (birth weight 2500 grams or less) and premature (gestational age 37 weeks or less) infants. The low birth weight of the former is generally assumed to be due to a shortened gestational period (i.e., prematurity), a reduced rate of intrauterine growth, or both (McKay, 1969). Low birth weight and prematurity generally occur concomitantly, especially in infants weighing less than 1500 grams.

Prematurity and/or low birth weight are associated with delayed motor development. Infants classified as such are not only smaller, but also perform consistently poorer on developmental tests, most of which include gross and fine motor development scales. This depression in early motor (and also mental) development is frequently related to the neurological damage associated with low birth weight (Illingworth, 1967). In an early study, Drillien (1948) related the age of attainment of three motor development milestones to birth weight, noting a later attainment of sitting, standing and walking behavior in low birth weight infants. Cutler, Heimer, Wortis and Freedman (1965) noted significantly lower gross motor scores in premature boys and girls at two and one-half years of age compared to full-term children. The foregoing would seem to indicate a persistence of early gross motor deficiencies in low birth weight children at later ages.

Motor performance data for premature and/or low birth weight infants at school ages are lacking. Other data indicate that such children may not catch-up to their more mature (full term, normal birth weight) age and sex peers in both physical and intellectual growth (Weiner, 1968, 1970). Since body size, maturation, strength and performance are related during growth (see below) one might possibly expect lesser motor performance levels in children who were premature at birth or of low birth weight. The foregoing suggests a need for the study of the motor development and performance of children categorized according to maturity status at birth. Children are usually classified according to chronological age, but the data suggest growth and development differences between premature and full term children of the same chronological age.

SIZE, PHYSIQUE, AND COMPOSITION

Although the preceding data suggest an independence of early motor development and birth weight in full term infants, the relationship of motor development and other physical characteristics needs to be examined. Studies including measures of size, build, and composition indicate some relationship between these indices of physical growth and motor development in infancy.

Body weight at six, nine and 12 months of age is not related to the age at sitting, the age at standing and the age at walking respectively, suggesting an independence of these motor milestones and body weight around the age at which these milestones are generally attained (Peatman and Higgons, 1942). Body weight, however, is a gross measure of mass and using it alone provides little information on body build and composition which might affect the course of motor development. Weight relative to body length (height) is frequently used to assess physique-associated variation in motor development during infancy and early childhood. Bayley (1935), for example, noted considerable variation and little consistent relationship between an index of stockiness (weight/length^2; W/L^2) and motor test scores from three through 36 months of age. The relationship between the motor scores and the W/L^2 index appeared curvilinear, suggesting poorer motor scores for children having extreme physiques; i.e., the very thin and the very chubby children. In contrast to observations for the W/L^2 index, the ratio of stem length to total body length (SL/L), an index of the relative contribution of the head, neck and trunk to total length, indicated a slight tendency for children with longer legs; i.e., shorter stem lengths, to have better motor test scores.

With regard to specific developmental milestones of infancy, Bayley (1935) and Shirley (1931) noted that infants with relatively long legs (lower SL/L ratios) walk earlier than those with relatively short legs. Shirley (1931) also noted a tendency for muscular and small-boned infants to walk at an earlier age. In Bayley's (1935) analysis, relationships between the W/L^2 index and the age at walking, though low, indicated a tendency for the relatively heavy infant at one year of age to walk later than the rather slender infant. Norval (1947) reported a similar relationship; i.e., infants relatively long for their body weight tended to walk at an earlier age. On the other hand, Peatman and Higgons (1942) found essentially no relationship between two height/weight indices of body build (weight/height; weight/height^3) at 12 months of age and the age at walking alone. These two indices at six and nine months of age were likewise unrelated respectively to the age at sitting and the age at standing.

Using bony chest breadth as an index of lean body mass, Garn (1966) noted that infants with a greater lean body mass attain better scores on early motor development tasks. Garn also noted that a larger leg muscle mass is significantly related with earlier standing and walking, while a smaller muscle mass is associated with later attainment of these two developmental milestones.

Garn further suggests that leg muscle mass at six months of age is predictive of walking unaided at one year, which would seem to indicate a developmental rather than an activity-mediated relationship.

The preceding discussion of body build and composition relative to early motor development indicates some relationship between these factors and motor development. The relationship, however, is not a simple one, and is most apparent at the extremes of the physique continuum. Analyses of physique and body composition relative to motor development during the preschool years are lacking (see Malina and Rarick, 1973; Malina, 1975). This lack and the limited observations on infants emphasize the need to extend studies of size, physique, and body composition relative to motor development to infancy and the preschool ages. Subcutaneous fat, for example, decreases from about one year of age through early childhood, the years when basic motor skills are developing at a rapid rate. During this time, muscle and bone mass gradually increase. Unfortunately, we know very little about the impact of the body's changing composition on the development of motor skills early in life. Relative to motor performance, fat represents dead weight that must be moved, and studies of older children clearly indicate a negative effect of excess fatness on performance (Malina, 1975).

At older ages, a child's level of strength and motor performance is in part related to age, size, physique, body composition and biological maturity status. These biological correlates of performance have been treated elsewhere in depth (Malina, 1975), and only a summary of the general direction of the relationships will be presented. Evidence suggests negative effects of excess body weight, fatness and endomorphy (over-weight, obesity) on motor performance items involving movement of the entire body, and positive effects of body size, especially weight, on strength. Correlations of body weight, mesomorphy (muscularity) and lean body mass with strength are not appreciably different. The magnitude of correlations of size, physique, body composition and maturity status with strength and motor performance, however, are generally low and at best moderate. As such, they are not meaningful in a predictive sense. Further, size, physique and maturity effects on strength and performance are generally more apparent at the extremes of physique, composition and maturity; i.e., extreme endomorphs relative to extreme ectomorphs, or early-compared to late-maturing children, and so on.

Many factors, either directly or indirectly related to body build and composition, are apparently operating on performance during middle childhood. Strength and motor performance improve with age. Generally bodily growth, strength and performance appear to progress in a parallel fashion during these ages. Performance is only moderately related to skeletal maturity (Seils, 1951), though the maturity effect can be partialed out when chronological age, skeletal age, height and weight are considered as multiple factors affecting performance (Rarick and Oyster, 1964). In the latter study, however, the extremes of the performance continuum, i.e., the best versus the poorest performers, showed maturity differences. The best performers were advanced, while the poorest were retarded in skeletal maturation.

Over-all body size and physique are to some extent inherited; i.e., are dependent upon size and physique of one's parents. Hence, the parental size and body build might possibly be parameters affecting the growth and development of offspring. Grouping children according to the size and build of parents, Garn (1962, 1966) noted that children born of large parents both in terms of stature and build, tend to be not only taller and heavier, but also advanced in motor development (Gesell scale) at 6, 12, and 18 months of age. Using Garn's approach, Malina, Harper and Holman (1970) attempted to assess the relationship between parental stature and the growth, strength and motor performance of children of elementary school age in Philadelphia. With parents classified as tall, medium, and short, the growth status of the children was assessed. Tall parents tended to have tall children, while short parents tended to have short children. This was true for both Black and White children 6 through 13 years of age. Then, taking the extremes of parental stature-mating combinations; i.e., tall X tall, short X short, the children's performance status in three gross motor and four static strength items was assessed. In the performance events, the result of Malina *et al.* (1970) for children were in the opposite direction to those reported by Garn (1962, 1966) for infants. Children of the short X short parental stature combination tended to perform somewhat better in the 35-yard dash, standing broad jump and throw for distance. Among white children, there was a slight tendency for offspring of tall X tall parental stature combinations to perform better on the jump and throw. Hence, factors other than size alone are important in determining motor performance levels during the elementary school ages. A large size, for example, might be associated with excess body fat, which is negatively related to performance, especially in items in which the body is projected as in the jump and dash.

In the strength items, the data of Malina *et al.* (1970) indicate a parent size-related trend for girls, but no consistent pattern for boys. Size is a factor in strength, and tall parents tend to have tall children. The sex difference suggests that factors other than size alone are related to muscular strength in boys, while size *per se* is an important variable affecting strength in girls (recognizing, of course, the fact that size and strength are related). The significance of strength and power in the male cultural ideal, a sex role learned early in life, would seem to suggest the importance of extraneous factors affecting performance in strength tests in boys. The words of Kagan (1968, p. 87) summarize the role of strength in children: "The uncorrupted sign of power for all children is strength. Strength is the only legitimate currency of power which cannot be corrupted, and children recognize this principle."

The foregoing limited observations suggest that the effects of parent size differences on the strength and performance of their offspring, an indirect size and build effect, are not as clear cut in the middle childhood as the parent size effects on gross motor items during the first three years of life. There is more to performance than size alone, although size and performance are generally positively correlated at these ages. Behavioral correlates of size, physique, and composition also need to be investigated. Do parents expect and/or encourage certain forms of behavior from children differing in physique, for example, the fat as opposed to the thin, muscular child? Conversely, how does the motor progress of the child influence parental rearing attitudes and expectations? The effects of child rearing conditions and related factors on motor performance, though frequently cited as exerting an influence on motor development during infancy and early childhood (see Chapter 24), have gone largely unexamined in the elementary school ages.

Nutrition. An adequate nutritional intake is essential to support the needs of normal growth and development, including of course motor development (see Jelliffe, 1966; Malina, 1979). The quality and quantity of food eaten by a child, however, is determined to a large extent by the culture in which he is reared, i.e., culturally determined habits, attitudes, preferences, and avoidances. Thus, the nutritional status of a child, which influences his growth and development, is virtually dependent upon cultural factors, emphasing the interaction of biological and cultural factors in development.

Much of the preceding discussion of growth and performance concerned children from developed, industrialized countries which offer children a reasonably adequate growth environment. Note, however, that the population of developed countries accounts for a little more than one-fourth of the world's population, while the population in developing areas of the world, on the other hand, are increasing more rapidly in number and in rate of growth (Demeny, 1974). Hence, the childhood population of the developing world, characterized by high mortality, morbidity (disease), and malnutrition, deserves more detailed consideration relative to growth and performance.

Perhaps the most significant growth influencing factor affecting children in the developing world is the widespread incidence of nutritional deficiencies and imbalances. Although undernutrition can occur any time during the life cycle, its effects are marked early in life, and the number of individuals so affected throughout the world is stagger-

ing. It is estimated, for example, that approximately 350 million children, or 7 out of 10 children under six years of age in the world have deficient diets (Keppel, 1968).

Interest in nutrition as a critical correlate of physical growth and psychomotor development is considerable. Severely undernourished infants and young children are retarded in motor development and show neuromuscular involvement, e.g., reduced nerve conduction velocities. It must be recognized that there are a variety of environmental factors in addition to nutritional factors, that may negatively influence early development. Severe undernutrition is accompanied by stunted physical growth and skeletal maturation, muscle wasting, general psychomotor change, and reduced levels of physical activity. Further, retarded motor development is indicated as one of the "constant" signs of kwashiorkor (Jelliffe, 1966). Kwashiorkor is a form of severe protein-calorie malnutrition most commonly occurring during the pre-school years.

When nutritional stress is considered, the role of organic changes in the central nervous system as underlying retarded development is usually emphasized. However, disturbances in social experiences also accompany malnutrition, and may interact with organic changes. In other words, there is more to the relationship of malnutrition and retarded development than food alone. As summarized by Birch (1968, p. 596):

Children who are ill-nourished are reduced in their responsiveness to the environment, distracted by their visceral state, and reduced in their ability to progress and endure in learning conditions.

The persistence of detrimental changes associated with severe undernutrition may be dependent upon the timing, severity, and duration of the nutritional stress. Children put on nutritionally adequate diets show some catch-up in growth and development. Nevertheless, it is difficult to assess how much of the child's potential is affected by the nutritional stress. In a three to six year follow-up of 14 severely malnourished children after nutritional recovery, Monckeberg (1968) noted that motor development was still retarded. Two long-term follow-up studies of infants hospitalized for severe protein-calorie malnutrition during the first two or three years of life indicate persistent effects on perceptual motor-development into adolescence. Stoch and Smythe (1976) noted deficits in visual-motor perception, which reflected deficits at the central neurosensory integration level, in 13 to 18 year old Cape Town (South Africa) youths (n=20) followed since hospitalization for marasmus during infancy. Hoorweg and Stanfield (1976) reported lower Lincoln-Oseretsky motor development scores in 11 to 17 year old Kampala (Uganda) children (n=60), who were hospitalized for protein-calorie malnutrition between 8 and 27 months of age. Interestingly, there was no relationship between subsequent motor performance and the age at hospital admission, and both "acute malnutrition" and "chronic undernutrition" had similar relationships to motor development.

The influence of nutritional inadequacy early in life on motor development may be related to the brain growth spurt described by Dobbing and Sands (1973). The spurt is a period of rapid brain growth which begins at about mid-pregnancy and continues through three or four years of age. The early part of the spurt, from mid-pregnancy to about 18 months, is characterized by rapid multiplication of glial cells, while the latter part which lasts to three or four years is characterized by myelinization. The extent of the spurt, however, varies with region of the brain, and the unique pattern characteristic of the cerebellum is relevant to motor development. The cerebellum starts its growth spurt later than the other parts (forebrain and stem), but completes the spurt earlier, i.e., it is getting its growth faster and over a shorter period of time.

Functions of the cerebellum include the development and maintenance of neuromuscular coordination, balance and muscle tone. Hence, potential interference with the growth spurt of the cerebellum through nutritional inadequacy prenatally and early postnatally might possibly interfere with normal motor development. Studies of adult rats undernourished during most of gestation and all of lactation indicate poor motor performance, which was attributable to impaired motor coordination. The undernourished rats also had smaller cerebella (Lynch, Smart, and Dobbig, 1975). These data thus suggest a differential vulnerability of the cerebellum to early nutritional stress, with resulting impairments in motor coordination. Implications for motor development in infants and young children are obvious.

The preceding has considered severe nutritional inadequacy early in life, primarily due to the widespread prevalence of protein-calorie malnutrition, associated mortality, and physical and behavioral consequences. Such observations also have implications for motor development in general. What level of development might we expect from children reared at marginally adequate nutritional levels (as compared to those who have been hospitalized for severe nutritional inadequacy)? The question can also be extended to children of school age in those areas where undernutrition is a chronic problem. School age children in these areas are somewhat special, in the sense that they have survived an infancy and early childhood characterized by undernutrition and infectious disease. Functional implications of the growth retardation (i.e., smaller body size and reduced muscle mass) characteristics of these children warrant concern. There is thus a need to consider the implications of a childhood characterized by undernutrition on the development and refinement of motor skills, the acquisition of new skills, the development and expression of muscular strength, and so on.

Studies evaluating the effects of mild-to-moderate malnutrition during the school ages usually concentrate upon measures of intellectual function to the omission of motor characteristics. Cravioto and De Licardie (1968) considered intersensory development in children 6 through 11 years of age relative to nutritional status. Intersensory integration is ordinarily measured via visual, haptic (relates to the sense of touch) and kinesthetic sense modalities. It is an indicator of neurointegrative development or the ability to integrate sensory information from several different modalities (see Birch and Lefford, 1967). Measures of intersensory function emphasize the central role of intersensory organization in the child's adaptive behavior. Efficient intersensory organization can thus be viewed as important in the child's motor behavior, which is in turn an important aspect of the individual's adaptive repertoire. After a detailed analysis of social and anthropological factors in the intersensory integrative performance of rural Guatemalan and Mexican school children, Cravioto and DeLicardie concluded that the inadequacy in intersensory integration was due primarily to earlier and perhaps present malnutrition.

Although the preceding observations on neurosensory integrative development are perhaps only inferential for motor performance during the elementary school ages, they serve to emphasize the need to view nutrition more closely when assessing the motor status of children. Nutrition influences all aspects of growth and development, and in all probability influences motor development and learning both directly and indirectly. Periodic bouts of acute nutritional stress are quite common in the life of individuals of developing countries, particularly children. The cumulative effects of such bouts, in addition to chronic mild-to-moderate malnutrition, on the growth and development of children and on motor learning and performance may be significant, and have not been thoroughly investigated.

The foregoing has concerned primarily undernutrition and its effects on motor development and performance. At the other end of the nutritional continuum, overnutrition must also be considered. Overnutrition ordinarily manifests itself in the form of a gross overweight condition and obesity. The detrimental effects of excess body weight, which is comprised essentially of fat, on motor performance have been indicated earlier. Overweight and/or obesity may also function to limit the physical activity pursuits of children, and thus indirectly influence their developing motor capacities.

References

Bayley, N. "The Development of Motor Abilities during the First Three Years." *Monographs of the Society for Research in Child Development* Number 1, 1935.

Birch, H. G. "Health and the Education of Socially Disadvantaged Children." *Developmental Medicine and Child Neurology* 10 (1968):580-99.

Birch, H. G. and Lefford, A. "Visual Differentiation, Intersensory Integration, and Voluntary Motor Control." *Monographs of the Society for Research in Child Development* 32 serial no. 110 (1967).

Bouchard, C. "Genetics, Growth and Physical Activity." In *Physical Activity and Human Well-Being,* edited by F. Landry and W.A.R. Orban. Miami, Florida: Symposia Specialists, Inc., 1978, pp. 29-45.

Cravioto, J. and De Licardie, E. R. "Intersensory Development of School-Age Children." In *Malnutrition, Learning, and Behavior,* edited by N. S. Scrimshaw and J. E. Gordon. Cambridge, Mass.: MIT Press, 1968, pp. 252-68.

Cutler, R., Heimer, C. B.; Wortis, H.; and Freedman, A. M. "The Effects of Prenatal and Neonatal Complications on the Development of Premature Children at Two and One-Half Years of Age." *Journal of Genetic Psychology* 107(1965):261-76.

Dales, R. J. "Motor and Language Development of Twins during the First Three Years." *Journal of Genetic Psychology* 114(1969): 263-71.

Demeny, P. "The Populations of the Underdeveloped Countries." *Scientific American* 231 (September 1974):148-59.

Dobbing, J. and Sands, J. "Quantitative Growth and Development of Human Brain." *Archives of Disease in Childhood* 48(1973):757-67.

Drillien, C. M. "Development and Progress of Prematurely Born Children in the Preschool Period." *Archives of Disease in Childhood* 23(1948):69-83.

Edwards, N. "The Relationship between Physical Condition Immediately after Birth and Mental and Motor Performance at Age Four." *Genetic Psychology Monographs* 78(1968): 257-89.

Garn, S. M. "Determinants of Size and Growth in the First Three Years." *Modern Problems in Pediatrics* 7(1962):50-54.

Garn, S. M. "Body Size and Its Implications." In *Review of Child Development Research,* edited by L. W. Hoffman and M. L. Hoffman. New York: Russel Sage Foundation, 1966, pp. 529-61.

Gesell, A. "The Ontogenesis of Infant Behavior." In *Manual of Child Psychology,* 2nd ed., edited by L. Carmichael. New York: John Wiley and Sons, Inc., 1954, pp. 335-73.

Hoorweg, J. and Stanfield, J. P. "The Effects of Protein Energy Malnutrition in Early Childhood on Intellectual and Motor Abilities in Later Childhood and Adolescence." *Development Medicine and Child Neurology* 18 (1976):330-50.

Illingworth, R. S. *The Development of the Infant and Young Child, Normal and Abnormal,* 3rd ed. London: E. & S. Livingstone Ltd., 1967.

Jelliffe, D. B. *The Assessment of the Nutritional Status of the Community.* Geneva: World Health Organization, 1966.

Kagan, J. "His Struggle for Identity." *Saturday Review* (December 7, 1968):80-82, 87-88.

Keppel, F. "Food for Thought." In *Malnutrition, Learning and Behavior,* edited by N. S. Scrimshaw and J. E. Gordon. Cambridge, Mass.: MIT Press, 1968, pp. 4-9.

Komi, P. V.; Klissouras, V.; and Karvinen, E. "Genetic Variation in Neuromuscular Performance." *Internationale Zeitschrift fur Angewandte Physiologie Einschliesslich Arbeitsphysiologie* 31(1973):289-304.

Kovar, R. "Prispevek ke studiu geneticke podminenosti lidske motoriky." *Autoreferat disertace k zizkani vedecke hodnosti kandidata biologickych ved,* Praha, Czechoslovakia, 1974.

Laughlin, W. S. "Hunting: An Integrating Biobehavior System and Its Evolutionary Importance." In *Man the Hunter,* edited by R. B. Lee and I. Devore. Chicago: Aldine, 1968, pp. 304-20.

Lynch, A.; Smart, J.L.; and Dobbing, J. "Motor co-ordination and cerebellar Size in Adult Rats Undernourished in Early Life." *Brain Research* 83(1975):249-59.

Malina, R. M. "Anthropometric Correlates of Strength and Motor Performance." *Exercise and Sport Sciences Reviews* 3(1975):249-74.

Malina, R. M. "Development, Aging, and Nutrition." In *Anthropological Aspects of Human Nutrition,* edited by F. E. Johnston. Albuquerque: University of New Mexico Press and the School for American Research, 1979 (in press).

Malina, R. M.; Harper, A. B.; and Holman, J. D. "Growth Status and Performance Relative to Parental Size." *Research Quarterly* 41 (1970):503-9.

Malina, R. M. and Rarick, G. L. "Growth, Physique, and Motor Performance." In *Physical Activity: Human Growth and Development, edited by G. L. Rarick.* New York: Academic Press, 1973, pp. 125-53.

Marisi, D. Q. "Genetic and Extragenetic Variance in Motor Performance." *Acta Geneticae Medicae et Gemellologiae* 26(1977):197-204.

McKay, R. J. "The Fetus and the Newborn Infant." In *Textbook of Pediatrics,* 9th ed., edited by W. E. Nelson; V. C. Vaughan; and R. J. McKay. Philadelphia: Saunders, 1969, pp. 347-410.

Mead, M. and Macgregor, F. C. *Growth and Culture: A Photographic Study on Balinese Childhood.* New York: Putnam, 1951.

Monckeberg, F. "Effect of Early Marasmic Malnutrition on Subsequent Physical and Psychological Development." In *Malnutrition, Learning, and Behavior,* edited by N. S. Scrimshaw and J. E. Gordon. Cambridge, Mass.: MIT Press, 1968, pp. 269-78.

Norval, M. A. "Relationship of Weight and Length of Infants at Birth to the Age at Which They Begin to Walk Alone." *Journal of Pediatrics* 30(1947):676-78.

Peatman, J. G. and Higgons, R. A. "Relation of Infants' Weight and Body Build to Locomotor Development." *American Journal of Orthopsychiatry* 12(1942):234-40.

Penrose, L. S. "Genetics of Growth and Development of the Fetus." In *Recent Advances in Human Genetics,* edited by L. S. Penrose. London: J. & A. Churchill, Ltd., 1961, pp. 56-75.

Pineau, M. "Development de L'enfant et Dimension de la Famille. *Biotypologie* 22 (1961):25-53.

Rarick, G. L. and Oyster, N. "Physical Maturity, Muscular Strength, and Motor Performance of Young School-Age Boys. *Research Quarterly* 35(1964):523-31.

Richards, T. W. and Newbery, H. "Studies in Fetal Behavior." III. "Can Performance in Test Items at Six Months Postnatally Be Predicted on the Basis of Fetal Activity?" *Child Development* 9(1938):79-86.

Rosenblith, J. F. "Prognostic Values of Neonatal Assessment." *Child Development* 37(1966):623-31.

Seils, L. G. "The Relationship between Measures of Physical Growth and Gross Motor Performance of Primary-Grade School Children. *Research Quarterly* 22(1951):244-60.

Shirley, M. M. *The First Two Years: A Study of Twenty-Five Babies. Postural and Locomotor Development,* vol. 1. Minneapolis: University of Minnesota Press, 1931.

Sklad, M. "Similarity of Movements in Twins." *Wychowanie Fizycznie i Sport,* nr. 3 (1972): 119-41.

Sklad, M. "The Genetic Determination of the Rate of Learning Motor Skills." *Studies in Physical Anthropology* (Wroclaw, Poland), 1(1975):3-19.

Solomons, G. and Solomons, H. C. "Factors Affecting Motor Performance in Four-Month-Old Infants." *Child Development* 35(1964): 1283-95.

Stoch, M. B. and Smythe, P. M. "Fifteen-Year Developmental Study on Effects of Severe Undernutrition during Infancy on Subsequent Physical Growth and Intellectual Functioning." *Archives of Disease in Childhood* 51(1976):327-36.

Tanner, J. M. "Variability of Growth and Maturity in Newborn Infants." In *The Effect of the Infant on Its Caregiver,* edited by M. Lewis and L. A. Rosenblum. New York: Wiley, 1974, pp. 77-103.

Vickers, V. S.; Poyntz, L.; and Baum, M. P. "The Brace Scale Used with Young Children." *Research Quarterly* 13(1942):299-308.

Walters, C. E. "Prediction of Postnatal Development From Fetal Activity." *Child Development* 36(1965):801-8.

Weiner, G.; Rider, R. V.; Oppel, W. C.; and Harper, P. A. "Correlates of Low Birth Weight: Psychological Status at Eight to Ten Years of Age. *Pediatric Research* 2 (1968):110-18.

Weiner, G. "The Relationship of Birth Weight and Length of Gestation to Intellectual Development at Ages 8 to 10." *Journal of Pediatrics* 76(1970):694-99.

Witherspoon, R. L. "Selected Areas of Development of Twins in Relation to Zygosity." In *Methods and Goals in Human Behavior Genetics,* edited by S. G. Vandenberg. New York: Academic Press, 1965, pp. 187-97.

Environmentally Related Correlates of Motor Development and Performance during Infancy and Childhood

24

Robert M. Malina
University of Texas

In addition to physical characteristics of the child that may influence motor development and performance early in life and during middle childhood, the child's environments must be considered. The environments in which a child is reared also represent a substrate. The term environment is used in the plural, for an individual's environments are many. They can be subdivided into three broad, but interrelated categories: the natural, the man-made, and the human environments. Environments are likewise cumulative, exerting their influences early in life, in many instances prenatally, and throughout life. The cumulative as well as complex nature of an individual's environments thus renders extremely difficult the partitioning of effects due to specific factors, for example maternal care, nutrition, and the physical development of the child.

A child must adapt to the stresses imposed by the environments, and as such, these environments in turn will undoubtedly have an impact on the child's developmental progress, including motor development. The accurate delineation, definition, and assessment of such correlates in the motor development of the child is thus a difficult task.

The child's family, siblings, spontaneous peer groups, ethnic group, socio-economic background, and institutionally based peer groups must be considered relative to motor development and performance. The influences of these environments represent antecedent conditions whose consequences are seen in the behavior of the child. How are these conditions translated into behavior? Or, more specifically, how do they affect the child's motor development and behavior?

Between birth and school age, the child is experiencing rapid development in the motor sphere of his/her behavioral repertoire. The child is like-wise undergoing dramatic psychological and personality changes. Most studies of preschool children, however, have examined the impact of parent-child relationships, ethnic group membership and socio-economic status on psychological, cognitive, and personality development so that the effects of these conditions and related factors on motor development have gone largely unexamined.

REARING AND SOCIAL CLASS

Studies of child rearing practices across social class, ethnic groups, and different cultures have primarily concerned socialization and personality development. Emphasis is generally placed upon feeding practices, toilet training, age at weaning, independence and aggression training, mother-infant attachment, and so on. More recently, attention has been given to cognitive development and academic motivation relative to the child rearing environment, especially in minority, lower class, and/or disadvantaged children. Rearing studies are also limited to a large extent to infancy and early childhood, and have generally not been concerned with motor development and behavior as the central focus of study, except for walking behavior.

One can thus inquire as to the effects of child care practices on motor development and motor activity during infancy and childhood. More specifically, how are child rearing practices translated into different motor development levels. Do children reared in over-protective or restrictive atmospheres develop and behave differently in motor activities than children reared in permissive, less protective atmospheres?

Child rearing practices vary across social class and ethnic group (see, for example, Bronfenbrenner, 1958; Waters and Crandall, 1964; Hess, 1970; Jackson, 1973; Chamberlin, 1978). In a review of child care practices over a 25 year period between 1930 and 1955, Bronfenbrenner (1958) reported a shift in the rearing attitudes of middle class and working class mothers. From about 1930 to the end of World War II, working class mothers were generally more permissive, but after World War II, the middle class mothers became more permissive in practices relating to eating, sleeping and toileting. Similarly, middle class mothers became more permissive towards the child's expressed desires, but with greater expectations for the child. Working class mothers tended to demand obedience and discipline, while middle class mothers emphasized the importance of self direction on the part of

their children. Waters and Crandall (1964), evaluating maternal behavior between 1940 and 1960, noted that mothers, regardless of social class, showed a tendency to be less coercive and more permissive than before. Hence, these observations suggest child rearing practices vary among social classes, as well as within social classes, with much overlap. Child rearing practices, however, should not be viewed as being stable; we are living in an age of relatively rapid change, which undoubtedly affects the relationships between parent and child. Also, it should be carefully noted that the predictive and explanatory power of observed rearing practice differences on the child's motor development and performance are not yet established.

Several studies have examined social class criteria relative to early motor development. Bayley and Jones (1937), for example, reported no relationship between socio-economic variables and age of first walking independently. There was, however, a tendency for an increased number of negative correlations between motor scores and socio-economic variables, implying somewhat more rapid motor development in children from the lower social strata. Neligan and Prudham (1969) also reported a social class difference in the age of independent walking among a sample of Newcastle (England) children, the social class difference favoring the lower class children. Neligan and Prudham (1969, p. 417) interpreted the observations as possibly reflecting ". . . deprivation of the opportunity to learn resulting from overprotection . . ." in the upper social class. Hindley, Filliozat, Klackenberg, Nicolet-Meister and Sand (1966), on the other hand, did not find any social class difference in the age of walking among five European longitudinal samples. There were, however, significant differences between the five samples in the mean age of walking alone.

During early childhood socioeconomic background is often implicated as an important factor affecting the activity pursuits of children and presumably their development in motor spheres (see Malina, 1973a). In general, data suggest greater freedom to move about the neighborhood among lower socioeconomic background children. Such an atmosphere might be conducive to greater freedom of motor activity and opportunity for practice. It should be noted that many of these studies consider ethnic variation in rearing, life style, patterns of socialization, and so on, with little, if any, consideration for motor development and activity (ethnic aspects of motor development are considered below).

REARING AND SEX DIFFERENCES

It is well known that cultural conditioning for specific sex-associated roles begins early in life. Mothers, for example, treat sons differently than daughters, and this sex difference begins early in infancy (Moss, 1967; Goldberg and Lewis, 1969). Behavioral differences are also apparent early in life. One year old boys, for example, already spend more time in gross motor activity, while girls of the same age spend more time in fine motor activity (Goldberg and Lewis, 1969). Boys are also more vigorous in their play and show more exploratory behavior than girls, who are more dependent and prefer a more quiet style of play. Observations on nursery school children two to five years of age offer similar evidence. Boys spend more time in "rough and tumble" gross motor activities, while girls spend more time in activities requiring fine motor manipulation (Blurton

Jones, 1967; Clark, Wyon and Richards, 1969). In a related study, Walker (1962) compared behavior of mesomorphic boys and girls. Although similar in physique, mesomorphic girls tend to channel their energies into social activities, while mesomorphic boys channel their energies into gross motor activities. Walker suggests that variations in physical energy and in body sensitivity to energy needs may thus be important mediating links between physique and behavior. It would appear, however, that at these early ages, the expectations of our culture already have an impact on what children sense is appropriate behavior for each sex.

The translation of such descriptive data into specific correlates of motor development of preschool boys and girls is difficult and needs a finer approach relating generalized observations to the development of specific motor patterns. Sex differences in motor development during infancy are not systematically apparent (Bayley, 1935, 1965; Frankenburg and Dodds, 1967), although sex differences in rearing practices and play behavior are apparent. Sex differences in motor development and performance, however, are evident during early childhood. From about two to five years of age, girls, on the average, excel in tasks requiring jumping, hopping, rhythmic locomotion and balance, while boys generally perform better in tasks requiring strength and speed (Frankenburg and Dodds, 1967; Sinclair, 1971; Espenschade and Eckert, 1974; Welon and Sekita, 1976). From the age of five or six years on, boys generally perform better in running, jumping, and throwing activities, while girls excel in hopping (Keogh, 1965; Espenschade and Eckert, 1974). Balancing activities show no consistent pattern of sex difference, although girls show better performances at some ages (Keogh, 1965).

Such observations as the preceding are based on group averages and mask the considerable overlap that does exist. The observations, however, need to be related to sex differences in activity interests, opportunity for practice, opportunity and frequency of participation, requirements of specific activities, and so on. Govatos (1966), for example, suggests that the motor performance advantage of boys during middle childhood is related to their greater interests in and more frequent opportunities for participation in activities requiring ball handling, throwing and jumping. On the other hand, Govatos relates the performance superiority of girls in balance beam activities to a combination of factors including advanced maturity, better balancing ability, and a closer attention to the performance of the task.

The cultural socialization or exclusion of the young girl from activities requiring physical strength and skill is perhaps an important underlying correlate of sex differences in motor performance. The significance of western cultural influences on the differential acquisition of motor skills by boys and girls during early childhood thus needs consideration. Observations considered above suggest, perhaps, differences in cultural expectations and opportunities for boys and girls. These may be viewed in terms of available models to mimic (e.g., father, athletes, etc.), the models that are encouraged, opportunities for practice, parental motivation, sibling relationships, and so on. Motor skill development and acquisition are an integral part of the child's socialization process and they have not received detailed study. These topics are discussed in more detail in the next chapter.

REARING AND BIRTH ORDER

A child's position in the family and sibling-sex status are also factors that influence early motor development. Some data suggest that first born children perform slightly better on motor tasks early in life (Solomons and Solomons, 1964; Bayley, 1965), an observation generally related to greater maternal indulgence and therefore stimulation of the first born compared to later born. Descriptions of play behavior in nursery school children indicate that first born children spend more time alone, engage in more non-specific activity, and are generally more dependent upon adults (Clark *et al.*, 1969). Rearing studies of single child families suggest overprotection, greater restriction on physical mobility, and a strong tendency to keep close track of the child on the part of mothers (Sears, Maccoby, and Levin, 1957). In contrast to an only child, studies of siblings indicate that children with opposite sex siblings have more of the characteristics of the opposite sex than children with siblings of the same sex (Rosenberg and Sutton-Smith, 1964, 1968; see also Sutton-Smith, Roberts, and Rosenberg, 1964). It would be interesting to relate such observations to the motor development and performance of children. For example, does a girl with an older brother develop differently in motor activities or have different activity interests than a girl who has an older sister as a sibling? The same question can be raised for boys with female and male siblings respectively. On the other hand, the role of a younger sibling in possibly influencing the motor behavior of an older child also warrants study.

We attempted to look at some of these possibilities in a cross-sectional sample of elementary school children 6 to 12 years of age (Malina and Estrada, unpublished data). Stature and weight did not vary with the number of children in these middle to upper middle class families. Strength and motor performance also did not vary significantly and consistently with family size. For example, boys in small families (one and two children) ran faster (35 yard dash) than boys in medium sized (three children) and large (four and five children) families. In contrast, boys from larger families jumped (standing long jump) slightly better than boys in smaller families. For girls, those in medium size families (three children) performed better in the running and throwing tests. Grip strength decreased slightly with an increase in family size for boys; in contrast, however, it showed a slight increase with an increase in family size for girls. Pushing and pulling strength showed no consistent pattern of differences relative to the number of children in the family. Note that these observations are based on group means with considerable overlap between them.

Since it is often hypothesized that females with brothers would have greater sport participation and interests than females with sisters, we compared the performance of girls with an older brother to that of girls with an older sister. We chose to limit our analysis to girls with older brothers or sisters since this was an elementary school sample and some of the children had younger, preschool siblings. Girls with older brothers or sisters did not differ in height and weight, and showed no consistent pattern of differences across the three motor tasks. Girls with an older sister ran slightly faster, those with an older brother threw a ball slightly farther, while the two groups did not differ in jumping. Running and jumping are perhaps more phylogenetically based motor skills than throwing, and might not be markedly influenced by sibling-sex status, while overhand throwing, being a somewhat more culturally sensitive motor skill, is influenced favorably in young girls having an older brother. In contrast to these observations on motor performance, the four strength measurements were slightly and consistently greater in girls having an older brother. Interpretation of these trends suggests, perhaps, that interaction with an older brother demands greater physical prowess from a young girl. Although our results are only suggestive, they do imply a role for sibling-sex-status combinations in the strength and motor performance of elementary school age children, and obviously emphasize the need for more detailed investigations of sibling-sex-status in children.

ETHNIC CONSIDERATIONS

Available data comparing the early motor development of American black and white children indicate advanced motor development in black children during the first two or three years of life. The differences are more apparent at the younger ages, and superiority in any one class or motor behavior is not responsible for the black motor precocity (Bayley, 1965; Malina, 1973a). These generalizations are not without exception as several studies indicate minor or inconsistent differences in early motor development of black and white children (Knobloch and Pasamanick, 1958; Walters, 1967). Explanations offered for the observations vary. Some implicate genetic factors, while others indicate socioeconomic variables as affecting the results (Bayley, 1965; Malina, 1973a). Note that social class and ethnicity are closely related in the United States. The socioeconomic hypothesis suggests that a more permissive rearing atmosphere characterizes lower socio-economic classes and enhances motor development (Scott, Ferguson, Jenkins and Cutter, 1955; Williams and Scott, 1953). Results concerning a socioeconomic interpretation, however, are conflicting. Social class differences in motor development have been reported among American black (Knobloch and Pasamanick, 1958; Walters, 1967) and white infants (Willerman, Broman and Fiedler, 1970). In these studies, contrary to the suggestions of Scott *et al.* (1955) and Williams and Scott (1953), infants from higher socioeconomic backgrounds had significantly higher motor development scores than those from lower socioeconomic strata. More detailed considerations of the growth, maturation, motor development and performance of American black and white children have been reported elsewhere (Malina, 1969, 1973a, 1973b).

Thus, the socioeconomic hypothesis is by no means clear-cut in accounting for observed motor development differences during infancy and early childhood. Further, the hypothesis is not consistent with the child rearing studies reviewed by Bronfenbrenner (1958). His review indicated a shift towards greater permissiveness in the middle class mothers (presumably higher social class than the working class mothers) after World War II. This appears to be in accord with the observations of Knobloch and Pasamanick (1958) and Walters (1967), but contrary to Williams and Scott (1953) and Scott *et al.* (1955). Yet, all samples are post-World War II, and the last two mentioned studies attributed advanced motor behavior among lower class black infants to more permissive child rearing practices. Perhaps the trends in child care practices derived from studies of eating, sleeping and toileting are not applicable to motor development. Or, perhaps child rearing trends based upon white American families do not necessarily apply to black American

families? Or, the social class criteria for black and white samples might be different. It should be noted that the number of black families that can be classified as middle class is probably very small, but steadily increasing today. Further, the data of Frazier (1948), Baughman and Dahlstrom (1968), Schulz (1969) and Young (1970) suggest somewhat different black family life styles, values and patterns of socialization compared to the white family cultural tradition (although aspirations of black and white parents for their children are reasonably similar).

Nevertheless, the fact that differences in early motor development between samples of American black and white children are apparent in most, but not all studies, is significant in itself. Why do findings of separate studies differ? Sampling variation and testing procedures, of course, must be recognized. One may ask, however, whether the socioeconomic explanation, particularly the permissiveness theme, operates by permitting the full development of the infant's genotype, which might in fact differ between populations? Knobloch and Pasamanick (1958, p. 131) seem to imply this trend of thought by commenting that ". . . child-rearing makes no difference in gross motor development in infancy, except when certain biological or cultural thresholds are exceeded." What are these thresholds and how are they affected by the child rearing situation?

Comparisons of motor development and performance of children with Spanish surnames (Mexican-American, Puerto Rican) are quite limited. Using the Denver Developmental Screening Test, Frankenburg, Dick, and Carland (1975) noted few differences in fine and gross motor items between anglo (white) and Spanish-surnamed children when controlling for social class (all fathers were unskilled workers). Anglo children were significantly advanced in four motor tasks (all in the first year of life), while the Spanish-surnamed children did not show advancement in any motor tasks. Comparisons of Spanish-surnamed and black children showed the black children significantly advanced in ten fine and gross motor test items. All items were tasks measured during the first year of life. However, after about three years of age, the Spanish-surnamed children excelled in two fine motor and one gross motor task. Interpretation of the results is difficult, and may be related to ethnic differences in rearing style. The authors did not consider specific motor items, but only considered components of the Denver Developmental Screening Test as a whole.

The correlates of permissiveness and acceptance which might function to enhance motor development obviously need further explanation, specifically in terms of correlation, causation and related problems. Detailed study of child rearing practices within the context of the social and/or sub-cultural units within the vast American culture complex is also needed, especially with motor development and performance as the central problem of observation. Much that can and has been said about child rearing practices and motor development must be inferred from general rearing studies, which have traditionally concerned themselves with personality development and socialization within a psychoanalytic framework. It is beyond the scope of this chapter to delve into the details and possible inferences for motor development and performance contained in such studies. A review by the author (Malina, 1973a) has considered these studies relative to performance in infancy, childhood, and adolescence.

Related to the preceding discussion are problems associated with the "disadvantaged child." There is, however, no such thing as a typical "socially disadvantaged child"; rather, there are probably a great variety of such children, black, Spanish-surnamed and white. Descriptive reviews of problems associated with disadvantaged children generally do not include their motor characteristics and possible correlates in the environments of the children. Hence, observations are limited and sketchy. Pavenstedt (1967), for example, noted superior gross motor coordination but a lack of "motoric caution" in pre-school children from lower class "disorganized" families. The motor characteristics of these children, however, are only described generally with little, if any, supporting quantitative data. Evaluating the effects of nursery school experiences on these children of disorganized families, Pavenstedt noted beneficial effects on motor development, gross motor skills becoming "functionally excellent." Hodges and Spiker (1967) made similar reports. Motor deficiencies in pre-school disadvantaged children improved after a special instructional program. Hodges and Spiker, however, emphasized the importance of opportunities for running, climbing, jumping, and so on, in the child's home and neighborhood as sufficiently important for the development of gross motor skills, compared to changes observed in fine motor skills with the special instructional program.

CROSS-CULTURAL CONSIDERATIONS

Cross-cultural observations of early motor development are available for a number of cultural groups. These generally include data for developmental tests. However, after the age of two, the cross-cultural motor development data are scanty at best, with little formally collected motor ability information. This probably reflects the orientation of the researchers, which commonly focuses on cognitive development, mother-infant attachment, infant-caretaker interactions, and so on. Since the focus of many studies is cognitive development, motor items on the infant scales are less emphasized as they show reduced correlations with mental items with increasing age (see, for example, Bayley, 1951). The early motor skills are perhaps developing functional specificity as they become more unrelated to cognitive development.

Examples of early motor development data are considered subsequently for samples of children within several cultural groups. Most data are available for sub-Saharan African populations, while less extensive data are available for Jamaica, Mexico, Guatemala, and Japan (see Malina, 1977). Samples of African children are generally precocious in motor development compared with infants of the United States. Precocity against the norms, however, commonly declines with age. Whether this precocity is evident at birth is not entirely clear; however, it is apparent during the first month of life and continues during the first year. There are methodological weaknesses in the African studies (see Warren, 1972), but critical evaluation does not exclude the phenomenon of precocity of African infants in motor development.

The rapid motor development of the African infant in several cultural groups has been attributed to environmental influences, especially to the kinds of mothering and caretaking received, and lack of physical restriction. Early rearing is characterized by physical closeness between mother and child, a constant supply of kinesthetic and tactile stimulation. Observations on five and six month old American Black infants show a low to moderate relationship between kinesthetic stimulation and the Bayley psychomotor development index, and fine and gross motor scores (Yarrow, Pedersen and Rubenstein, 1977). Based upon observations in a Kenyan community, Super (1976) relates African infant motor precocity only to those tasks which are specifically taught by caretakers and/or which are incidental effects of daily caretaking practices. Further, among Kenyan communities, encouragement of motor development is a widespread practice. The observations of Leiderman, Babu, Kagia, Kraemer, and Liederman (1973) on Kikuyu infants suggest significant relationships between motor development during infancy and the number of individuals in the household past 40 years of age and the economic status of the father.

These positive correlations are interesting, first in that they suggest an effect for kinesthetic stimulation and for additional caretaking of the infant by an older woman and/or grandmother in contributing to early motor development, second in that they indicate a role for specific teaching, and third in that they indicate a small, positive economic effect. The latter is contrary to the earlier observations of Geber and Dean (1958), who suggested that motor precocity was inversely related to social class in Uganda. Interestingly, the Kikuyu data also indicate a low, negative relationship between motor scores of infants and the number of household members less than three years of age.

Three studies of Mayan infants from Mexico and Guatemala provide somewhat different results. Solomons and Solomons (1975) observed consistently accelerated

Bayley motor scores during most of the first year of life in Mayan infants in Yucatan. The infants were especially precocious in fine motor items, and slightly delayed in locomotor skills and gross coordination towards the end of the first year. Interestingly, there was no difference in the early motor behavior among three sociocultural groups comprising the Yucatecan infant samples — working and middle class Mestizos and rural Mayan. On the other hand, Brazelton (1972, 1977) reported well-organized neonatal motor responses at birth and shortly after among rural Zinacanteco Indians (Mayan), which were followed by a level of motor development that lagged consistently behind U.S. standards by about one month throughout the first year of life. De Leon, de Licardie, and Cravioto (1964) noted a similar delay in the motor development of rural Guatemalan Mayan infants. The development of the independent sitting as well as the development of prehension during the first year showed a progressive delay of one or two months relative to the Gesell standards. Development of locomotor abilities showed a similar delay relative to the standards. The children progressed in reasonable accord (one to two months) with the standard through 15 months, but became progressively delayed through 48 months. Performance on items of the Gesell adaptive scale also showed a pattern of progressive delay relative to the norms.

Mayan infants are held constantly and are commonly carried on the back during most of their first year of life. Infants, especially lower class and rural, are tightly wrapped in a shawl with head and eyes covered most of the time to protect them from the "evil eye." Brazelton (1972, 1977) relates the mother/child interaction to the imitation and conformity emphasized by the local culture. Such early care, tightly swaddled and covered most of the time, apparently fosters ". . . quiet alertness conducive to imitation and conformity." It should be noted that among rural Zinacantecos imitation is the chief mode of learning in older children, such that children are not confronted with the choice of roles as are children in our cultural complex.

The developmental lag in motor test items towards the end of the first year and during the second and third years in African and Mayan infants is likely related to the break in continuity of rearing at weaning and to the effects of undernutrition. After weaning children do not get the adult treatment and attention they had before, while delayed motor development and reduced levels of physical activity accompany protein-calorie malnutrition. It is also at these ages that stunting in physical growth becomes especially apparent.

The preceding cross-cultural comparisons suggest culturally distinct environmental and child rearing practices that are related to early motor behavior. Relationships, however, do not imply a cause-effect sequence in motor development. Note also that the infants are generally compared to western standards, which raises the possibility that some of the observed differences in motor behavior might relate to test items per se. For example, if an infant is never placed in the prone position, it is difficult to elicit a response for test items requiring this position. Placing an infant in this position generally elicits a stress response, which masks the motor performance being tested. In addition, some test items require objects that are not familiar to the particular cultural group, e.g., cubes, rattles, spoons, cups, etc. These can perhaps be substituted with culturally appropriate items. Superimposed upon the preceding are problems of stranger-anxiety in older infants and young children, which may make testing or observing motor behavior quite difficult.

Comparisons of motor performance, usually by means of physical fitness test items, indicate some mean differences among several cultural groups, for example, Japanese, Danish, South African Black (see Malina, 1977). Social and cultural factors are commonly cited as possible influences on the observed average differences in motor performance. However, the operation or translation of these factors into performance variation is generally not considered and/or perhaps not known with certainty. Some possible explanations are obvious. Proficiency of European and Latin American children in soccer skills compared to United States children, for example, undoubtedly reflects greater emphasis on soccer in these two cultures. Recent emphasis on soccer programs for children in the United States over the past few years may reduce the apparent differences.

OVERVIEW

The pattern of motor development and performance during infancy and childhood has been briefly considered. Biologically and environmentally related factors that may influence motor development and performance were also considered. Environmental correlates are related to a large extent to the cultural group within which the child is reared. Hence, the term "biocultural influences" on motor development and performance should perhaps be used (see Malina, 1976, 1978).

Motor development is obviously a plastic process. There is variation in the timing and rate of development which can be related to a variety of biocultural correlates. The significance of variation in early motor de-velopment for later motor proficiency, however, is not known with certainty, nor is the significance of the effects of both biological and cultural correlates.

The motor activity of the infant and young child presumably represents the foundation upon which subsequent motor proficiency is built. However, the predictive significance of early motor assessments for later, more mature motor patterns is not clear, and not ordinarily investigated. One may ask whether differences in timing and sequence during the first year or two of life lead to parallel differences at later ages. Answers to this question are not available. In other words, it is difficult to extend observations from infancy and early childhood to older ages.

It is within the interaction of the motor and other aspects of development that factors underlying and modifying the course of motor development during infancy and childhood are manifest. Motor activities constitute an essential component of the child as a biological organism, and are also an important aspect of the child's daily life pattern, which is carried on in a variety of settings including the home, school, spontaneous peer groups, organized groups, and so on.

Many interacting and covarying factors impinge upon the motor development and motor behavior of children during infancy and childhood. The preceding chapters are not intended as a comprehensive review of these factors. It is hoped that the student will have a better awareness of the many factors which may influence a child's motor progress, and the difficulties involved in understanding the process. Available data are derived from many disciplines asking different questions and using different methods. Very frequently, the study of the child's motor development is not the primary objective in these studies. Also, the significance of early motor development for subsequent motor behavior in early and middle childhood needs further clarification.

Obviously more questions have been raised than answers provided. Nevertheless, this is a good sign. The time is ripe for and there is a need for more comprehensive studies of motor behavior during infancy and childhood. Because motor activities are an integral part of the developing child's behavior, it is important for him or her to meet some degree of success in the motor domain. If success is to be assisted, an understanding of the factors underlying and modifying motor processes is essential.

References

Baughman, E. E. and Dahlstrom, W. G. *Negro and White Children: A Psychological Study in the Rural South.* New York: Academic Press, 1968.

Bayley, N. "The Development of Motor Abilities during the First Three Years." *Monographs of the Society for Research in Child Development* (1935):number 1.

Bayley, N. "Development and Maturation." In *Theoretical Foundations of Psychology,* edited by H. Helson. New York: Van Nostrand, 1951, pp. 160-65.

Bayley, N. "Comparisons of Mental and Motor Test Scores for Ages 1-15 Months by Sex, Birth Order, Race, Geographical Location, and Education of Parents." *Child Development* 36(1965):379-411.

Bayley, N. and Jones, H. E. "Environmental Correlates of Mental and Motor Development: A Cumulative Study from Infancy to Six Years." *Child Development* 8(1937): 329-41.

Blurton Jones, N. G. "An Ethological Study of Some Aspects of Social Behaviour of Children in Nursery School." In *Primate Ethology,* edited by D. Morris. Chicago: Aldine Publishing Co., 1967, pp. 347-68.

Brazelton, T. B. "Implications of Infant Development among the Mayan Indians of Mexico." *Human Development* 15(1972):90-111.

Brazelton, T. B. "Implications of Infant Development among the Mayan Indians of Mexico." In *Culture and Infancy,* edited by P. H. Leiderman; S. R. Tulkin; and A. Rosenfeld. New York: Academic Press, 1977, pp. 151-87.

Bronfenbrenner, U. "Socialization and Social Class through Time and Space." In *Readings in Social Psychology,* 3rd ed., edited by E. E. Maccoby; T. M. Newcomb; and E. L. Hartley. New York: Holt and Company, 1958, pp. 400-25.

Chamberlin, R. W. "Relationships between Child-Rearing Styles and Child Behavior Over Time." *American Journal of Diseases of Children* 132(1978):155-60.

Clark, A. H.; Wyon, S. M.; and Richards, M. P. M. "Free-Play in Nursery School Children." *Journal of Child Psychology and Psychiatry* 10(1969):205-16.

De Leon, W.; de Licardie, E.; and Cravioto, J. "Operacion Nimiquipalg: VI. Desarrollo psicomotor del nino en una poblacion rural de Guatemala, perteneciente al grupo Cakchiquel." *Guatemala Pediatrica* 4(1964):92-106.

Espenschade, A. and Eckert, H. "Motor Development." In *Science and Medicine of Exercise and Sport,* 2nd ed., edited by W. R. Johnson and E. R. Buskirk. New York: Harper and Row, 1974, pp. 322-33.

Frankenburg, W. K. and Dodds, J. B. "The Denver Developmental Screening Test." *Journal of Pediatrics* 71(1967):181-91.

Frankenburg, W. K.; Dick, N. P.; and Carland, J. "Development of Preschool-Aged Children of Different Social and Ethnic Groups: Implications for developmental Screening." *Journal of Pediatrics* 87(1975):125-32.

Frazier, E. F. *The Negro Family in the United States,* rev. and abridged ed. New York: Dreyden Press, 1948.

Goldberg, S. and Lewis, M. "Play Behavior in the Year-Old Infant: Early Sex Differences." *Child Development* 40(1969):21-31.

Govatos, L. A. Sex Differences in Children's Motor Performances." Collected papers, the Eleventh Interinstitutional Seminar in Child Development. Greenfield Village, Michigan: Education Department of the Henry Ford Museum, 1966, pp. 55-75.

Hess, R. D. "Social Class and Ethnic Influences upon Socialization." In *Carmichael's Manual of Child Psychology*, vol. 2, 3rd ed., edited by P. H. Mussen. New York: Wiley, 1970, pp. 457-557.

Hindley, C. B.; Filliozat, A. M.; Klackenberg, G.; Nicolet-Meister, D.; and Sand, E. A. "Differences in Age of Walking in Five European Longitudinal Samples." *Human Biology* 38 (1966):363-79.

Hodges, W. L. and Spiker, H. H. "The Effects of Preschool Experiences on Culturally Deprived Children." In *The Young Child*, edited by W. W. Hartup and N. L. Smothergill. Washington, D.C.: National Association for the Education of Young Children, 1967, pp. 262-89.

Jackson, J. J. "Family Organization and Technology." In *Comparative Studies of Blacks and Whites in the United States*, edited by K. S. Miller and R. M. Dreger. New York: Seminar Press, 1973, pp. 405-45.

Keogh, J. *Motor Performance of Elementary School Children*. Los Angeles: University of California, Department of Physical Education, 1965.

Knobloch, H. and Pasamanick, B. "The Relationship of Race and Socioeconomic Status to the Development of Motor Behavior Patterns in Infancy." *Psychiatric Research Reports* 10(1958):123-33.

Leiderman, P. H.; Babu, B.; Kagia, J.; Kraemer, II. C.; and Leiderman, G. F. "African Infant Precocity and Some Social Influences during the First Year. *Nature* 242(1973):247-49.

Malina, R. M. "Growth and Physical Performance of American Negro and White Children." *Clinical Pediatrics* 8(1969):476-83.

Malina, R. M. "Ethnic and Cultural Factors in the Development of Motor Abilities and Strength in American Children." In *Physical Activity: Human Growth and Development*, edited by G. L. Rarick. New York: Academic Press, 1973a, pp. 333-63.

Malina, R. M. "Biological Substrata." In *Comparative Studies of Blacks and Whites in the United States*, edited by K. S. Miller and R. M. Dreger. New York: Seminar Press, 1973b, pp. 53-123.

Malina, R. M. "Physical Anthropology, Physical Activity and Sport." *Canadian Journal of Applied Sport Sciences* 1(1976):155-61.

Malina, R. M. "Motor Development in a Cross-Cultural Perspective." In *Psychology of Motor Behavior and Sport*, vol. II, edited by R. W. Christina and D. M. Landers. Champaign, Illinois: Human Kinetics Publishers, 1977, pp. 191-208.

Malina, R. M. "Growth, Physical Activity and Performance in an Anthropological Perspective." In *Physical Activity and Human Well-Being*, edited by F. Landry and W.A.R. Orban. Miami, Florida: Symposia Specialists, 1978, pp. 3-28.

Moss, H. "Sex, Age and State as Determinants of Mother-Infant Interaction." *Merrill-Palmer Quarterly* 13(1967):19-36.

Neligan, G. and Prudham, D. "Norms for Four Standard Developmental Milestones by Sex, Social Class and Place in Family." *Developmental Medicine and Child Neurology* 11 (1969):413-22.

Pavenstedt, E., ed. *The Drifters*: *Children of Disorganized Lower-Class Families*. Boston: Little, Brown and Company, 1967.

Rosenberg, B. G. and Sutton-Smith, B. "Ordinal Position and Sex-Role Identification." *Genetic Psychology Monographs* 70(1964): 297-328.

Rosenberg, B. G. and Sutton-Smith, B. "Family Interaction Effects on Masculinity-Feminity." *Journal of Personality and Social Psychology* 8(1968):117-20.

Schulz, D. A. *Coming Up Black*: *Patterns of Ghetto Socialization*. Englewood Cliffs, N. J.: Prentice-Hall, Inc., 1969.

Scott, R. B.; Ferguson, A. D.; Jenkins, M. E.; and Cutter, F. F. "Growth and Development of Negro Infants." "Neuromuscular Patterns of Behavior during the First Year of Life." *Pediatrics* 16(1955):24-30.

Sears, R. R.; Maccoby, E. E.; and Levin, H. *Patterns of Child Rearing*. New York: Harper and Row, 1957.

Sinclair, C. B. *Movement and Movement Patterns of Early Childhood*. Richmond, Virginia: State Department of Education, 1971.

Solomons, G. and Solomons, H. C. "Factors Affecting Motor Performance in Four-Month-Old Infants." *Child Development* 35(1964): 1283-95.

Solomons, G. and Solomons, H. C. "Motor Development in Yucatecan Infants." *Developmental Medicine and Child Neurology* 17 (1975):41-46.

Super, C. M. "Environmental Effects on Motor Development: The Case of 'African Infant Precocity.'" *Developmental Medicine and Child Neurology* 18(1976):561-67.

Sutton-Smith, B.; Roberts, J. M.; and Rosenberg, B. G. "Sibling Associations and Role Involvement." *Merrill-Palmer Quarterly* 10 (1964):25-38.

Walker, R. N. "Body Build and Behavior in Young Children." I. "Body Build and Nursery School Teacher's Ratings." *Monographs of the Society for Research in Child Development* 84(1962).

Walters, C. E. "Comparative Development of Negro and White Infants." *Journal of Genetic Psychology* 110(1967):243-51.

Warren, N. "African Infant Precocity." *Psychological Bulletin* 78(1972):353-67.

Waters, E. and Crandall, V. J. "Social Class and Observed Maternal Behavior from 1940 to 1960." *Child Development* 35(1964):1021-32.

Welon, Z. and Sekita, B. "Physical Fitness, Body Size, and Body Build in Preschool Children." *Studies in Physical Anthropology* (Wroclaw, Poland) 2(1975):25-32.

Willerman, L.; Broman, S. H.; and Fiedler, M. "Infant Development, Preschool IQ, and Social Class." *Child Development* 41(1970): 69-77.

Williams, J. R. and Scott, R. B. "Growth and Development of Negro Infants." IV. "Motor Development and Its Relationship to Child Rearing Practices in Two Groups of Negro Infants." *Child Development* 24(1953):103-21.

Yarrow, L. J.; Pedersen, F. A.; and Rubenstein, J. "Mother-Infant Interaction and Development in Infancy." In *Culture and Infancy,* edited by P. H. Leiderman; S. R. Tulkin; and A. Rosenfeld. New York: Academic Press, 1977, pp. 539-64.

Young, V. H. "Family and Childhood in a Southern Negro Community." *American Anthropologist* 72(1970):269-88.

Social-Psychological Correlates to Motor Development

25

Jacqueline Herkowitz
Ohio State University

In the previous chapter you learned about many of the environmentally related correlates to motor development of children. Among these were rearing and social class, rearing and sex differences, rearing and birth order, and ethnic considerations. All of these are social-psychological correlates to motor development. However, these factors were discussed primarily with reference to early childhood development. These factors, and other social-psychological factors which influence motor development, particularly in the elementary school years, will be discussed in this chapter. To some extent there is repetition, however, social-psychological factors play a very significant role in the motor development of children and for this reason some duplication is warranted.

INTRODUCTION

Socialization is the process by which society trains children to behave as adults. Through this process children learn that society has certain values or ideas about what is right and wrong. They learn patterns of behavior common in our society, or what we call norms. And, they come to realize that our society has a social structure in which people are assigned different roles and statuses. A role is the behavior expected of a person who occupies a particular status and status is a position of relative esteem in the social structure. Each child assumes certain statuses and roles within the social structure and quickly becomes aware of the privileges and responsibilities of each.

The goal of society, to be realized through the socialization process, is the creation of socially competent people. Competence in this sense means the ability to socially and physically interact with one's environment in ways that are in keeping with society's expectations. In order to possess such an ability, people must acquire many skills and a good deal of knowledge. The keys to the acquisition of these skills and this knowledge are social learning and maturation. Social learning is learning about a society's culture through the processes of modeling, social reinforcement, and social comparison. Maturation is a process by which the potentialities of an organism demonstrate themselves more or less automatically. Maturation, to a large extent, determines when and to what extent social learning will occur.

The culture of a society encompasses all of the beliefs, institutions, art forms, socially transmitted behavior patterns, and other societal products, that are passed from one generation to the next. Culture provides people with a social reality that lends coherence to their outlook and approach to life. Influenced by cultural forces such as race, social class, ethnic and religious differences, agencies such as the family, peer group, community, and school, through their agents, transmit and teach our culture. These socialization agents include all members of society, but for children the primary agents are parents, teachers, siblings, and peers.

The degree to which the socialization process is effective may be evaluated by assessing a person's ability to function successfully in many social roles. A person who can function successfully in many social roles is said to be socially competent. Competence may be defined as effective role performance in terms of how society defines competence.

A frequent misconception about the socialization process is that it is concerned only with developing interpersonal skills. The socialization process is not only concerned with the development of interpersonal skills, but many other skills and knowledges, all of which help make a person a socially competent member of society. It is important to distinguish between interpersonal competence and social competence. Interpersonal competence refers to certain attitudes and interpersonal skills that facilitate relations between two or more persons. However, a great many other skills and a good deal of additional knowledge must also be acquired by a person in order to be socially competent. Motor skills, writing skills, and speaking skills facilitate effective functioning in society.

These two facets of the socialization process are interdependent. For example, many young children who are poor climbers, throwers, and runners have difficulty developing the interpersonal skills that normally arise through peer group interaction.

This is because many peer group interaction opportunities occur within gross motor play situations which unskilled children avoid. Conversely, children may be skilled in running, throwing, and climbing, but their lack of interpersonal competencies may cause them to be rejected by their peer groups.

INTERPERSONAL COMPETENCE

Interpersonal competence refers to the ability to effectively interact with others. Participation in physical activity, including games, play and sport, provides children with the opportunity to engage in considerable social interaction in a wide variety of settings.

Play Behavior

A number of scholars have suggested that sports were developed by societies in order to develop interpersonal competence in young members (Helanko, 1957), while other have taken the position that societies use physical activity as an important means of socializing the young. Moore and Anderson (1969) hypothesized that each society has developed relatively abstract models in order to socialize their young. These models help familiarize new members with man's relation to the environment. They view: (1) puzzles as models of the relationship between man and nature that are not due to chance or luck, (2) games of chance as models of the relationship between man and uncertain aspects of existence, (3) games of strategy as models of the relationship between man and other men, and (4) art forms as giving man the opportunity to evaluate his/her experiences.

Roberts, Arth, and Bush (1959) have provided evidence to indicate that various games serve as opportunities to master various aspects of the environment. They hypothesized that games of strategy were associated with mastery of the physical environment, and that games of chance were related to familiarization with the supernatural. Roberts and Sutton-Smith (1962) used these same game categories in analyzing the child-rearing practices of over 100 societies. Their findings in part confirmed the study of Roberts, Arth, and Bush (1959) as well as suggesting additional themes. They found that societies which stressed obedience training emphasized games of strategy, societies which emphasized responsibility training stressed games of chance, and that societies which were most concerned with achievement training emphasized games of physical skill. Sutton-Smith, Roberts, and Kozelka (1963) then used these findings to predict game preferences among segments of our society that could be differentiated on these three dimensions of child rearing. They confirmed the prediction within our society for boys and girls, and among adults who differed by sex, education and occupation. Taken together these studies do suggest a positive relationship exists between games and the development of interpersonal competence. They do not give much insight, however, into how such games are used to help children acquire interpersonal competence, nor whether societies are successful through these games in developing interpersonal competence in their young members.

Leadership

Leadership is one area of interpersonal competence. Proficiency in motor behavior as reflected by the motor development process is thought by some to be related to leadership. Evidence concerning this relationship is presented in this section.

Between one and three years of age, physical prowess is usually not an important factor in gaining leadership because the social organization of children at those ages is not complex. Children in this age group usually imitate and engage in parallel play, perhaps with one other individual. Forming groups and deciding upon a leader does not occur until about age four. As the child reaches five or six years of age, play units grow larger. At that time leadership and social recognition are often gained through effective physical performance. Studies by Parten (1933) and Hardy (1937) indicate that group leaders among five- and six-year-olds who are identified by teachers and pupils as "most liked" and "popular," are children who demonstrate high levels of physical skill. According to Hardy, social recognition during the elementary school years is closely related to a child's ability to distinguish oneself from his/her peers. If this is true, it is reasonable to assume that excellence in physical performance situations would contribute in part to the ability of a child to capture and maintain a leadership position.

A number of attempts have been made to experimentally induce leadership behavior in children at play. Jack (1934), for example, surveyed children's play groups and selected those children who exhibited a lack of leadership. (i.e., low "ascendant" scores). These children were given specific training in using specific types of play materials by the experimenter, and then were placed in new groups. Their interactions were again recorded. Significant changes in these children's ascendant behaviors in the new groups were exhibited. Children trained in this manner exhibited impatience at the mistakes of their companions while a "control" group within the investigation who had received no training in using specific play materials exhibited no comparable changes in behavior. It would seem, therefore, that children may learn leadership behaviors as a result of group esteem as well as by an outcome of their own perceived proficiencies within play situations. When they begin to perceive their own potential for leadership, they begin acting as leaders, assuming a role that reflects ascendent behavior (including gestures and verbalization as well as specific and general leadership skills).

As adolescence is reached and youngsters play within more absolute rules, leadership may be bestowed for different reasons that were apparent during early, middle, and late childhood. Jones and Bayley (1950) found that physically accelerated boys were more accepted, and were treated more favorably, by both peers and adults. Such status leads to positions of leadership and persists in measurements of personality traits made during adulthood. Several studies seem to indicate that as boys progress from the elementary school years social status increases as a function of athletic ability (Anastasiow, 1965; Coleman, 1961; Hunt and Solomon, 1942; Nelson, 1966). At the same time, other studies (Davitz, 1955; Jones, 1948) indicate that with increased interaction the effects of athletic ability on social status may be diminished. Boys begin to look for less obvious personality qualities on which to base their friendships. Nelson (1966) studied the personality traits and social attributes of captains of basketball teams and found that leadership on these teams was not always attained by the best-liked boys. Boys who became captains of these teams were often rated as selfish by their peers. However, at the same time, the student leaders' proficiencies and social skills had somehow gained them the grudging respect of their teammates. Adolescent boys who are more accepted and who become leaders are those who tend to carry impulses into action (Pigors, 1933) and who desire to lead (Puffer, 1905). Leaders of adolescent teams are generally more interested in people and tend to be aware of others' needs for social recognition. They are talkative and socially expressive, adventurous and relatively impervious to social criticism (Nelson, 1966).

As girls grow older less emphasis is placed upon excellence in physical activity. Differentiation based upon sex role occurs regarding the acquisition of leadership via physical prowess. This sex difference becomes most pronounced as adolescence is reached. Tyron (1939) found that girls at ages 12 and 15 possessing ability at "active games" gained little prestige and were at times looked upon with disfavor. By the age of 15 it seemed that girls who were classified good at games benefited from it in terms of prestige only if they were not successful in heterosexual relations.

As early adulthood is reached, emphasis on athletics and the resultant prestige diminishes. However, even in adult life, outstanding athletic endeavor coupled with other leadship qualities important to the mature community (e.g., intelligence) can enhance the extent to which an individual achieves some leadership role.

Outlining trends relative to the assumption of social success, status, or leadership as a function of age and sex is a somewhat tenuous undertaking. At the preent time it is not possible to find direct causal relationships between sociality and physical proficiency during infancy, childhood, and adolescence. The presently available evidence which suggests that a relationship exists between interpersonal skills and physical activity is largely correlational and does not indicate that participation in physical activities causes that development of interpersonal competence. This does not mean, however, that generalizations based on existing correlational evidence are not valid. It simply means that they must be interpreted cautiously until causal evidence is available. It would be foolish for an educator to ignore the marked influence that game success has on the social acceptance of children.

Interpersonal Competence and Physical Activity. It may be that the relationship between physical activity and interpersonal competence may be a circular spiraling relationship. Those children who are emotionally healthy and socially better adjusted engage in a good deal of physical activity and social interaction because they have higher levels of physical skillfulness. Because of their higher levels of physical skillfulness they receive favorable evaluation by their peers. Poorly adjusted children probably elect to engage in more individualized, less demanding physical activities, or in fewer physical activities. They are, therefore, in a less favorable position for obtaining desirable evaluation by their peers.

There is some research which suggests that one way to help children in attempting to improve motor skills is to break the circular spiral previously eluded to. A number of investigators (Brown, 1970; Haley, 1969; Johnston, Kelley, Harris, and Wolf, 1966) have provided evidence to indicate that improvement in motor skills via participation in special motor skill development programs results in increased peer acceptance and self-concept. However, the type of activity selected, the instructional techniques to be used in the program, and the specific interpersonal skills to be developed all need careful consideration if such motor skill development programs are to be successful in increasing interpersonal competence. Not all physical activity programs automatically result in improved interpersonal competencies (Olson, 1968).

CULTURAL FACTORS INFLUENCING MOTOR DEVELOPMENT

As discussed in the preceding chapter, cultural factors are important to the motor development process. Among the more important cultural forces operative in any society are social class, ethnicity, race, and religion. Different groups possess unequal amounts of prestige, opportunity, wealth, and influence. Social class is often divided into upper, middle, and lower class, based on family income, occupational level of the father, educational level, or location of residence. Social class is important because differences among classes differentially influence the socialization of member children. The types of learning experiences to which children are exposed, children's self-concepts, the manner in which personality dispositions and attitudes are developed, and the goal-setting behavior of children, differ from one social class to another.

Social Class

Unfortunately too little is known about the relationship between social class and physical activity. It may be that social class interacts with other variables to influence physical activity. For example, social approval has been found to facilitate the performance of lower class boys and disapproval impair their performance more than it does for middle class boys (Rosenhan, 1966). It may well be that different social classes use different forms of social reinforcement, and it is this fact that directly influences motor skill acquisition. Many questions regarding the relationship between differences in social class and motor behavior need to be asked. Is the amount of physical activity engaged in by children of a particular social class associated with encouragement by adult members of that social class? Do differing social classes value different motor skills? Are peer groups in different social classes important encouragers of skill acquisition in child members? Do the families of different social classes provide more or less opportunity to participate in certain physical activities? But as noted in the previous chapter, few answers are available.

Ethnicity

Ethnic differences influence the socialization process because members of ethnic groups learn unique knowledges, skills, attitudes, and perspectives that are associated with that subcultural group. Frequently the unique cultural differences associated with an ethnic group are in conflict with the values and norms of the larger society. When they are, the ethnic group is generally assigned inferior status and roles in the social structure of society and subjected to unequal treatment. Minority groups are often denied equal access to the material goods of society as well as many cultural opportunities and experiences. Such material and social deprivation generally restricts minority groups' opportunity to learn the norms and values of the larger society and influences minority members self-

concept, attitudes, and personality dispositions. Not only are the members of ethnic and minority groups socialized in a culturally distinct group, but they are discriminated against for their differences by other socialization agents of society who should be helping these people fit into the larger society.

Are ethnic differences and corresponding differences in socialization patterns related to differences in minority members' physical skillfulness or fitness? Most available evidence has been gained studying blacks. It appears that black infants are more precocious than whites (Bayley, 1965; Knobloch and Pasamanick, 1953, 1958; Scott, Ferguson, Jenkins, and Cutter, 1955; Solomons and Solomons, 1964; Walters, 1967; Williams and Scott, 1953). Black elementary school children seem to perform physical skills slightly better than white elementary school children. However, there are relatively few differences between whites and blacks in physical performance at all other ages (Barker and Ponthieux, 1965; Lambert and Lanier, 1933; Moore, 1941; Ponthieux and Barker, 1965; Stone, 1966). Unequal access to various sport equipment, the impact of black athletes appearing on television frequently, and possible uniquenesses associated with child rearing practices, may, to some extent, explain whatever differences exist.

AGENTS AND AGENCIES

Just as evidence related to the influence of cultural forces is meager, our understanding of the influence of such agencies as the family, peer group, and school, and of such agents as parents, siblings, peers, and teachers, on motor skill learning is largely intuitive or based on experience.

Family

The family is the first and most important socialization agency. Parents attempt to socialize their children in a manner that reflects what they believe the child ought to be like. Their efforts, in turn, are influenced by the social settings in which the family operates. Some of the behavior patterns that a child learns through the family are characteristic of the larger culture and others are unique of the particular family. It is through interaction with family members that a child learns values, attitudes, self deportment, and something of the child's status in society. The family, through social mechanisms of reinforcement, modeling, and comparison processes, provides children with their first rewards and punishments, their first models, and their opportunities to make comparisons.

The child's development of physical skillfulness, knowledges, and attitudes regarding physical performance are enormously influenced by the family. The amount of physical control exerted by parents appears influential in the acquisition of motor skills by children between the ages of two and six years. The amount of physical mobility permitted by mothers varies markedly between parents. Sears, Maccoby, and Levin (1957) found that about 50 percent of the mothers studied in their investigation restricted children of five and six years to their immediate' neighborhood, and 11 percent restricted their children to the yard. Only 1 percent of the parents surveyed admitted imposing no restrictions on their child's geographical play areas.

The same study also evaluated the amount of physical restriction which was imposed on the child's motor behavior in the home. About half the parents did not permit children to jump from furniture or engage in other vigorous activity within the home. However, 30 percent indicated that they permitted their children to move in the home in a moderate fashion within certain restricted areas.

Montemayor (1974) has shown that sex-labeling a neutral toy as inappropriate or appropriate for a certain sex child very much influences the amount of use and preference that the child shows to the toy. Goldberg and Lewis (1969), watching 13-month-old boys and girls in interaction with their mothers, have found that girls were more dependent than boys, showed less exploratory behavior, and demonstrated quieter play behaviors. Boys played with toys that required more gross motor activity. They tended to be more vigorous and to run more in their play. Girls proved more reluctant than boys to leave their mothers, staying near them during play, and seeking physical reassurance more often. Both of these studies suggest that the family plays a potent role in defining gender appropriate movement behavior for young children.

It seems apparent on consideration of the previous information that the parents exert early and direct influences that mold the child's inclinations for action and the amount of vigorous activity they consistently express in various structured and unstructured play situations. Whether parental influences are direct though reinforcement or modeling procedures, or whether they are indirect through the development of attitudes and personality dispositions is not always clear. More than likely it is a combination of both factors.

It would be interesting to know whether interest in physical activity and motor proficiency are associated with parental provision of space and equipment. It is correct to assume that parents who themselves engage in physical activity, who value physical fitness, and who reward the acquisition of motor skills, will have children who are more competent and interested in physical activity? Just what types of parent-child relationships foster the acquisition of accurate and positive concepts about oneself performing physical skills? Which parent is most influential in the development of such accurate and positive concepts? Do siblings, their sex, and birth order, influence the acquisition of motor skills and the development of interest in physical activity?

Peers

The peer group plays an increasingly important role in socializing the child as the child grows older. It provides the child with the opportunity to learn about "taboo" subjects, expand social horizons, establish self-concept, participate in egalitarian types of relationships, and participate in situations involving group expression.

The peer group has its own norms and values. Acceptance in and rejection from peer groups are largely determined by a child's ability to learn these norms and accept these values. These norms and values strongly influence a child's behavior, attitudes, and personality. The peer group can provide important reinforcers and models for the acquisition of motor skills and knowledges regarding physical activity.

School

The school is a formal institution of society designed to socialize its members. Its basic function is to transmit basic skills and knowledges to children. In addition to the "three R's," many less obvious skills, knowledges, and dispositions are intended

to be transmitted by the school. The teacher, as the agent of the school, obviously serves as an important model and reinforcer for the development of a wide range of skills, knowledges, and dispositions.

Physical education is a unit of the school whose primary socialization function is the transmission of skills and knowledge about physical fitness and movement. Other agencies of society, of course, are also important in teaching these skills and knowledges, however, the acquisition of such skills and knowledges is more frequently a secondary function of these agencies. An important question then is, "How successful is physical education in accomplishing its primary socialization function?" Do other agencies such as the family, peer groups, and other sport or recreational organizations contribute more or less than physical education to accomplishing this function?

Obviously, physical education programs have been somewhat successful in achieving their primary socialization function. However, no attempt has been made to compare the contributions of physical education with those of other cultural forces, agencies, and agents of society that most directly influence the development of social and motor competence.

OTHER SOCIAL-PSYCHOLOGICAL FACTORS

In addition to the social-psychological factors already discussed, there are others which influence motor development or are influenced by the motor development process. Social reinforcement, social facilitation, social evaluation, observational learning, and sex role stereotyping are five that will be discussed in this section.

Social Reinforcement

Social reinforcements are nonverbal and verbal messages sent by one individual to another that increase the strength of the latter's behavioral responses. Praise and censure, smiles and sneers, and friendly and hostile gestures are some of the forms that social reinforcements often take. Social reinforcements are able to energize and direct the motor learning and motor performance of children.

A number of factors mediate the influence of social reinforcement on social and verbal behaviors, and on very simple motor tasks. One of the most consistent findings in the social reinforcement literature has been the cross-sex effect; the finding that females who act as social reinforcers have more influence on male subjects and vice versa (Gewirtz, 1954; Gewirtz and Baer, 1958). This is not true with children under five years of age, however. Both boys and girls in this age group are consistently most influenced by social reinforcements delivered by females (Stevenson, 1961).

Another interesting difference is that younger children are more affected by social reinforcement than older children. The period of childhood during which verbal encouragement and various other kinds of social reinforcers appear to affect performance most is between six and about ten or eleven years. After this age, children seems to be able to block off various kinds of social re-inforcers, becoming more sensitive to the intrinsic interest and difficulty of the task itself (Murphy and Murphy, 1935; Lewis, Wall, and Aronfreed, 1963).

Baron (1966) recently found that when social reinforcement is considerably above or below a person's expectation, that the individual will vary task performance in a manner that is likely to result in receiving reinforcement which is more in keeping with expectations. The implication of this is that if you expect an average amount of positive reinforcement but receive a great deal of praise, you may attempt to perform less well in order to bring reinforcements more in line with your expectations.

A final issue deals with the relative influence of positive and negative social reinforcements. On simple tasks where only two responses are possible, punishments alone tend to be more effective short-term reinforcers than rewards (Brackbill and O'Hara, 1958; Curry, 1960; Meyer and Seidman, 1960, 1961). However, on tasks such as complex motor skills where more than two responses are possible, rewards appear more effective than punishments (Crandall, Good, and Crandall, 1962).

It appears that at least some positive reinforcement is essential to the motor development process for all people. While a proper balance of praise and criticism appears to be essential to effective motor performance, it is clear that positive social reinforcement is critical to early motor development. Further, though praise and positive reinforcement may provide the learner with little information which is of value in learning a skill, it may be of value in motivating children to learn motor skills. This is especially true for simple skills and for skills which have already been overlearned.

Social Facilitation

Children are often asked to learn and perform motor tasks in front of parents, peers, and teachers. It is natural to ask whether the presence of these people facilitates or impedes their efforts. Social facilitation refers to any increment or impairment of motor behavior that is the direct consequence of the presence of one or more other individuals. Zajonc (1965) popularized the term social facilitation as a general term that referred to both positive and negative effects that were a consequence of the presence of others. He included two conditions under the social facilitation rubric. The audience effect refers to the behavioral effects occurring due to the presence of passive spectators. The coaction effect refers to the behavioral effects due to the presence of other individuals who are doing the same thing at the same time, independently.

Zajonc (1965) distinguished between learning and performance, and interpreted social facilitation effects in terms of drive theory. He hypothesized that on simple tasks that required little learning, the presence of others resulted in improved performance. However, on complex tasks which required considerable learning, task performance decreased in the presence of others. He also hypothesized that the presence of others increases arousal and concluded that the mere presence of others impairs learning because the aroused individual more frequently emits incorrect responses, but the presence of others facilitates the performance of well-learned tasks because the aroused person more often emits the correct response. Investigations of audience effects and coaction effects have generally supported Zajonc's social facilitation theory. (Cottrell, Rittle, and Wack, 1967; Ganzer, 1968; Martens, 1969; Rosenquist, 1972; Zajonc and Sales, 1966), (Ader and Tatum, 1963; Burwitz and Newell, 1972; Carment and Latchford, 1970; Martens and Landers, 1969; Martens and Landers, 1972; Schachter, 1959; Seidman, Bensen, Miller, and Meeland, 1957).

Evaluation apprehension studies provide a potential explanation for why the mere presence of others has proven to be arousing (Cottrell, Wack, Sekerak, and Rittle, 1968; Henchy and Glass, 1968; Klinger, 1969; Martens and Landers, 1972). They have shown that the presence of an audience or coactor who was blindfolded and could not evaluate an individual's performance did not produce the expected social facilitation phenomenon. Only when the audience was in a position to evaluate the subject's performance did impeding or facilitory effects occur. The mere presence of others is not a sufficient condition for social facilitation to occur. The audience or coacters must be perceived as having the potential to evaluate the subject's performance. However, the potential for evaluation is present in the presence of others. It is children's learning to associate desirable and undesirable outcomes with these particular evaluative situations that makes social facilitation an important phenomenon.

A variety of individual and situational variables seem to influence the degree to which the presence of others effects performance. Some of these factors are the nature of the task, the nature of the audience, the relationship of the audience or coactor to the performer, and the personality and ability of the performer. Maturation may also mediate social facilitation effects. Prior to the age of six, children, when confronted by an audience, seem to become generally excited and aroused. But this increase in activation does not usually translate itself into improved motor performance scores on simple tasks as it does for older subjects. Missiuro (1964) examined the social facilitation effect as it influenced the behavior of children and adults. Electromyographic changes of muscular tension in children of various ages were compared with those of adults. Two types of tasks were employed in the investigation. One involved the performance of long, rhythmical work on an ergograph. The load of the ergograph was varied by age. The second involved maximal isometric contractions of the upper-arm muscles during which electric potentials were recorded. Both activities were performed and recorded in the presence of an experimenter and later in the presence of other children. Missiuro found, when only an experimenter was present, that younger children evidenced a spread of electrical excitation throughout muscle groups not directly involved in the volitional contractions. Older children and adults evidenced electrical excitation specifically located in the arm under volitional control. Missiuro's findings of excitatory processes over inhibitory processes in the central nervous system in early stages of development. The same general excitation was exhibited by the younger children again when an audience was present during the performance of the finger ergograph task. The younger children failed to exhibit any improvement in the presence of the audience due to general excitation, which manifested itself in behavior inappropriate to the task. Children who were older than six years of age and adults exhibited improvement when asked to perform in the presence of an audience. In addition, Missiuro also found that boys over six years of age were more favorably influenced by the presence of an audience than were girls of the same age.

The influence of coactors and audiences (social facilitation) on the motor development of children is not totally understood. Many factors mediate the social facilitation effect. However, it is generally acknowledged that the presence of others is detrimental when initially learning motor tasks, but facilitates performance once tasks are

well-learned. It appears that the evaluation apprehension associated with the presence of others who have the potential to evaluate the individual positively or negatively, rather than the mere presence of others, is responsible for the operation of these phenomena. It would seem that when teaching motor skills, particularly to children who become nervous in the presence of others, instruction in nonevaluative situations is more desirable than instruction in evaluative situations. Additionally, when one wishes to facilitate the performance of motor skills that are well-learned by children, the presence of an evaluative audience may help.

Observational Learning (Modeling)

We have just examined how the presence of others in the form of audiences or coactors influences an individual's behavior. We will now consider how observing others influences the behavior of an audience of one. Observational learning is said to occur when an individual approximates his/her behavior to that of a model in order to learn some behavior. Social cues, rather than impersonal cues, guide the selection of particular behaviors to be approximated. The young child watches a brother mount and ride a bicycle and tries to do the same thing. A teacher demonstrates an underhand volleyball serve in a fifth grade physical education class and asks his/her children to "do it this way." Demonstrations frequently provide an economical means of sharing information. Learning by observation is of great significance in the socialization process through which culture is transmitted. It is through this process that children learn to speak, gesture, and perform a large variety of specialized sport skills.

Some of the important information about observational learning is summarized below:

1. If a child is exposed to an inferior model, that child will tend to adopt relatively low standards. Conversely, if a child is exposed to a more competent model, the child will establish relatively high standards of performance for self-reinforcement. Therefore, it is important that those who model motor skills be relatively highly skilled. However, if the model is very superior to the child, the child tends to reject the very high standards set by that model and adopt relatively lower standards for themselves. Because of this it is effective to make use of peer models in physical skills learning settings.

2. Observers more frequently imitate models who are successful, who have high status, who control resources valued by the observer, and who are perceived competent. The more frequently a model's responses are rewarded, the more the observer tends to imitate those responses. Reinforcement given to peer models tends to encourage imitative behavior on the part of other students.

3. Live models may be most effective, but filmed or televised exposure to models can also be impactful. The use of recognized tennis and basketball professionals as models has not only impact on the motor skill learning of children, it may also influence children's interpersonal skills. Both desirable and undesirable observational learning is occurring as a direct result of television. Both incorrect and correct behaviors can be modeled in learning situations. Incorrect models may impair performance. Therefore, it is essential that models demonstrate accurately.

4. A teacher models all the time he or she is before a class. Not only are specific skills fair game for the observer, but the teacher's general behavior is also influencial. Teachers who demonstrate rational control of their behavior, respect for others, interest in students as individuals, good listening and communicative skills, emotional control, logical thinking and problem solving behavior, and curiosity and interest in learning for its own sake, encourage those behaviors in the children who observe them.

The presence of others both energizes behavior (social facilitation) and influences the direction of behavior (observational learning). Thus far the impression has been given that observational learning is always desirable and is an all-encompassing phenomenon. This is not true. Although imitation is desirable in many facets of motor learning and performance, it is not in others. It may be a powerful technique and most appropriate when certain skills need to be introduced to a group of children. However, modeling is of limited value when skills need to be performed in a great variety of settings and under a variety of conditions. Complex tasks require practice as well as observational learning. Creative performances rarely benefit from extensive observational learning opportunities alone.

Social Evaluation

Social evaluation is the appraisal of one's ability through receiving information from other persons. The developing child has little past experience upon which to draw and consequently is very dependent on others for information about reality and the adequacy of his or her abilities for dealing with this reality (Jones and Gerard, 1967). There are at least three separate processes of social evaluation of ability including comparative appraisal, reflected appraisal, and consultation.

Comparative appraisal is the process of comparing with others to determine one's own relative standing on some ability (Jones and Gerard, 1967). Comparative appraisal occurs when the comparison standard is another individual's performance rather than a past or idealized performance standard. Developmental literature indicates that this comparative appraisal process becomes extremely important to children at about four or five years of age and intensifies as children progress through the elementary school years (Master, 1972; Veroff, 1969; White, 1960).

Very young children do not compete or compare themselves with others (Greenberg, 1932, 1952: Masters, 1972; Veroff, 1969; White, 1960). They spend their time autonomously collecting considerable information about their own personal abilities through solitary play, exploration, mastery attempts, and striving to attain autonomous achievement goals (Cook and Stingle, 1974; Veroff, 1969; White, 1959, 1960). Eventually, however, personal ability has to be placed into a larger relative framework through comparative appraisal in order to achieve an accurate assessment of ability. Children appear to engage in this process at about four or five years of age (Cook & Stingle, 1974; Greenberg, 1932, 1952: Leuba, 1933: Masters, 1972; Veroff, 1969). Comparative and competitive behavior increase with age throughout the elementary school years with a peak reached around grades four, five or six (Cook and Stingle, 1974; Kagan and Madsen, 1972: McClintock and Nuttin, 1969; Nelson, 1970; Veroff, 1969). It is during this age period that many children engage in competitive youth sport activities

and it is in this arena that much of the comparative appraisal process occurs. Further, since the appraisal is of motor ability and to excel in physical skills is an esteemed commodity of children, the comparative appraisal involves a potentially very potent group of outcomes.

The second social evaluation process is reflected appraisal. This is the process by which the child "derives an impression of his position on some attribute through the behavior of another person toward him" (Jones and Gerard, 1967). For example, a teacher might unintentionally transmit reflected appraisal cues to a child after the child has failed in performing a motor task. Many different people can potentially provide reflected appraisal. These include teachers, parents, as well as peers. Many evaluative cues may be unintentionally emitted, but easily detected by the child. For example, parents may provide cues of pride and approval after successful motor performance, or embarrassment and disapproval after failure. Other examples include the nonverbal behaviors indicating elation by coaches, teammates, and supporting fans when a highly skilled player steps up to bat with bases loaded or the nonverbal behaviors indicating chagrin by these same individuals when a relatively unskilled player is faced with a similar situation. Reflected appraisal can represent an evaluation that is based on many observations rather than on a one time occurrence. In such a situation the potency of reflected appraisal is increased.

A third social evaluation process is termed consultation. This involves the child directly asking another person for an ability appraisal or directly receiving an evaluation without having necessarily asked for one (Jones and Gerard, 1967). The consultation process usually involves evaluation from parents, teachers, or peers. For example, parents frequently provide children with information about how well they are throwing a ball, batting, or performing a gymnastics stunt. Teachers have the job of evaluating ability and providing extensive information that indicate the strengths, weaknesses, and progress of a chid.

It is not difficult to see that all aspects of the social evaluation process are important to the motor development of the child. As the child develops he/she relies on social evaluation to obtain information about motor performance. It is through social evaluation that children determine their ability (perceived ability) and set motor performance goas for themselves. Anyone concerned about the motor development of children should understand the social evaluation process and should be concerned with helping children mediate the social evaluation information to set realistic motor performance goals.

Sex-Role Stereotyping

As previously outlined, physical activities and their perceived appropriateness for the different sexes is established early in life. Within each society certain stereotypes develop concerning appropriate physical activity behaviors for males and females. As early as the second year of life, American boys have adopted more vigorous play styles than girls and girls are more dependent on their mothers than are boys. (Goldberg and Lewis, 1969). Early studies by Sutton-Smith and Rosenberg (1961) and Rosenberg and Sutton-Smith (1960) indicate that play preferences and activities appropriate for each sex have changed in recent decades. Based on data from 1896, 1921, 1929, and 1959, it is clear that game preferences have changed

over time. Findings indicate that the game preferences of girls are becoming more like those of boys, and boys tend to be more limited in the games in which they participate. Though more activities are becoming identified as "'boy-girl" activities, "boy" activities as characterized by children are becoming more clearly identified. These data are somewhat dated, though more recent studies tend to support these general findings.

Herkowitz (1976), on the basis of a study of 360 school children of different ages, arrived at four basic conclusions concerning sex typing of motor activities. First children tended to perceive most motor activities as appropriate for both sexes. Second, as children grow older the sex groups were more likely to sex-type activities similarly. The third finding related to the nature of the differences in choices between sexes. The most noticible differences were the tendencies for very young boys to select boy-girl ratings less often than older groups. Finally, it was found that the most strongly sex-typed activities were overwhelmingly perceived as "boy" activities. Those activities requiring strength, power, and speed or "force production" were most frequently perceived to be "boy" activities.

As previously noted, it is likely that the exact nature of the activities perceived as male and female have changed over the decades. However, it also seem clear that more activities are becoming "non-sex" activities. That is, increasingly more activities are rated by both boys and girls as appropriate for either sex. At the same time, the activities that are not classified as boys-girls are becoming more strongly sex stereotyped, especially for "boy" or male activities.

Cratty (1967) noted that males gain leadership roles and recognition through activities requiring physical strength and prowess while females earn leadership and recognition through verbal abilities and manipulative skills. Methaney (1970) noted that some activities, namely those requiring body contact, strength, and explosive power are perceived in our society as "categorically unacceptable" for females. Activities involving light resistance, use of a light object or implement, and a barrier such as a net are perceived as "generally acceptable" for females. Corbin and Nix (1979) classified three different motor tasks using a scheme similar to that outlined by Metheny. Results indicated that both boys and girls rated the task requiring strength, muscular endurance, and power as a "boy" activity. Of the three tasks the one which was fine muscle manipulative was most frequently rated as a "girls" task though the manipulative task and a gross body balance task were both perceived to be basically "boy-girl" activities. This study supported the general notion that most types of activities are rated as "boy-girl" though as previous studies have indicated, and as movement theorists have suggested, certain types of activities are still perceived to be "for males only." Interestingly, both boys and girls tend to perceive the strength, power, speed activities to be male in orentation.

One study (Brawley, Landers, Miller, and Kearns, 1979) indicates that both males and females may be prejudiced against female performers when making subjective evaluations on a motor task. In their study, both male and female subjects rated the performance of females to be worse than the performance of males when in fact the actual performance was identical.

It appears that sex-role stereotyping does exist. Though the rapid increase in sport's opportunities for females has already resulted in a changed perception of the female in physical activity, the early socialization of children in "appropriate sex-roles" is too powerful to offset recent changes in behavior of females in activity. It may be that in some activities, because of structural and physiolgical sex differences, females may not as a group equal males in absolute performance. However, there is no convincing scientific evidence to indicate that any activity is the exclusive domain of the male. As the past has seen changes in sex-role expectations, the future will see continued change. It docs appear that females, as well as males, will have to change their attitudes about "appropriate" activities for females if the future is to see the elimination of sex-role stereotypes in physical activity.

SUMMARY

As the child develops various social-psychological factors most certainly influence that development. Motor development, as one important aspect of total development, is infuenced by these social-psychological factors. The child must receive positive social reinforcement and must learn to use social evaluation to set realistic goals and to make accurate assessments of his or her own ability. The social environment (observational learning and social facilitation) will also influence the child's motor development as will sex-role stereotypes which may result in perception of "I can't or I shouldn't" in activity if the child feels that the activity is inappropriate. In addition it is important to know that optimal motor development may, under certain circumstances, influence social and personal development in areas such as interpersonal competence and leadership. Regardless, a knowledge of the interrelationships between motor development and social-psychological factors is essential to the study of motor development.

References

Ader, R. and Tatum, R. "Free-Operant Avoidance Conditioning in Individual and Paired Human Subjects." *Journal of Experimental Animal Behavior* 6(1963):357.

Anastasiow, N. J. "Success in School and Boys' Sex Role Patterns." *Child Development* 33 (1965):1053.

Barker, D. G. and Ponthieux, N. A. "Relationships between Race and Physical Fitness." *Research Quarterly* 36(1965):468.

Baron, R. M. "Social Reinforcement Effects as a Function of Social Reinforcement History." *Psychological Review* 6(1966):527.

Bayley, N. "Comparisons of Mental and Motor Test Scores for Ages 15 Months by Sex, Birth Order, Race, Geographical Location, and Education of Parents." *Child Development* 36(1965):379.

Brackbill, Y. and O'Hara, J. "The Relative Effectiveness of Reward and Punishment for Discriminative Learning in Children." *Journal of Comparative and Physical Psychology* 51(1958):747.

Brawley, L. R. et al. "Sex Bias in Evaluation Motor Performance." *Journal of Sex Roles* 1(1979):15.

Brown, J. B. "The Influence of a Motor Development Program on the Social Performance of Preschool Males." Paper presented at the Second Canadian Psycho-Motor Learning and Sports Psychology Symposium, University of Windsor, 1970.

Burwitz, L. and Newell, K. M. "The Effects of the Mere Presence of Coactors on Learning a Motor Skill." *Journal of Motor Behavior* 4 (1972):99.

Carment, D. W. and Latchford, M. "Rate of Simple Motor Responding as a Function of Coaction, Sex of the Participants, and the Presence or Absence of the Experimenter." *Psychonomic Science* 20(1970):253.

Coleman, J. S. *The Adolescent Society.* New York: Free Press of Glencoe, 1961.

Corbin, C. B. and Nix, C. "Sex Typing of Physical Activities and Success Predictions of Children Before and After Cross-Sex Competition." *Journal of Sport Psychology* 1(1979): 43.

Cook, H. and Stingle, S. "Cooperative Behavior in Children." *Psychological Bulletin* 81 (1974):918.

Cottrell, N. B. "Performance in the Presence of Other Human Beings: Mere Presence, Audience, and Affiliation Effects." In *Social Facilitation and Imitative Behavior,* edited by E. C. Simmel; R. A. Hoppe; and G. A. Milton. Boston: Allyn & Bacon, 1968, p. 91.

———; Rittle, R. H.; and Wack, D. L. "The Presence of an Audience and List Type (Competitional or Noncompetitional) as Joint Determinants of Performance in Paired-Associates Learning." *Journal of Personality* 35 (1967):425.

———; Wack, D. L.; Sekerak, G. J.; and Rittle, R. H. "Social Facilitation of Dominant Responses by the Presence of an Audience and Mere Presence of Others." *Journal of Personality and Social Psychology* 9(1968):245.

Crandall, V. C.; Good, S.; and Crandall, V. J. "The Reinforcement Effects of Adult Reactions and Non-Reactions on Children's Achievement Expectations: A Replication Study." *American Psychologist* 17(1962): 299.

Cratty, B. J. *Social Dimensions of Physical Activity.* Englewood Cliffs, N. J.: Prentice-Hall, 1967.

Curry, C. "Supplementary Report: The Effects of Verbal Reinforcement Combinations on Learning in Children." *Journal of Experimental Psychology* 59(1960):434.

Davitz, J. R. "Social Perception and Sociometric Choice of Children." *Journal of Abnormal and Social Psychology* 50(1955):173.

Ganzer, V. J. "Effects of Audience Presence and Test Anxiety on Learning and Retention in a Serial Learning Situation." *Journal of Personality and Social Psychology* 8(1968):194.

——— and Baer, D. M. "Deprivation and Satiation of Social Reinforcers as Drive Conditions." *Journal of Abnormal and Social Psychology* 57(1958):165.

Goldberg, S. and Lewis, M. "Play Behavior in the Year-Old Infant: Early Sex Differences." *Child Development* 40(1969):21.

Greenberg, P. J. "Competition in Children: An Experimental Study." *American Journal of Psychology* 44(1932):221.

———. "The Growth of Competitiveness during Childhood." In *Psychological Studies of Human Development,* edited by R. G. Kuhlen and G. G. Thompson. New York: Appleton-Century-Crofts, 1952, p. 337.

Haley, B. B. "The Effects of Individualized Movement Programs upon Emotionally Disturbed Children." Doctoral Dissertation, Louisiana State University, 1969.

Hardy, M. C. "Social Recognition at the Elementary School Age." *Journal of Social Psychology* 8(1937):365.

Helanko, R. "Sports and Socialization." *Acta Sociologica* 2(1957):229.

Henchy, T. and Glass, D. C. "Evaluation Apprehension and the Social Facilitation of Dominant and Subordinate Responses." *Journal of Personality and Social Psychology* 10 (1968):446.

Herkowitz, J. "Sex-Role Expectations and Motor Behavior of Young Children." In *Motor Development: Issues and Applications*, edited by M. V. Ridenour. Princeton, N. J.: Princeton Book Company, 1978.

Hunt, J. M. and Solomon, R. L. "The Stability and Some Correlates of Group Status in a Summer Camp Group of Young Boys." *American Journal of Psychology* 55(1942): 33.

Jack, L. M. "An Experimental Study of Ascendant Behavior in Preschool Children." *University of Iowa Studies in Child Welfare* 9 (1934):7.

Johnston, M. K.; Kelley, C. S.; Harris, F. R.; and Wolf, M. M. "An Application of Reinforcement Principles to Development of Motor Skills of a Young Child." *Child Development* 37(1966):379.

Jones, M. C. "Adolescent Friendships." *American Psychologist* 3(1948):352.

——— and Bayley, N. "Physical Maturing among Boys as Related to Behavior." *Journal of Educational Psychology* 41(1950):129.

Jones, E. E. and Gerard, H. B. *Foundations of Social Psychology.* New York: John Wiley and Sons, Inc., 1967.

Kagan, S. and Madsen, M. C. "Rivalry in Anglo-American and Mexican Children of Two Ages." *Journal of Personality and Social Psychology* 24(1972):214.

Klinger, E. "Feedback Effects and Social Facilitation of Vigilance Performance: Mere Coaction Versus Potential Evaluation." *Psychonomic Science* 14(1969):161.

Knobloch, H. and Pasamanick, B. "Further Observations on the Behavioral Development of Negro Children." *Journal of Genetic Psychology* 83(1953):137.

——— and Pasamanick, B. "The Relationship of Race and Socioeconomic Status to the Development of Motor Behavior Patterns in Infancy." *Psychiatric Research Reports* 10 (1958):123.

Lambert, M. and Lanier, L. H. "Race Differences in Speed of Reaction." *Journal of Genetic Psychology* 42(1933):255.

Leuba, C. "An Experimental Study of Rivalry in Children." *Journal of Comparative Psychology* 16(1933):367.

Lewis, M.; Wall, M.; and Aronfreed, J. "Developmental Change in Relative Values of Social and Non-Social Reinforcements." *Journal of Experimental Psychology* 66(1963): 133.

Martens, R. "Effect of an Audience on Learning and Performance of a Complex Motor Skill." *Journal of Personality and Social Psychology* 12(1969):252.

——— and Landers, D. M. "Coaction Effects on a Muscular Endurance Task." *Research Quarterly* 40(1969):733.

———and Landers, D. M. "Evaluation Potential as a Determinant of Coaction Effects." *Journal of Experimental Social Psychology* 8 (1972):347.

Masters, J. C. "Social Comparison by Young Children." *The Young Child* 2(1972):320.

McClintock, C. and Nuttin, J. "Development of Competitive Game Behavior in Children across Two Cultures." *Journal of Experimental Social Psychology* 5(1969):203.

Metheny, E. "Symbolic Forms of Movement: The Feminines Image in Sports." In *Sport and American Society*, edited by G. H. Sage. Reading, Mass.: Addison-Wesley, 1970.

Meyer, W. J. and Seidman, S. B. "Age Differences in the Effectiveness of Different Reinforcement Conditions on the Acquisition and Extinction of a Simple Concept Learning Problems." *Child Development* 31(1960): 419.

Missiuro, W. "The Development of Reflex Activity in Children." In *International Research in Sport and Physical Education*, edited by E. Jokl and E. Simon. Springfield, Illinois: Charles C. Thomas, 1964, p. 372.

Montemayor, R. "Children's Performance in a Game and Their Attraction to It as a Function of Sex-Typed Labels." *Child Development* 45(1974):152.

Moore, J. "A Comparison of Negro and White Children in Speed of Reaction on an Eye-Hand Coordination Test." *Journal of Genetic Psychology* 59(1941):255.

Murphy, L. B. and Murphy, G. "The Influence of Social Situations upon the Behavior of Children." *Handbook of Social Psychology,* Worcester, Massachusetts: Clark University Press, 1935.

Moore, O. K. and Anderson, A. R. "Some Principles for the Design of Clarifying Educational Environments." In *Handbook of Socialization Theory and Research,* edited by D. A. Goslin. Chicago: Randy McNally, 1969, p. 571.

Nelson, D. O. "Leadership in Sports." *Research Quarterly* 37(1966):268.

Nelson, L. L. The Development of Cooperation and Competition in Children from Ages Five to Ten Years Old: Effects of Sex, Situational Determinants, and Prior Experiences." Doctoral Dissertation, University of California at Los Angeles, 1970.

Olson, D. M. "Motor Skill and Behavior Adjustment: An Exploratory Study." *Research Quarterly* 39(1968):321.

Parten, M. B. "Leadership among Preschool Children." *Journal of Abnormal and Social Psychology* 27 (1933):430.

Pigors, P. "Leadership and Domination Among Children." *Sociologus* 9(1933):140.

Ponthieux, N. A. and Barker, D. B. "Relationships between Race and Physical Fitness." *Research Quarterly* 36(1965):468.

Puffer, J. A. "Boys' Gangs." *Pedagogical Seminar* 12(1905):175.

Roberts, J. M.; Ash, M. J.; and Bush, R. R. "Games in Culture." *American Anthropology* 61(1959):597.

——— and Sutton-Smith, B. "Child Training and Game Involvement." *Ethnology* 2(1962):166.

Rosenberg, B. and Sutton-Smith, B. "A Revised Conception of Masculine-Feminine Differences in Play Activities." *Journal of Genetic Psychology* 96(1960):165.

Rosenquist, H. S. "Social Facilitation in Rotary Pursuit Tracking." Paper presented at the Midwest Psychological Association, 1972.

Schachter, S. *The Psychology of Affiliation.* Stanford: Stanford University Press, 1959.

Scott, R. B.; Ferguson, A. D.; Jenskins, M. E.; and Cutter, F. F. "Growth and Development of Negro Infants." V. "Neuromuscular Patterns of Behavior during the First Year of Life." *Pediatrics* 16(1955):24.

Sears, R. R.; Maccoby, E. E.; and Levin, H. *Patterns of Child Rearing.* Evanston, Illinois: Row, Peterson and Company, 1957.

Seidman, D.; Bensen, S. B.; Miller, I.; and Meeland, T. "Influence of a Partner on Tolerance for Self-Administered Electric Shock." *Journal of Abnormal and Social Psychology* 54(1957):210.

Solomons, G. and Solomons, H. C. "Factors Affecting Motor Performance in Four-Month-Old Infants." *Child Development* 35(1964):1283.

Stevenson, H. W. "Social Reinforcement with Children as a Function of CA, Sex of E, and Sex of S." *Journal of Abnormal and Social Psychology* 63(1961):147.

Stone, W. J. "The Influence of Race and Socioeconomic Status on Physical Performance." *Dissertation Abstracts International* 27/03A:661(1966).

Sutton-Smith, B.; Roberts, J. M.; and Kozelka, R. M. "Game Involvement in Adults." *Journal of Social Psychology* 60(1963):15.

Tryon, C. M. "Evaluation of Adolescent Personality by Adolescents." *Child Development Monographs* 4(1939).

Veroff, J. "Social Comparison and the Development of Achievement Motivation." In *Achievement-Related Motives in Children,* edited by C. P. Smith. New York: The Russell Sage Foundation, 1969, p. 46.

Walters, C. E. "Comparative Development of Negro and White Infants." *Journal of Genetic Psychology* 110(1967):243.

White, R. W. "Competence and the Psychosexual Stages of Development." In *Nebraska Symposium on Motivation,* edited by M. R. Jones. Lincoln, Nebraska: University of Nebraska Press, 1960.

———. "Motivation Reconsidered: The Concept of Competence." *Psychological Review* 66 (1959):297.

Williams, J. R. and Scott, R. B. "Growth and Development of Negro Infants." IV. "Motor Development and Its Relationship to Child Rearing Practices in Two Groups of Negro Infants." *Child Development* 24(1953):103.

Zajonc, R. "Social Facilitation." *Science* 149 (1965):269.

——— and Sales, S. M. "Social Facilitation of Dominant and Subordinate Responses." *Journal of Experimental Social Psychology* 2(1966):160.

Section 9

The Motor Development of Children: Practical Applications

Motor Learning and Motor Development during Infancy and Childhood

26

Aileene S. Lockhart
Texas Woman's University

The preceding chapters have presented much information concerning the motor development of the child. This chapter is intended to synthesize some of this information and to discuss some of the implications of the information for helping children effectively learn motor skills. For ease of discussion the basic information is presented for different age groups.

INFANT DEVELOPMENT AND LEARNING: AGES 0-2

Characteristics

The average infant triples in birth weight within the first year, and height increases by about 33 percent. The teeth have erupted and the bones have started to ossify.

The amount of motor activity during infancy is associated with the baby's stage of motor development. From reflex responses gross and undifferentiated movements evolve. Some reflex responses drop out or are inhibited in time. Others are the basis for developing generalized patterns of movement which eventually make it possible for the child to learn to move about in the environment and to handle objects. Before the end of this period the child has improved uncoordinated and random movement to the point that he/she can, in the following general developmental sequence, hold the chin up, the chest up — thus raise the head —, reach, sit with support, grasp, sit alone, stand with help, creep, walk when led, pull up to a stand when holding onto something, climb stairs, stand alone, and then walk alone. Learning to walk is a very important milestone because thereby the child's sensory, perceptual, motor, and intellectual world is enlarged. The basis for all forms of locomotion is begun and the arms and hands are freed for exploration of the environment and manipulation of objects.

The mechanisms that make learning possible (physical and neurological) are inherent, so during this two year period the bases for all future learning and behavior are already present. The baby *begins* to develop those functions on which later cognition, personality and socialization depend. The child *begins* to perceive, comprehend, interpret, interact, use words, and develop consciousness of other members of the family.

Motor Learning

A baby achieves a tremendous amount of improvement during this period: developments in motor, adaptive, language, and personal-social behavior. Most development emerges, and is then improved upon, by the very active motor experimentation and exploration in which the child engages.

Development which is genetically induced and controlled (phyletic) cannot be speeded up but an environment which offers appropriate experiential opportunity can somewhat improve ontogenetic learnings. The infant should be given the opportunity to reach, grasp, and release objects and to sense form, shape and color. A young child should be free to move and experience, if human functions are to develop properly and completely. A comfortable, secure environment with love and attention should be provided.

Skills per se cannot be taught in any formal or specific sense until the child is more mature. Verbal instructions at this age have very little if any effect on motor behavior. Nevertheless the most necessary and important role of informal practice and learning is obvious to anyone who observes an infant. If a child is deprived of opportunities to experiment with emerging abilities, if nothing is available to play with, and if there is little social contact and concern, learning may be permanently impaired.

THE YOUNG CHILD: AGES 2-6

Characteristics

Now able to move about, the young child wants to go everywhere. The child wants to explore everything: to see, touch, feel, hear, taste, know, and to be exposed to almost all the situations that the social environment will allow.

The rate of growth of the upper body slows down but the length of the child's legs increases rather rapidly, so that by age six overall proportions and appearance are similar to those of an adult. By the end of this period the child cannot only walk well, but can run, jump, climb and hop, and can possibly gallop and skip.

Perceptions and comprehensions increase strikingly during this period and the child can talk about experiences which are no longer confined completely to the family but have extended out into the neighborhood and possibly to preschool. To the extent that this is true self-confidence is developed. The young child moves from an understanding of 272 words on the average, at age two, to 2562 at age six. Social experiences are very important to language development and if there has been a rich environment, one in which fear has not developed, then motor ability is advanced. If on the other hand, the child has been overly protected and every wish has been anticipated and fulfilled, the child probably will not investigate, explore and experiment as he/she should and, as a consequence, motor development and learnings will have suffered.

The young child enjoys participating in symbolic play, a tricycle becoming a fire engine or a sports car, blocks a castle or a fort. Although understanding has improved amazingly the child is not able to generalize much or reason logically. During this period the child moves in his/her associations with others, without regard for sex or race, from the simplest kind of parallel play (alongside but independent of others) to a small amount of very elementary cooperative play.

Motor Learning

A happy start is what children need most to propel them without fear and with enthusiasm into all learning. If a child is allowed to set the pace, is encouraged, and if motor learning is left as play, the child will *want* to develop skills. Children two to six do not respond well even to simple rules and regulations if these are imposed upon their games. These children learn fast if they are mature enough to handle that with which they are confronted. The story of Johnny and Jimmy confirms the fact that it doesn't take as long to learn when children are allowed to wait until they are ripe for specific learning.

Young children need a good environment, one that provides them with the chance to develop many motor skills. They will spontaneously make up their own play from the raw materials with which they should be provided: barrels, boxes, slides, blocks, paint, clay, sand boxes, tricycles, wagons, water, balls, ropes, and toys. It has been suggested that it would be best if each child has at least a few toys chosen from each of the following categories (1) creative toys which allow the child to construct and invent; (2) toys which can be used for dramatic purposes; (3) toys that develop the artistic sense; (4) toys that will develop strength; and (5) toys that will challenge the child intellectually. The kind of toys provided for a child can affect both physical and psychological development, imagination and creative abilities. Toys should be simple and sturdy, and not overly realistic. They should be moved and manipulated by the child, not by a battery.

The child's improvement in locomotion and manipulation is marked. As the child improves the basic requirements of walking, running, climbing, jumping, hopping, kicking, throwing, catching, galloping and skipping the child will invent all sorts of variations of these abilities. Experimenting and exploring can be aided and stimulated by informal and individual teaching and help. Because balance and strength are so important the child should be given numerous opportunities to develop these requirements

of skillful performance. The child needs help and much practice in learning to throw (which is typically at first performed with a same arm-leg pattern), and catch (which is typically accomplished with arms and trunk), in learning to start and stop and turn quickly. The child is not without the persistence which is required and may try the patience of the adult who is attempting to help with learning. The normal child will repeat motor skills joyfully over and over and will take great pride in accomplishments; these should be praised by adults.

Most children like to play in water. They may not automatically learn to swim but a normal four- or five-year-old can learn; there are examples of such learning as early as two months.

It is through play that children two to six develop their abilities to move, talk, and work with others; develop their curiosity and self-assurance; develop their attitudes about learning, about objects and people; develop their concepts of self; and extend the length of their attention spans.

No hard and fast rules can be enunciated regarding when an individual child is ready for any specific experience. The child is ready when there is evidence of voluntary involvement. The child is not ready if the learning takes more time and interest than he/she displays or if more experience or ability is required than the child has to offer. Children vary widely in readiness but the alert adult cannot miss when the time comes: the child has ways of letting the adult know when he/she is wanting to talk, wanting to read, wanting to skip. The adult's challenges and responsibilities are to lend a hand when it is needed, to "capture the moment when learning comes easy," and to provide the environment and materials for learning.

THE ELEMENTARY SCHOOL CHILD: AGES 6-12

Characteristics

At age six the child understands simple concepts and enjoys engaging in imagery. Imagination is a joy! The child can group or categorize items in a very elementary fashion but the attention span is short. Behavior is not always exemplary. The child always wants to be "first" and is apt to be noisy and not always cooperative. He/she has to learn to wait his/her turn on apparatus, and is not always too good about sharing with others. The center of life as the child enters school is *I*. Learning to write and to use crayons, in the acceptable manner seems to require tension in the whole body. Fine manipulative skills are still very difficult. While these must be practiced, the need for active movement requiring use of large muscles is great. School is enjoyable and gradually the child is able to cooperate in small groups.

By age *seven* real progress has been made in all directions. The child is becoming more involved socially, works better with small groups, and is improving in skill. By *eight* the child is assured at school and with friends. Adaptive behavior has greatly expanded, self control is much improved, language can be used well, the child can work long and hard, and move gracefully, fast, and well.

The *nine*-year-old is full of curiosity and realism. Eye-hand coordination is at last good, but much more experience is needed with ball handling skills, and practice on balance and general body control. The child is eager, ready, and will persist in perfecting skills. The child is highly self-motivated and independent and wants to make independent decisions. Boys and girls begin to play in separate groups.

Girls on the average become a bit taller and heavier than boys at about age *ten* but later boys overtake the girls in height and muscular growth. A few biologically advanced girls may reach puberty. Girls do reach this stage before boys. Self responsibility is good in both sexes. Both like group activities and body control is developing fast. The competitive urge is growing and the capacity to learn all kinds of skills is marked.

Around ages *eleven* and *twelve* boys and girls may prefer segregation in their play activities. Their behavior has become rather well integrated. They have developed considerable social intelligence and personal organization. They can concentrate. An amazing number of skills have been acquired and many perfected. The good adjustment and general happiness may be short-lived because these children are about to become adolescents. The transition can bring problems.

The person who works with children between the ages of six to twelve should realize the impact that physique makes both on a child's peers and on adults. A few youngsters who are only six or seven years old may be as tall as the smallest eleven-year-olds, and some eleven and twelve-year-olds may be as tall as some who are seventeen. Physical size may affect a child's behavior and personality, partly because society imposes its own expectancies which are largely based on size. Children who are large and well built for their ages are expected to act more mature, yet these children may feel pressured to act more assured and poised than they really feel. The small child may withdraw because of feelings of inadequacy. Children tend to judge each other with reference to their physical abilities and achievements. A child who is awkward, incompetent motorly, or obese may lead a hard life with peers, and one's estimation of self and level of aspiration may be seriously affected unless adult guidance is sensitive and wise. There are wide variations in all abilities but those that are displaced via motor performance are so observable that they may be the direct cause for pride or shame in youngsters.

Social relationships are widely extended during the six to twelve age period. Beginning as a very individualistic and egocentric, the child gradually can work cooperatively with a few children. Later as a member of the gang there is growing pressure to conform and such groups become highly influential in terms of attitude development.

Motor Learning

The years between six and twelve are ideal for skill learning. The range and depth of a child's motor interests are largely determined by available opportunities, since the neurological prerequisites for the learning of the normal child are present. It is crucial that the child should find, therefore, many suitable motor experiences and be given the aid, the coaching and the encouragement to develop the motor skills which mean so much to self-esteem and body image, to acceptance with peers, and to social behavior. Children are naturally so active, so interested in play and so ingenious in initiating their own play that it is easy to assume that "free play" is sufficient for their needs. Motor learning opportunities, however, must not stop. Never are they needed more, and at this period of growth and development learning is almost un-

limited. That which has been developed between birth and age twelve is of infinite importance in determining interests and abilities at later ages. Systematic instruction in motor skills is probably more important than at any other age level. A broad array of activities, increasingly complex in nature and progressive in presentation should be planned so that health related and skill related aspects of fitness as well as specific skills can be developed.

Children can become amazingly proficient in some sports. However, the danger of specialization is that in so doing they may be cheated by not receiving, as they should, the variety of opportunities which are necessary for developing a wide range of skills. True specialization should come later, based on enough experiences so that choice can be made wisely and realistically. Variety is important at this age level.

The younger learners like rhythmic and dramatic activities, movement exploration, simple stunts and games of low organization. They progress best with individualized instruction and individualized challenges. Beginning with the younger learners and then continuing throughout the six to twelve period, youngsters should be taught how to use force and space, how to improve balance and stability, and how to improve timing and coordination. This means that they should be helped to gain "good form" in their movements for this makes possible the greatest amount of precision, force, ease and poise. Instruction in golf, tennis, and diving can be appropriately begun with some children at age nine or ten, swimming even earlier.

Children begin with great flexibility but American children, boys in particular, are not proficient in this component of fitness. Children are taller and heavier than they used to be; their strength, however, has not developed in proportion. These facts should be remembered for they are important to appropriate curriculum planning.

There are some sex differences in growth and *performance,* the greater strength and endurance of boys becoming more and more evident during later childhood. Potential strength, however, is only about 30 to 50 percent attained by age twelve, and endurance is not great. It is only after puberty that boys develop significantly greater strength than girls and superior levels of motor performance.

By age twelve children have achieved a large amount, from 85 to 90 percent of their potential speed of reaction and mobility. Therefore it is not surprising that, particularly those from nine to twelve years of age, are especially challenged by races, stunts, and self-testing activities. Development of strength, balance, speed and coordination occur partly as a function of time. A child automatically gets better in these requirements of skillful performance as a result of growth and appropriate experience. But further improvement and refinement of *skill* require years of practice and experience, and systematic progression from the simple to the more complex. All of the prerequisites of good development and of good performance (health related and skill related fitness factors), and all of the bases of good body mechanics can be improved through physical activity. These should be continuously and progressively worked on during this entire period.

Individual differences between the performances of boys and girls are overshadowed by the very great variability within each sex. Actually there is great overlapping in performance, and sex differences per se

in growth have very little effect on the potentialities for skill *learning* at the early age levels. It appears that boys and girls can learn motor skills about equally well. The observable differences in the way boys and girls play, what they play, the importance they attach to their motor achievements, and their skill in moving are at least partly due to sex typing and socially induced motivation. This type of stereotyping is now beginning to diminish.

Skill learning is an active process and learning is always best if it is individualized. Though it is the child who does the learning, the teacher should provide the opportunities for learning and the occasions for practice. The teacher should see that experiences are appropriate to the readiness of the child. Adequate motor learning equipment and materials must be available. Children should not be forced to wait in long lines in order to practice.

Emphasis should be put on the child's own progress, not on comparing achievements with those of others. So great are individual differences that even by the fourth grade there may be a gulf between youngsters as wide as a six year span. Approaches and expectancies for motor learning therefore must differ from individual to individual.

Elementary school children need hours of daily physical activity. It is impossible to meet the need of this requirement in the required physical education class. Good intramural programs should be supervised by school personnel, and children should be encouraged to participate in out-of-school play of a vigorous kind.

New motor learning should be practiced often, but not for too long a period at one time. As skill, and the motivation which results from success, increase then practice periods can be extended. The problem is to challenge enough to stimulate real efforts toward learning but to realize when the child begins to become fatigued and when interest begins to lag learning becomes inefficient. The problem is to challenge, but not to overstimulate and not to put a lid on the child's level of aspiration by expecting too much, too fast.

References

Bayley, Nancy. "The Development of Motor Abilities during the First Three Years." *Society for Research in Child Development* Monograph No. 1 (1935).

Bernstein, N. *The Coordination and Regulation of Movements*. Oxford: Pergamon Press, 1967.

Cole, Luella, and Hall, Irma Nelson. *Psychology of Adolescence*. New York: Holt, Rinehart and Winston, Inc., 1970.

Dohrmann, Paul. "Throwing and Kicking Ability of Eight-Year-Old Boys and Girls." *Research Quarterly* 35(December 1964):464-71.

Espenschade, Anna S. and Eckert, Helen M. *Motor Development*. Columbus, Ohio: Charles E. Merrill Books, Inc., 1967.

Galambos, Robert and Morgan, Clifford T. "The Neural Basis of Learning." *Handbook of Physiology, edited by John Field*. Washington: American Physiological Society. Chapter 61, 3(1960):1471-99.

Gesell, Arnold and Ilg, F. L. *The Child From Five to Ten*. New York: Harper and Brothers, 1946.

Gessell, Arnold. *The First Five Years of Life*. New York: Harper and Bros., 1940.

Goodenough, F. L. and Brian, C. B. "Certain Factors Underlying the Acquisition of Motor Skill by Pre-School Children." *Journal of Experimental Psychology* 12(1921):127.

Gutteridge, Mary V. "A Study of Motor Achievement of Young Children." *Archives of Psychology* 244(1939).

Halverson, Lolas. "Development of Motor Patterns in Young Children." *Quest*, May 1966.

Halverson, H. M. "The Acquisition of Skill in Infancy." *Journal of Genetic Psychology* 43 (1933):3.

Hellebrandt, F. A.; Rarick, G. L.; and Carns, M. L. "Physiological Analysis of Basic Motor Skills." I. "Growth and Development of Jumping." *American Journal of Physical Medicine* 40(1961):14-25.

Hilgard, J. R. "Learning and Maturation in Preschool Children." *Journal of Genetic Psychology* 41(1932):31.

Jenkins, L. M. "A Comparative Study of Motor Achievements of Children Five, Six and Seven Years of Age." Teachers College, Columbia University, New York, 1930.

Johnson, Robert. "Measurements of Achievement in Fundamental Skills of Elementary School Children." *Research Quarterly* 33 (March 1962):94-104.

Kawin, E. *The Wise Choice of Toys*. Chicago: University of Chicago Press, 1934.

Lawther, John D. *The Learning of Physical Skills*. Englewood Cliffs, N. J.: Prentice-Hall, Inc., 1968.

Lawther, John D. "Directing Motor Skill Learning." *Quest*, May 1966.

Lockhart, Aileen S. "Conditions of Effective Motor Learning." *Journal of Health, Physical Education and Recreation* 38(1967):36-39.

McCandless, Boyd R. *Adolescents Behavior and Development*. Hinsdale, Illinois: The Dryden Press Inc., 1970.

McCaskill, C. L. and Wellman, B. L. "A Study of Common Motor Achievements of the Pre-School Ages." *Child Development* 9(1938):141-50.

Mussen, Paul H. *The Psychological Development of the Child*. Englewood Cliffs, N.J.: Prentice-Hall, Inc., 1963.

Nash, John. *Developmental Psychology: A Psychobiological Approach*. Englewood Cliffs, N.J.: Prentice-Hall, Inc., 1970.

Paillard, Jacques. "The Patterning of Skilled Movements." *Handbook of Physiology*, edited by John Field, Chapter 67, Vol. 2, 1679-1708. Washington, D.C.: American Physiological Society, 1959-1960.

Rarick, G. Lawrence, ed. *Physical Activity: Human Growth and Development*. New York: Academic Press, 1973.

Shirley, M. M. *The First Two Years: A Study of Twenty-Five Babies,* Vol. 1. Minneapolis, Minn.: University of Minneapolis Press, 1931.

Watson, Ernest H. and Lowrey, George H. *Growth and Development of Children.* Chicago: Year Book Medical Publisher, 1967.

Wellborn, Beth. "Motor Achievements of Pre-School Children." *Childhood Education* 13 (1937):311-16.

Wild, Monica. "The Behavior Pattern of Throwing and Some Observations Concerning Its Course of Development in Children. *Research Quarterly* 9(3)(1938):20-24.

Practices and Principles Governing Motor Learning of Children

27

Aileene S. Lockhart
Texas Woman's University

CONDITIONS WHICH IMPROVE MOTOR LEARNING AND PERFORMANCE

Some circumstances make motor learning easier, more efficient and more effective. A considerable body of information has been gleaned through the years both through observation and research about the conditions which attend best learning and about the factors which influence behavior, attitudes and interests. Some of these are presented briefly below:

1. Learning should be a happy experience. It is much more important for young children to find that learning is satisfying and pleasurable than it is for them to learn predetermined and specific skills. Furthermore, learning and attitudes achieved under pleasant circumstances seem to be better retained.

2. A relatively free and flexible learning environment should be maintained during the beginning stages of learning a new skill. A certain amount of experimentation is necessary for motor learning, and a relaxed and undemanding atmosphere is conducive to learning. The learning-teaching situation should be kept calm, controlled and steady.

3. If the child's abilities are used to set the pace and his/her interests used as a guide in program planning, motivation and determination of needs are not staggering problems. A close correlation apparently exists between the ability to learn and the young child's interests.

4. Adequate space must be available in which to move; there must be time to practice, and enough equipment of suitable quality and choice with which to practice.

5. Movement should not be analyzed excessively during early learning. Beginners cannot perceive the details and subtleties of complex movement patterns nor understand involved verbal instructions or analyses. The learning of young children is richest when approached by problem solving methods. Learning to ask good questions and learning to find answers are perhaps the two greatest capabilities that can be developed. Children can learn how to solve movement problems.

6. Vigorous activity should be alternated with less demanding activity; both because of inefficient effort-benefit ratios (see Section 6) and short interest spans of children of this age.

7. Children should not be pressed to try to learn motor skills that appear to be too difficult for them. Children must be sure of themselves, have the required capacity before accepting a challenge, and must want to participate if their learning is to bring them satisfaction. If they are overly anxious or too frustrated or try too hard to please parents and others who pressure them, they will not learn readily. Anxious persons usually

perform poorly and therefore find no pleasure in the learning. Behavior deteriorates fast when pressure results in near panic. There is a proper time for learning. Overwhelming learners with too much, to fast and too intense challenges retards and may even prevent further learning. Intense pressures threaten development.

8. Play is the *way* that much of the learning of children is achieved. Children eventually may learn to relate the knowledges, attitudes and interests which surround their immediate motor experiences to broader and later situations. Children's concepts of time, force, speed, direction, space, quantity, magnitude, cause and effect, and their relationships with other persons often are originally developed and tested in motor experiences. The good teacher, cognizant of the integrated nature of the total organism with its delicate combination of the physical, the emotional and the intellectual is able to broaden the scope and significance of the child's motor successes.

9. Child behavior should not be strictly channeled. If it is, a child can learn only one of two things. Either the child learns to be complacent, submissive, unimaginative and unquestioning, or learns to be defiant, uncooperative, rebellious, and overly aggressive.

10. All learners will eventually "balk" if their efforts appear to bring no success or recognition. There is no need to attempt to speed up the learning of youngsters to the point of risking repeated failure and discouragement. What is important is for them to find learning fun and desirable. Give them encouragement, understanding, support, experiences that they can deal with, and experiences that are meaningful to them.

11. Learning and expectancies regarding performance should be individualized because of the great inter- and intraindividual differences within and among children. Children start school with differences in abilities, differences in the degree of control and coordination of abilities, and differences in interests, attitudes and self-direction. Instead of becoming more and more alike, differences among children become greater and greater with experience and advancing years. Children simply are not of the same mold. They should not be held to the same specific performances and predetermined expectancies. But this is not to say that they should not be held for the level of achievement of which they are individually capable.

12. There is no need to classify children less than eight years of age for their motor learning except for helping them to learn qualitative fundamental skills at their own rate.

13. Teachers who have basic information about the development and functioning of the nervous system, who understand the concepts of growth and development, and who have conceptions about the nature and potential of children should be understanding, perceptive and sympathetic leaders of elementary school children.

14. It is most important for children to have sound and competent motor learning instruction. Attitudes regarding physical activity and abilities which are basic to the later learning and use of motor skills are largely determined by the time a child is twelve years old. The years between six and twelve have repeatedly been described as the skill learning and refining years; no more accurate description of this crucial period can be given here. During these years a child

should develop a large repertoire of skills; if not, the chances of ever doing so are small.

15. The adult's job is to establish a good climate for learning, to provide a variety of experiences which are appropriately progressive in complexity, to help the learner find good methods of moving and practicing, and to sensitively and patiently guide the learner's efforts when needed.

PRINCIPLES WHICH GOVERN MOTOR LEARNING

Although the exact process of how learning is achieved is not known, from that which is understood about the total growth and development of children and about the conditions which appear to affect their learning, it is possible to derive some principles of motor learning. Some of these which seem especially important and appropriate to learners who are in the beginning stages of acquiring motor skills are suggested now.

1. The development of motor ability in children proceeds in accordance with the laws of physiological maturation. The motor learning of children depends upon the interaction between maturation and learning.

2. The development of phylogenetic activities are controlled chiefly by maturation, whereas ontogenetic skills result primarily from experience and practice.

3. The motor learning of the youngest learners begins with movement exploration and experimentation. Although the amount of time devoted to these methods differs, actually all motor learning begins this way.

4. Demonstration should be held to the minimum during children's motor exploration sessions; if it is not, problem solving possibilities are lessened. Demonstration, however, is of great value in the presentation and practice of formalized skills, at all levels of learning.

5. Progressive adaptation describes motor learning. The learner gradually establishes a pattern of movement, the pattern and its execution gradually becoming more accurate and more effective as the result of well directed practice.

6. There are critical periods for learning and during those times motor learning can best be achieved. When the child is "ready," maturationally and psychologically, learning is most efficient.

7. Insufficient motor learning may retard general development and certainly will retard more complex motor learning.

8. Motor learning progresses from the simple to the complex, from the gross to the refined, and from large to small. Motor learning should be planned to conform to these developmental patterns.

9. Undifferentiated movement occurs before specific patterns can develop. Voluntary control of large muscles must be achieved before smaller muscles can be controlled.

10. A most important aspect of a skill is its "wholeness." In keeping with concepts of developmental trends and with what is known about the psychology of perception, skills can best be practiced and learned as "wholes." If success is then not forthcoming, practice smaller individual subskills.

11. Changes in strength and balance in young people are associated with growth, and are evidenced in improved motor ability.

12. To acquire skill requires practice, but practice does not automatically result in improved proficiency. Practice does not necessarily make perfect.

13. Significant improvement in movement abilities comes only when the learner

intends to learn and tries to improve. Merely "going through the motions" is no guarantee of learning.

14. Distributed or spaced practice is more effective than massed practice during initial learning.

15. Frequent practice is most effective if practice periods are short.

16. How long practice can be profitably maintained depends on the maturity of the learner, the extent of interest, the reason or purpose for the learning, the movement background or experience of the learner, and the complexity of the thing to be mastered.

17. Short and frequent practice favors high motivation and concentrated effort, two absolute requirements for motor learning. This practice arrangement seems best for young and immature learners, and for those who are in the beginning stages of motor learning, no matter the age level.

18. There are large individual differences in the rate and extent of motor learning and motor development. Great variability among children and within any one child characterizes initial motor learning and performance.

19. Complicated movement patterns are not mastered suddenly; motor learning is a slow process which requires much practice in order to learn to control the sequential and temporal aspects of movement and in order to develop the appropriate quality and quantity of movement. These are requirements of good coordination and effective action.

20. Motor learning at any age is characterized by the gradual elimination of superfluous and tense movement.

21. Learning and the motivation to learn demand knowledge of results. Any learner wants to know how he/she is progressing and if there is no way to find out, interest will lag.

22. In order to master specific skills (which is one way of defining motor learning), learning must be goal-directed. Unless the goal is understood and desired, activity will lack direction and improvement will probably not occur.

23. Specific motor learning begins with a very generalized concept of what is to be done and vague ideas of how to do it. If a child has the desire to learn a specific skill he/she already has some concept about it. Let the child try it. He/she will then be ready to accept suggestions.

24. Achievement leads to further achievement. A reasonable amount of success is necessary to maintain effort and interest.

25. The better perceived and learned, the more accurately and longer a skill will be remembered. The probability of retention is also enhanced if the learning has been achieved under conditions of high drive.

26. Specific motor skill learning is the result of progressive differentiation, subtlety and control of function. This takes time, exploration, and practice.

27. Motor learning begins with a movement idea which probably cannot be conceptually verbalized.

28. The teacher's responsibility is to help to evoke new movement ideas. He/she should remember that the *goal* is much more important than specific methods of achieving it. When a learner knows *what* is to be accomplished, he/she already is started on how to go about it.

Organizing Sports for Children 28

Charles B. Corbin
Kansas State University

Recent years have seen an unprecidented growth in organized children's sports. Though most programs were originally planned for boys, increasing numbers of girls have become involved in organized sports and all indications are that the number of participating girls will continue to increase. Some (Thomas, 1977) estimate the numbers of participants in children's sports for children age 8 to 16 to be as high as 20 million. Martens (1978) indicates that as many as 19 million boys and 12.5 million girls between 6-16 participate in organized sports each year. Of course these figures are somewhat inflated since many children participate in more than one sport. Children who participate in more than one sport are counted more than one time. Regardless, it can be seen that participation in youth sports is extensive.

This chapter is designed to examine the children's sports phenomenon. Specifically it is important to determine the extent to which participation in these programs affects or influences motor development and it is important to determine how the body of knowledge in motor development (as presented in the previous pages) can be helpful in effectively administering programs which are truely designed to meet the needs and interests of the child participant.

PURPOSES OF CHILDREN'S SPORTS

The originators of most youth sports programs, regardless of the exact sport to be played, have supported the need for these activities based on social, physical, intellectual, and personal benefits which are purported to come to the child who participates. To a great extent the organizers and proponents of children's sports programs have argued that sports are a "means" of accomplishing these "ends" or benefits. In recent years critics of youth sports programs have suggested that sports may not be the most effective means of achieving goals such as physical fitness, good sportsmanship, and others outlined to be the "ends" of the programs.

Perhaps most often overlooked in the continuing debate over the pros and cons of youth sports are two basic points. First, it just may be that for many children the desired "end" may be fun or the mere enjoyment of participation. If fun is the sole goal, the means for accomplishing it should be designed with this goal in mind. Secondly, a frequently asked question resulting from the debate over children's sports is, "What is wrong with sports for kids?" What often is not realized is that this is the wrong question! If we are concerned with the total development of children, including motor development, the correct question is "What is the *best* way of helping children achieve important developmental goals and how can youth sports programs contribute?" In the final analysis one can see that sports and sports competition are neither good nor bad. It is how they are used that is important. If we can more clearly outline our developmental goals or "ends", then we can be much more effective in designing youth sports programs to meet these goals. The foregoing is true whether the intent is to plan a program just for "fun" or to design programs for meeting more elaborate goals such as sportsmanship, physical fitness, etc.

PHYSICAL RISKS OF SPORTS PARTICIPATION

The attitudes of the public and professional people in areas which relate to organized sport's competition for children under age 12 have varied over the years. Early objections of professional people to involvement of children in organized sports were largely based on the strenuous nature of competitive sports (Berryman, 1978.). The information presented in the previous sections of this book clearly indicate that school age children are quite capable of strenuous physical involvement in activity. Except for absolute performances such as comparing children's performances with adults, we now know that children are able to learn skills and to manage their own bodies in vigorous physical activity.

A second objection is the risk of injury which may result from participation in organized sports. Results of two comprehensive studies of injuries in youth baseball (Gugenheim, et al., 1976; Larson, 1976) indicate that the number of organized sports injuries may not be as extensive as some have thought. However, it should be pointed out that there is still a significant risk associated with participation in youth sports, particularly in collision sports for older children.

Little League elbow does pose some risk to the child involved with frequent ball throwing, but like other sports injuries, the risk of this malady is not as great as once thought. After reviewing the studies cited above and other recent studies concerning sports injuries associated with involvement in youth sports Martens concluded, "I am of the opinion that most sports can be made sufficiently safe so that the benefits far outweigh the risks. What we must do is concentrate our efforts on making children's sports as safe as possible (Martens, 1978, p. 196). Martens' point is a good one. However, inherent in his statement is the need to establish the benefits to be achieved in a specific sports program. Some sports programs are more risky than others, but there is no way that we can know if the benefits outweigh the risks if we do not have a clear understanding of the benefits. If we can first define what benefits we hope will come to the child then we can decide if the benefits are greater than the risks. Also we can determine if there are alternative methods of achieving the same benefits with lesser risk. Given the risks associated with boxing, there appears to be little reason for including this activity in youth sports programs. The risks exceed the benefits. Collision sports, especially when children are not grouped for maturation, should be scrutinized closely as should wrestling programs where children are allowed or encouraged to participate in weight loss programs to "make weight." At all times methods for reducing the risk of youth sports involvement should be considered as paramount.

In recent years the objections to children's sports by professional sports have shifted somewhat from risk of physical injury and physical harm to psychological concerns. Some of these concerns will be more completely outlined in subsequent sections of this chapter.

INTENSE EARLY PARTICIPATION

In Chapter 18 effort-benefit ratios were discussed. It was noted that in some forms of physical activity, particularly tasks requiring strength, power, muscular endurance, and speed, children will not benefit from training in proportion to the effort expended. This is especially true when comparisons of the effort-benefit ratios of children are compared with those of adolescents. Harter (1978) has also shown that for young children, intrinsic motivation or interest in performing activity "just because I want to" decreases as the time necessary to achieve mastery of the task increases. In other words, children like to see something for their efforts. Within reason they will work to earn the fruits of their efforts. However, there appears to be a point of diminishing returns for learning a skill. If the skill requires a disproportionate amount of time, given the benefits, the child loses interest in the activity. The child apparently concludes, "It just isn't worth it."

The implications of the foregoing information to children's sports are significant. If one of the goals of children's sports is fun, we must make sure that the amount of effort we require is closely related to the benefits or fun which comes to the child participating. If our goals are such things as physical fitness development and skill learning we must be careful not to require so much effort that the child loses interest. We must also remember that the goals we have for children may not be the same goals as they have for themselves. Overemphasizing effort when the benefits or goals are unrealistic or remote may be one good way to help children lose interest in children's sports. It is not unreasonable to expect children to accomplish certain goals as long as the goals are realistic in terms of the effort expended.

Other possible disadvantages of intense early training of children are outlined by Martens (1978, p. 189).

1. The chances are great that the late maturer is likely to fail.

2. Early specialization usually is achieved at the expense of developing a broader base of fundamental movement skills such as balance, agility, and coordination.

3. Early specialization usually occurs at the expense of learning other sports, especially lifetime sports skills.

4. Early specialization may channel children into sports not best suited to their talents.

5. Frequently youngsters feel considerable adult-imposed pressure, especially after experiencing some initial success. This drives them to excel at one sport even though they find it work and devoid of fun, and would rather participate in a variety of other sports. Yet, fearing failure, they are hesitant to risk competing in other sports in which they are less experienced.

6. Specialization all-too-often means a heavy emphasis on winning and a de-emphasis on having fun.

OTHER FACTORS RELATING TO YOUTH SPORTS

Participation Leadership

Of all factors discussed by experts on youth sports, leadership is most frequently mentioned. If children's sports programs are to accomplish the goals for which they were intended, sound leadership is a must. First and formost, leaders should be well aware of the principles of motor development discussed in this text. Of secondary importance is a knowledge of the sport. Leadership training programs are essential, especially when those assuming leadership roles are untrained volunteers. In addition to information about motor development, including how to work with children, there should be instruction in the skills of the sport, and how to teach these skills effectively. Not to be overlooked is the need to make leaders aware of the purposes of the program. Perhaps one reason why leadership is not as good as we might like is our failure to clearly communicate the goals of the program to the leaders.

Success

Recent studies (Scanlan, 1977; Scanlan and Passer, 1977) indicate that success is important to children who participate in youth sports. Children who succeed are less anxious after sports participation than are those who are unsuccessful. Nonwinners tend to perceive the competitive sports situation as threatening. Roberts (1977) indicates that continued failure in sports can lead to "learned helplessness." In other words children who constantly lose in sports situations begin to feel as if they don't have a chance. They feel that no matter how hard they try, their efforts do not count. As a result many merely choose not to participate. If they don't participate, they cannot fail. As far as sports are concerned, these children are helpless. They have learned that "I can't do it."

To help more children in being successful in sports, the following suggestions may be helpful:

1. Adapt sports to meet the need of children rather than adapting children to meet the needs of sports. Make the tasks and skills easy enough that most children can master them. Some sports are so complex that few, if any, children can perform the skills properly.

2. Use praise and positive social reinforcement to give children the feeling of success in sports.

3. Reward children for mastery *attempts*. If we want children to feel that they can learn, reward effort not just performance. Let children know when you appreciate their efforts. Too often we reward only good performances (this says something to the child who never performs very well).

4. Help children learn to set realistic goals. Success and failure are relative. Some children feel that they have failed if they don't win every game or get a hit every time at bat. These are unrealistic goals which increase the chances of failure.

Cross-Sex Competition

Much has been said about the wisdom of boys and girls competing together in sports. The best evidence available at this time suggests that preadolescent boys and girls are capable of similar motor performances. Given equal opportunity to learn fundamental skills and to develop adequate levels of physical fitness, there is no reason why cross-sex competition is not appropriate at this age level. Regardless of sex, it is important that children be matched for participation according to maturation level. One successful program is called SCAM (Selection Classification Age Maturity Program). Included as factors in the classification system are physiological age as assessed by pubic hair development for males and menarche for females, height, weight, age, and results of four ability tests. This systems is currently in operation in the state of New York (Whieldon, 1978).

PREDICTION OF FUTURE ATHLETIC SUCCESS

Some have suggested that one reason why parents and coaches sometimes lose sight of the goals of children's sports is the desire to see a child become a champion. Most children, at one time or another dream of becoming a star athlete. Many parents and coaches share this dream, especially if a child shows outstanding performance ability in early sports involvement. If the child is a better performer than other children of the same age, it is easy to jump to the conclusion that this child will be a "star" with lots of practice and good coaching. Unfortunately, there is little evidence to indicate that early sports success is indicative of future success. Bar-or (1975) after considerable research, concluded that there is no "a priori test" which can be used to predict if a young athlete will respond favorably to training. As previously mentioned, the overzealous parent or coach who emphasizes intensive early training with the thought of developing a champion, may be making a serious mistake.

SPORTS FOR SPECIAL CHILDREN

For many years normal healthy school children were discouraged from vigorous physical activity because of our lack of understanding of the human's potential to adapt to physical activity. While the study of exercise physiology has presented scientific information to dispel many of the myths about exercise, there are still many children who are prohibited from activity who could benefit greatly from participation. Many children with special medical problems are still restricted from participation in sports even when they are quite capable of becoming involved. As noted in Chapter 15, many children with congenital and rheumatic heart defects are now able to become involved in sports participation. Recently, Katz (1976) noted that many asthmatics who were thought to be unable to participate do not have to be excluded from sports. Katz noted that asthmatics should have the same opportunities as normal children to learn and benefit from exercise. They should not, according to Katz, be treated as invalids. Etzwiler (1974) draws similar conclusions for the diabetic child. He indicates that with proper planning and medical attention, diabetics should be encouraged to enjoy sports involvement. Livingston and Berman (1974) also encourage participation of the epileptic child in activity and sports. They indicate that the epileptic child may be capable of participation in all types of activities including contact sports, noting that the risk of inferiority or differentness is greater than the risk of physical injury. Medical doctors and exercise physiologists are learning more every day about the potential for people with all types of medical problems for participation in sports. It goes without saying that participation by special children require proper medical supervision and the good principles which apply to normal children in sports should also apply to these children.

GUIDELINES FOR YOUTH SPORTS INVOLVEMENT

The question is not whether children will participate in organized sports, but under what conditions. Corbin, D. E. (1978) has outlined some basic guidelines which should be considered in organizing and implementing youth sports programs. If these guidelines are followed, a great step will have been taken toward eliminating such problems as unnecessary injuries and psychological trauma associated with some youth sports programs.

An effective sports program recognizes, first, that to be beneficial to a child sports must be fun. In addition, children who participate in sports are entitled to certain ethical, psychological and physical considerations.
Specifically, children should have:

1. *The right to participate regardless of skill, ability or sex.* It is obvious that too many sports programs cater only to the elite and are usually dominated by males. If sports and play are children's "work" then *all* children should have equal opportunity. Yet, many children (girls in particular) don't even have a program to enter.

2. *The right to decide whether they want to participate in sports at all.* Kids should be able to make their own decisions regarding participation. Parents should not humiliate or punish their children if they choose not to participate.

3. *The right to know that a failure in sports is not a failure in life.* The win-at-all-cost philosophies in sport imply that to lose in sport is to lose in life. Sports is only one aspect of life. In his book *Life on the Run,* Bill Bradley (former New York Knick) says: "It is unlikely that a basketball player contributes as much to the social good as a teacher, a doctor or a member of the clergy. He works just as hard and has a brief career that frequently leaves him crippled." This statement may help parents, coaches and children to keep sports in their proper perspective.

4. *The right to have a coach who is competent.* The coach should be knowledgeable in such areas as child growth and development, child psychology and first aid. Sports can provide the child a time to try out life, free of adult-imposed pressures to be a winner. If all sport situations are pressured then the child has little room to make mistakes. No one, especially children, can learn to grow without trial and error, and the less pressure in developmental stages, the greater the potential for growth.

5. *The right to safe facilities and properly maintained equipment.* Equipment and facilities used by children should be tested and checked regularly by competent personnel and care taken to insure proper fitting of uniforms and protective gear.

6. *The right to their fair share of public funds and facilities.* Because children do not pay taxes they often get the short end of public funds. Many communities dish out millions of dollars for public stadia that are used solely or primarily for professional athletes while recreation and sport facilities for the children in the community are meager.

7. *The right to be treated like children, not like miniature adults.* Games should be structured to suit the needs and skill levels of children. It is unrealistic for a coach to treat young players as if they were collegiate or professional athletes. The child's involvement in sport is for the benefit of the child. Sports may fail to accommodate the child if "official" size balls, baskets, bats and other equipment are used rather than equipment of a more manageable size.

8. *The right to competent medical treatment.* Pre- and post-season medical exams plus checkup procedures should be established for those who have been sick or injured. Provisions should be made to have a medically trained person on call—particularly in the higher risk sports.

9. *The right to stop playing when hurt or sick without fear of reprisals.* Children should be taught that it is not a sign of toughness to play when injured or sick. Rules should strictly prohibit the playing of an injured or ill player.

10. *The right to their own individuality.* Kids should have the right to question team rules and to voice personal opinions without fear of repercussion. This further suggests the right to individual attention for each child accompanied by a supportive environment for learning.

11. *The right to have compassionate organized sports programs.* The child must be more important than bureaucracy. Sports programs should make provisions for children who move to new districts in mid-season, and children who go on vacations with their parents should not be punished or excluded from programs as a re-

sult. Too often coaches present children with all-or-nothing alternatives when the choice is not even the child's—it's the parents.

12. *The right to play opponents who are carefully matched in age, weight and size.* This diminishes the chances of injury and makes play more fun.

13. *The right to have a wide variety of sports to choose from.* Too often children are faced with no options in selecting sports activities. In many communities, particularly smaller ones, boys can choose between football, baseball or nothing at all. Girls often have even less choice. A greater number of options and a wider range of activities would allow for more participation of children of all shapes, sizes and interests. It is unrealistic to think that all boys are interested in football and hockey and all girls are interested in gymnastics and cheerleading. Good school intramural programs are essential (Corbin, D. E., 1978, p. 2).

SUMMARY

Of principal concern to the parents, coaches, and organizers of children's sports programs, is meeting the goals or objectives for which the programs were intended. For this to be possible it is very important that the adults involved with the programs know the benefits to be gained from the programs and the possible risks. These adults should also be aware of the goals of the participating children, as well as the most effective methods for making sure that the benefits become realities and that the risks be diminished.

Information is presented in this chapter which should be of value in implementing an effective program designed to meet the needs of the children participating in youth sports. The information and the guidelines presented in this chapter are consistent with those presented in a joint policy statement of the American Alliance for Health, Physical Education and Recreation, the American

Academy of Pediatrics, The American Medical Association Committee on the Medical Aspects of Sports, and the Society of State Directors of Health, Physical Education, and Recreation (1968). This statement reinforces the need for proper leadership, proper equipment, proper training practices, proper maturation grouping, and proper medical care for all youth sports athletes. Perhaps Rarick (1978) offers the best advice with the following statement, ". . . the statement (joint policy statement) places well defined restrictions on the type of athletic competition appropriate for children and the conditions should be met before such programs are instituted. Throughout the report emphasis is placed on the need for exemplary supervision, both educational and medical, and unless this can be assured, schools and communities should neither initiate nor continue sports programs for children."

References

AAHPER. *Desirable Athletic Competition for Children of Elementary School Age.* Washington: AAHPER, 1968.

Bar-or, O. "Predicting Athletic Performance." *The Physician and Sportsmedicine* 4(1975): 80.

Berryman, J. W. "The Rise of Highly Organized Sports for Preadolescent Boys." In *Children in Sport: A Contemporary Anthology,* edited by R. A. McGill et al. Champaign, Ill.: Human Kinetics Publishers, 1978.

Corbin, D. E. "Kids and Sports-In Perspective." *Leftfield: FANS Newsletter* 1(1978):2.

Etzwiler, D. D. "When the Diabetic Wants to Be an Athlete." *The Physician and Sportsmedicine* 2(1974):45.

Gugrnheim, J. J. et al. "Little League Survey: The Houston Study." *The Journal of Sports Medicine* 4(1976):189.

Harter, S. "Effectance Motivation Reconsidered." *Human Development* 21(1978):34.

Katz, R. M. "Asthmatics Don't Have to Sit out of Sports." *The Physician and Sportsmedicine* 4(1976):45.

Larson, R. L. et al. "Little League Survey: The Eugene Survey." *The Journal of Sports Medicine* 4(1976):201.

Livingston, S. and Berman, W. "Participation of the Epileptic Child in Contact Sports." *Journal of Sports Medicine* 2(1974):170.

Martens, R. *Joy and Sadness in Children's Sports.* Champaign, Ill.: Human Kinetics Publishers, 1978.

Rarick, G. L. "Competitive Sports in Childhood and Early Adolescence." In *Children in Sport: A Contemporary Anthology,* edited by R. A. McGill et al. Champaign, Ill.: Human Kinetics Publishers, 1978.

Roberts, R. "Children in Competition: Assignment of Responsibility for Winning and Losing." *NCPEAM Proceedings* 78(1977):328.

Scanlan, T. K. "The Effects of Success-Failure on the Perception of Threat in a Competitive Situation." *Research Quarterly* 48(1977):144.

Scanlan, T. K. and Passer, M. W. "Factors Related to Competitive Stress among Male Youth Sports Participants." *Medicine and Science in Sports* 10(1978):103.

Thomas, J. R., ed. *Youth Sports Guide: For Coaches and Parents.* Washington: The Manufacturers Life Insurance Company and NASPE, 1978.

Whieldon, D. "Maturity Sorting: New Balance for Young Athletes." *The Physician and Sportsmedicine* 6(1978):127.

Section 10

Motor Development in
Adolescence and
Adulthood

Adolescent Growth, Maturity, and Development

29

Robert M. Malina
University of Texas

Adolescence is the period of transition from childhood to adulthood. It is most commonly viewed within the context of sexual maturation and statural growth. Adolescence begins with an acceleration in the rate of growth prior to the attainment of sexual maturity, and then merges into a decelerative phase, terminating with the cessation of statural growth, i.e., the attainment of adult stature. The growth and sexual maturation characteristic of adolescence ordinarily begins and ends during the second decade of life. Awareness of adolescence is usually indicated by outward manifestations of pubertal changes. However, physiological events underlying the growth and maturational changes have been in progress for some time prior to the appearance of physical changes, while statural growth may continue into the third decade. Thus, the time span which accommodates adolescence varies from 9 or 10 years through 21 or 22 years of age.

Adolescence comprises a complex series of biological events including changes in size, i.e., the adolescent growth spurt, alterations in proportions and physique, changes in body composition, maturation of primary and secondary sex characteristics, changes in the cardio-respiratory system, and changes in the nervous and endocrine systems that initiate and coordinate the somatic, sexual and physiologic changes (Malina, 1974, 1975a, 1978a; Tanner, 1962, 1969). This chapter provides a brief overview of the growth, maturity and performance characteristics of the adolescent years.

ADOLESCENT GROWTH

Sex differences in body size before the adolescent spurt are minor, although boys tend to be, on the average, slightly taller and heavier. During the early part of adolescence, girls are taller and heavier than boys, due to the earlier adolescent spurt, i.e., earlier maturation of girls. Girls, however, soon lose this size advantage as the male adolescent spurt starts. Male catch up and eventually surpass females in height and weight. Most external dimensions of the body, for example, sitting height, leg length, shoulder breadth, hip breadth, limb circumferences, and the like, follow the same general growth pattern for size attained and growth rate as height and weight. In general, prior to adolescence, sex differences are minor; in the early adolescent years, females have a temporary size advantage, but males eventually surpass females in size attained in most dimensions.

As for body size, sex differences in body proportions, though apparent, are relatively minor during the preadolescent years. Sex differences in the adolescent growth spurt produce the characteristic sexual dimorphism (morphological differences between males and females) seen in young adulthood. For example, the obvious broadening of the shoulders relative to the hips is characteristic of male adolescence, while the broadening of the hips relative to the shoulders and waist is characteristic of female adolescence. The same is true for estimated leg length relative to stature. Prior to the adolescent spurt, both boys and girls are proportionately similar in terms of the contributions of the lower extremities and the trunk to total height. However, during adolescence and in adulthood, females have, for equal stature, shorter legs than males. Thus, females are, on the average, relatively short-legged compared to males, who are relatively long-legged.

Comparisons of somatotype* ratings over adolescence illustrate the effects of the adolescent spurt on physique development. Male adolescence is characterized by major development in the mesomorphic component, a reduction in the endomorphic component, and an increase in the ectomorphic component. Female adolescence, on the other hand, involves primary development in endomorphy, slight increase in mesomorphy, and a reduction in ectomorphy.

The effects of adolescence on physique are such that in young adulthood, as in childhood, there are more endomorphic females than males and more mesomorphic males than females. Females are more concentrated in the high endomorphic sector of a somatotype distribution, while males tend toward the mesomorphic sector. However, males are more extensively distributed throughout the somatotype spectrum than are females.

Physique changes during adolescence provide some indication of underlying changes in body composition. Compositional changes during adolescence vary primarily on a leanness-fatness axis. Males increase in lean body mass, especially muscle mass, and decrease in fatness, especially in the extremities. Females, on the other hand, increase in both lean body mass and fatness. The male increase in lean body mass during adolescence is rather abrupt, generally occurring after the adolescent height spurt. The increase in females is more gradual. The increase in lean body mass in male adolescents is relatively greater than the increase in body weight, since body fat content decreases at this time. Mature lean body mass values are reached earlier in females compared to males. Thus, average lean body mass values for postadolescent girls are, approximately, only two-thirds of the male values. On the other hand, young adult females have almost twice the amount of body fat as males. The growth pattern for lean body mass parallels closely the pattern for height and weight. Body fatness changes are more variable than those for lean body mass. Absolute amounts of total body fat, generally increase during childhood, but show a decrease in accumulation or a reduced rate of accumulation during adolescence, especially in males. The range of variation within and between sexes, however, is considerable and should be carefully noted.

MATURITY VARIATION AND GROWTH

The preceding overview of adolescent growth concerned changes with age or over time. The measure of age used is the child's chronological age. Size, build, and composition, however, vary considerably with the child's biological age or maturity status as

---

*Somatotypes or body types are generally typically assessed using Sheldon's three types. Mesomorphy is a muscular characteristic, endomorphy is a predisposition to fatness, and ectomorphy is the tendency toward a lean or linear build.

indicated by skeletal age, age at menarche, development of secondary sex characteristics, or the timing of most rapid growth during adolescence (peak height velocity).

Maturity-associated variation, though apparent prior to adolescence, is most pronounced during this period of accelerated growth and sexual maturation. In girls, the first sign if impeding puberty is enlargement of the breasts, which is generally followed in sequence by the appearance of pubic hair, the height spurt, the final stages of pubic hair development, and menarche. In boys, the first sign of impending puberty is the beginning growth of the testes and scrotum, followed in sequence by the appearance of pubic hair, the height spurt and rapid growth of the penis, and the final stages of pubic hair development (Tanner, 1962, 1969). Although the sequence of maturational events is relatively uniform, children pass through adolescence at widely different chronological ages. Furthermore, the rate at which the events of the accelerated growth phase are passed through varies considerably.

Children are commonly grouped into maturity categories as "early," "average," and "late" maturing for growth studies. Early-maturing children are those in whom the maturity indicators are in advance of chronological age. For example, a child having a chronological age of 10 and a skeletal age of 12 would be early maturing, as would a girl experiencing menarche at 11 years of age. In contrast, late-maturing children are those in whom the maturity indicators lag relative to chronological age. For example, a child having a chronological age of 10 and a skeletal age of 8 would be late maturing, as would a girl experiencing menarche at 15 years of age. Average-maturing children make up the broad middle

range of normal variation, with the normal range in growth studies usually being defined as plus or minus one year of an individual's chronological age. For example, in a group of 10-year-old children, those with skeletal ages of between 9 and 11 years are in the average-maturing group. Those with skeletal ages in excess of 11 years are early maturers, and those with skeletal ages of less than 9 years are late maturers.

Early-maturing children of both sexes are generally heavier and taller for their age from early childhood through adolescence than their average- and late-maturing peers. The differences between the maturity groups are most apparent during adolescence. In late adolescence, late-maturing children generally catch up to the early maturers in stature, but not in body weight. Early maturers thus have more weight for their height, i.e., have stockier builds, than late maturers. Viewed in terms of physique, extreme mesomorphy is related to early maturation in boys, while endomorphy and early maturation are related in girls. On the other hand, extreme ectomorphy or linearity of physique is associated with lateness of maturity in both boys and girls. Many of the physique features which characterize early- and late-maturing children are apparent before adolescence and thus, are not entirely dependent upon the adolescent spurt. The differential timing and magnitude of the spurt, however, tends to magnify the apparent differences.

Maturity-associated variation in physique implies similar variation in body composition. Early-maturing children, as compared to late-maturing children, generally have larger amounts of fat, muscle, and bone tissue, and larger lean body masses, reflecting to a great extent their larger body size. On a relative basis, however, early-maturing children are fatter and not as lean as late maturers; that is, fat comprises a greater percentage of body weight in the early maturer. Differences between late-maturing children and those in the average, or middle, range of the maturity continuum are generally not as marked as the differences between these two maturity groupings and early-maturing children.

FACTORS INFLUENCING PERFORMANCE DURING ADOLESCENCE

Many of the factors viewed as influencing motor performance during childhood can be extended to performance during adolescence. The influence of size, physique and composition on motor performance during adolescence is affected by their relationships to maturity and the timing of the adolescent spurt. Strength and performance are also related. Further, during adolescence the role of nonbiological factors must be considered. These especially revolve about peer status, motivation, and culturally-dependent behavioral expectations.

The effects of size, physique and body composition on motor performance during adolescence are much the same as those apparent during childhood (Malina, 1975b). Relationships tend to be low to moderate, with little predictive significance. However, at the extremes of size, physique and composition, performance effects are apparent. The extreme endomorph is, for example, handicapped by the negative effects of excess fatness on performance items requiring the projection or movement of his body. The extreme ectomorph is handicapped by a deficiency in muscular strength necessary for power tasks. Data are more extensive for motor performance of boys,

while data relating growth, physique and performance of girls are more limited, especially during adolescence.

The seemingly small affects of size, physique and body composition on strength and performance during adolescence are related to the impact of variation in the timing and magnitude of the adolescent growth spurt and sexual maturation on these morphological indicators. During adolescence maturity relationships with strength are more apparent for boys than they are for girls. Early maturing boys are stronger age for age than their average and late maturing peers from pre-adolescence into adolescence (Jones, 1949; Carron and Bailey, 1974). Strength differences between early and late maturers are especially apparent between 13 and 16 years of age, and the strength advantage for the early-maturing boys reflects their larger body size and muscle mass. When the effects of body weight are removed in comparing early and late maturing boys, strength differences between the contrasting maturity groups are eliminated (Carron and Bailey, 1974).

Early maturing girls are stronger than their late maturing peers during early adolescence. They do not, however, maintain this advantage as adolescence progresses (Jones, 1949). Early and late maturing girls attain comparable strength levels in later adolescence by apparently different routes. The early maturer shows rapid strength development through 13 years of age and then improves only slightly thereafter. The late maturer, on the other hand, improves in strength gradually between 11 and 16 years, so that at 16 years of age, the contrasting maturity categories do not differ in strength.

During the adolescent years, boys advanced in biological maturity status also perform more proficiently in a variety of motor tasks than less mature boys. This, in part, is related to the greater muscularity and strength of the more mature boy. In girls, on the other hand, motor performance during adolescence is not related to measures of biological maturity (Espenschade, 1940). Correlations between skeletal maturity and age deviation from menarche and motor performance are low and in many tasks, negative. In fact, late maturation is commonly associated with outstanding motor performance of adolescent girls (see Malina, 1978b).

Thus, contrasting maturity-performance relationships during adolescence are apparent for boys and girls. The advent of male adolescence brings about marked improvements and, consequently, considerable differences in strength and performance of boys of contrasting maturity status. On the other hand, the advent of female adolescence brings about slight improvements in strength, but no marked changes in motor performance. Thus, variability in rate of maturation during adolescence exerts a significantly greater influence on the strength and performance of boys than of girls.

The changes in size, build and composition from pre-adolescence through adolescence result in an altered bodily configuration. The developing adolescent must adjust to his or her "new" body. The manner in which an adolescent boy or girl comes to terms with his or her altered morphology and physiology has significant behavioral correlates. The adolescent's body image, for example, is to a large extent revised, especially in terms of appearance, limits of strength, and perhaps coordination.

Variation in the timing of adolescent events adds to the complexity of changing relationships between body image and behavior during adolescence. Early and late maturation are associated with distinctive personality and behavioral characteristics, which in turn may have a strong influence on behavior during adolescence and in adult life.

It would be interesting to consider the relationships of biological and behavioral changes of normal adolescents. When for example, do certain behavioral changes occur in the cycle of biological events at adolescence? Are there particular behavioral changes that characterize the acceleration phase of growth at adolescence? Or, are there behavioral changes characteristic of the decelerative phase? Maximum strength development in males usually occurs after maximum growth in height and weight. How, for example, might such developmental changes relate to behavior modifications? Are they the same for early- and late-maturing adolescents? As indicated above, early- and late-maturing children differ in behavior and personality; however, more data are necessary concerning relationships between specific events and timing of the adolescent phase of growth and behavioral changes.

The role of societal expectations in determining the behavioral roles early- and late-maturing children assume must also be considered. In many studies of maturity, personality, and behavior, considerable importance has been placed on the fact that early maturers were expected to behave in an adult-like manner, and the late maturers were expected to assume less mature, defensive roles. Thus, the interaction between maturation and personality is influenced by another variable, cultural expectations. In the system of personality determination by maturational status, culture serves as the immediate directive force in shaping personality. The biology of the individual, i.e., his or her maturational status, acts through the individual's culture to shape personality differences. The interaction of the individual's maturity status, personality characteristics and cultural expectations is probably more complex than outlined. Nevertheless, it serves to illustrate the dynamic interaction of biology, culture and personality during development.

References

Carron, A. V. and Bailey, D. A. "Strength Development in Boys from 10 through 16 Years." *Monographs of the Society for Research in Child Development* 4(1974):39.

Espenschade, A. "Motor Performance in Adolescence." *Monographs of the Society for Research in Child Development* 1(1940):5.

Jones, H. E. *Motor Performance and Growth.* Berkeley: University of California Press, 1949.

Malina, R. M. "Adolescent Changes in Size, Build, Composition, and Performance." *Human Biology* 46(1974):117-31.

Malina, R. M. *Growth and Development: The First Twenty Years in Man.* Minneapolis: Burgess, 1975a.

Malina, R. M. "Anthropometric Correlates of Strength and Motor Performance." *Exercise and Sport Sciences Reviews* 3(1975b):249-74.

Malina, R. M. "Adolescent Growth and Maturation: Selected Aspects of Current Research." *Yearbook of Physical Anthropology* 21 (1978a):(in press).

Malina, R. M. "Physical Growth and Maturity Characteristics of Young Athletes." In *Children in Sport: A Contemporary Perspective,* edited by R. A. Magill; M. J. Ash; and F. L. Smoll. Champaign, Illinois: Human Kinetics Publishers, 1978b, pp. 79-101.

Tanner, J. M. *Growth at Adolescence,* 2nd ed. Oxford: Blackwell Scientific Publications, 1962.

Tanner, J. M. "Growth and Endocrinology of the Adolescent." In *Endocrine and Genetic Diseases of Childhood,* edited by L. I. Gardner. Philadelphia: Saunders, 1969, pp. 19-60.

Motor Performance and Physical Fitness in Adolescence

30

Charles B. Corbin
Kansas State University

The specific intent of this chapter is to present information concerning the motor performance and physical fitness of the adolescent.

FUNDAMENTAL SKILL LEARNING

Most studies indicate that the skill learning years are the years prior to adolescence. Nash (1960) indicated that 85% of motor skills and motor skill interests have been traced to an age of 12 or less. The implication is that childhood is a time for fundamental skill learning, while adolescence is a time for skill refinement, and learning a wide variety of motor skills. In general this is true. However, in spite of the fact that most fundamental skills can and should be learned in childhood, this is not always the case. Many children reach adolescence without the most basic abilities to perform fundamental skills such as throwing, catching, striking, etc. These people must be classified as remedial.

Just as the prognosis is not good for a 7th grade non-reader, the prognosis is not good for a 13-year-old who has little ability to perform fundamental skills. The fundamental skills can be considered the ABC's of motor behavior. The adolescent who does not know the alphabet and fundamental word construction has little interest in reading and often has little interest in school. Likewise, it is not surprising that adolecents who cannot perform basic fundamental skills have little interest in learning them. These people may have acquired "learned helplessness" as discussed in Chapter 28. They may feel that "I can't" or physical performance is "just not my thing." These people may totally opt out of physical activity.

It should be noted that "old dogs can learn new tricks", it's just harder than it is for the young. If adolescents, who cannot perform basic motor skills, are ever to learn them, several conditions are necessary.

1. Screening must be done. We must identify those adolescents who are having trouble.

2. Once identified, we must go back to the basics. It is important in doing this that we not call attention to the problem of the learner (see Chapter 25 for more details). Work with adolescents needing help in small groups and away from the view of those who do not have problems.

3. Do not evaluate learners on the quantity of their performance. To do so would place undue pressure on the learner. Concentrate on helping each learner improve the quality of his or her performance.

4. Help the learner understand that he or she may be able to perform (at first) the incorrect way better than the correct way. It took 12 or more years of practice to learn the incorrect skills. It may take some time to "unlearn" the incorrect method of performing and to learn the correct method.

PERCEPTUAL-MOTOR DEVELOPMENT

As noted in Section 7, the perceptual components of motor behavior are virtually fully developed in most individuals by adolescence. Of course there are obvious exceptions. Adolescents with perceptual-motor problems need special attention. It is beyond the scope of this text to deal with these special perceptual-motor development problems.

PHYSICAL FITNESS DIFFERENCES BETWEEN BOYS AND GIRLS

The figures presented in the preceding chapters concerning the physical fitness of children included information relevant to adolescents (See Figures 15.1, 16.1, 16.3, 16.4, 17.1). These figures illustrate the fact that health related fitness, in general, increases dramatically during adolescence. This is especially true for boys.

Although there are differences in performance curves within sexes for each separate factor of physical fitness, there is a pattern of performance for both boys and girls which typifies performance for each sex. That general pattern is presented in Figure 30.1.

One reason for the decreased performance for older girls relates to physical fitness testing procedures. Not only are girls less likely than boys to be encouraged to improve their physical fitness through regular vigorous exercise, they are often not motivated to score well on fitness tests, even though they could. Too few girls give an all out effort on a 600-yard run or even on a strength tests. Girls may have learned that, for them, high fitness test scores are not of great social value. The fact that laboratory test scores for girls on such measures a Maximal O$_2$ Intake and PWC, even when cor-

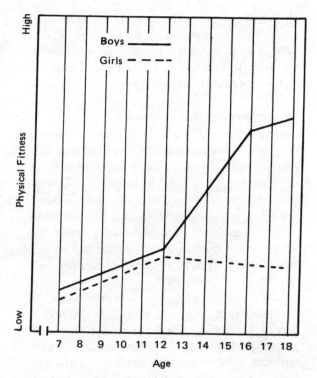

Figure 30.1. Physical fitness of performance differences between boys and girls.

rected for body weight, increase with age would tend to support the idea that girls *could* perform well if they would. Laboratory tests made on a one-on-one basis are not contaminated by the lack of motivation to perform as are the group administered field tests.

Fear of physical injury to female internal organs is another reason for limited physical fitness performance for girls after age ten. Many still cling to the wive's tale that performance of such activities as chin-ups, pull-ups, push-ups, and other strength feats will somehow damage the female internal organs. The myth suggests that heavy lifting, pushing, or pulling will force the neck of the uterus down into the vagina thus interferring with a girl's capability for bearing children. Physicians and researchers alike reject this myth; indeed, research indicates that women who exercise regularly have fewer cases of painful menstruation, fewer miscarriages, and easier labor and delivery (AAAU 1953; Erdelyi 1962; Clarke 1978). Nevertheless, girls may reject vigorous activity for fear of injury.

Fear of masculinization is another reason why girls may not perform well on physical fitness tests. Myths concerning the fear of developing "muscles like men" are prevalent among teenage girls. Though research does not support these myths, the performances of girls may be altered by them. To what extent this is a factor in the lack of improvement in physical fitness scores for girls can only be speculated.

Time and time again it was mentioned in the preceding chapters that performance of boys increases gradually with age until approximately age twelve. After that time performance increases dramatically with age. Girls on the other hand increase in performance up until ten or eleven and thereafter performance declines or at least levels off. Possible physiological reasons for this phenomenon are discussed in Chapters 15 and 16. The difference between performances of boys and girls cannot be explained away so easily, however. As already discussed, it is apparent that motivational factors of social origin are involved. Outstanding physical performance is often expected of boys but not girls in our culture. This is obvious for physical fitness tests which set a maximum allowable for girls sit-ups at 50 while boys are allowed to perform 100. Girls do not perform chins because it is expected that they can't. This writer suggests that performance curves for girls, though more gradual in slope, would more nearly approximate those of boys if societal values allowed for outstanding physical performances by girls. Girls can and would work to achieve physi-

cal fitness, even during adolescence, if this achievement was valued by society. To be sure, girls are now given greater opportunity to participate. For outstanding women performers there is increasing respect for physical competence. However, success in vigorous physical performance is not yet as acceptable for the "typical" girl as it is for the "typical" boy.

PHYSICAL ACTIVITY DURING MENSTRUATION AND PREGNANCY

In the preceding section it was noted that some girls may fail to perform well on physical fitness tests because of the fear of injury to the reproductive system. Not only has this been shown to be untrue, but evidence is now available which shows that girls who exercise regularly have fewer menstrual cycle and pregnancy problems than those who do not exercise (Clarke, 1978). The recently reported evidence has resulted in a significant statement by the Committee on the Medical Aspects of Sports of the American Medical Association:

The Committee on the Medical Aspects of Sports reiterates the beneficial aspects of sports and exercise participation for girls and women. Female participation in such programs previously was discouraged due to societal and cultural stereotypes that considered such participation a departure from the traditional role. Much to the contrary, physiological and social benefits are to be gained by girls and women through physical activity and sports competition. In many cases, vigorous physical activity improves the distinct biological functions of the female.

Usually, dysmenorrhea is unaffected by sports participation or subsides as a result of such participation. Exercise can also improve regulation of the menstrual cycle. Following active sports involvement of international caliber, female athletes have experienced a greater number of complication-free pregnancies and greater ease of delivery than recorded for a normal but less physically active control group. These specific benefits often accrue to female athletes quite apart from the normal physiological benefits to both males and females from regular exercise or sports participation, including improvement in muscle tone and strength, increased range of joint motion, and improvement in cardiovascular function. Thus, there is no medical or scientific rationale for restricting the normal female from participating in vigorous noncontact sports, and many reasons to encourage such participation. Physical activity and sports programs can contribute greatly to the personal fulfillment and healthful living of women (Corbitt, et al, 1975, p. 45).

It is important that every adolescent girl understand the information presented above. If performance scores of adolescent girls are to improve on tests of health related fitness, this is essential.

TRAINABILITY AND VARIATIONS IN HEALTH RELATED FITNESS OF ADOLESCENTS

Adolescence appears to be a time of optimal development of health related physical fitness. Developmental changes associated with increases in muscle mass and body size in both boys and girls result in increases in many gross performances. Optimal exercise in the threshold of training for a specific aspect of health related fitness will result in efficient effort-benefit ratios. For each unit of effort expended, the relative benefits will be great, especially compared to childhood. Though Ekblom (1969) suggests that the threshold of cardiovascular fitness training may be higher for adolescents than for adults, there is evidence that even cardiovascular fitness will develop rapidly with training in adolescence. Cooper et al. (1975) showed that a school aerobics program resulted in a 17.6% increase in cardiovascular fitness for normal adolescents. Landry (1973) notes gains in cardiovascular

fitness of up to 20% with training during the growth spurt.

All of the information presented in the preceding paragraph suggests that adolescence, in general, is a time when training for health related fitness is efficient. However, it should be noted that there is a wide variation in onset of adolescence and in age of achievement of physical maturity. Because of this wide variation, generalizations about trainability in adolescence must be tempered. For example, among boys 30% at age 12, 20% at age 13, 10% at age 14, and 5% from 15 to 17 cannot do one pull up (AAHPERD, 1976). While many boys are maturing physically and achieving fitness with training and normal developmental changes, there are still many even by the later teens who are not at a developmental stage where training is most efficient. For these people the effort-benefit ratios for fitness development are similar to those of children. For girls, because of earlier maturation this is less true. For the lesser number of girls to whom it applies, the potential for developing many aspects of gross health related fitness is not equal to the girls who are pubescent or postpubescent.

During adolescence it is especially important that information about individual differences in performance be discussed and taken into consideration in planning exercise programs. The evaluation of fitness, especially for grading, should take into account differences in maturation and ability levels of adolescents. It should also be noted that even though adolescence is a time when training may be efficient for many, it is a time of *development*. Absolute scores on many performance tasks are still not equal to adult standards and comparisons of adolescents to adult standards may be inappropriate.

THE MOTOR SKILL POTENTIAL OF ADOLESCENTS

Already established are the following facts: (a) adolescents with good motor experiences in childhood have acquired the basic or fundamental motor skills, (b) adolescents are experiencing a time of efficient learning in motor performance, (c) both boys and girls are capable of vigorous physical activity in adolescence, and (d) there is wide variation in the motor development of adolescents. Add to this the fact that adolescents often have the time and interest necessary to practice intensely, and it is not difficult to see why adolescence is a time of great motor accomplishment for many.

Though most fundamental motor skills are learned in childhood, it is during adolescence that many people achieve proficiency in many sports and games. Chourbagi (1973) noted that young children have neither the biological nor psychological characteristics necessary for outstanding performance. He noted that only 15% of all olympic champions started their sport prior to age 10. 45% started between the ages of 10 and 14 while 40% started between the ages of 15 and 19. Contrary to popular opinion, adolescents with good fundamental skills and a wide variety of motor experiences appear to be able to accomplish significant motor performance feats in spite of that fact that they did not train intensively as children.

Hirata (1973) also studied olympic champions and noted that adolescents were most likely to experience success in swimming, ice skating and skiing. These are "skill" sports which require intensive training and at least some prerequisite health related fitness. These are both factors present for many adolescents. Hirata also noted that adolescents do not do so well in sports requiring high absolute strength, power and muscular endurance. This corresponds to what exercise physiologists have noted for years, i.e. potential for optimal performance in strength, power and endurance activities occurs in the late to mid twenties. Teenagers do not do well in olympic events which require great amounts of strategy and experience. Examples are yachting, fencing, bicycle riding etc. Adolescence is a time of great potential for skill learning. However, as noted earlier, it is a time when development in many areas is far from complete. In some sports adolescents can and do excel, but for the person who continues to train, postadolescence may be the time of greatest accomplishment in many areas of motor performance.

It should be pointed out that the preceding discussion has dealt principally with the adolescent who trains vigorously to improve fitness and motor skill. Those who are less interested in superior performances such as those necessary for becoming an olympic champion may find adolescence to be a time for achieving their greatest motor skill accomplishments. With continued effort skills and fitness could improve until the late twenties. There is evidence to indicate that for many, if not most Americans, this is not the case. Because the teen years are, for many, the most active years, both young men and young women may achieve skill and fitness in adolescence which will never again be equaled in their lifetime.

SPORTS FOR ADOLESCENTS

For all intents and purposes, adolescence is the best time in life for active participation in sports. The time, interest and motivation necessary for involvement is often present.

Before making unreserved statements about sports for adolescents two basic factors deserved discussion. These factors are sports injuries, and sex and maturity matching for competition.

Sports Injuries

Many people expound on the risks associated with sports participation for children but few are as concerned about the risks of injury to the adolescent. In fact studies show that injuries are more severe and frequent between the ages of 15 and 18 than at any other age (Godshall, 1975). This may in part be due to the greater intensity with which adolescents participate and the greater size of the adolescent athlete, but it may also be due to the fact that less concern may be given for maturity or age matching at the higher levels. In schools where only gifted, mature, large individuals make the team this may not be a problem. It may, however, be a problem in smaller schools where smaller less mature adolescents participate to "fill out the team."

As with youth sports, leadership relates to sport's injuries. Blyth and Mueller (1974) note that teams with older coaches having athletic experience, coaching experience, and advanced degrees had less injuries than those with coaches not possessing these characteristics. Interestingly, coaches with a minor in physical education had fewer injuries than those with a physical education major.

Because of the risk of injury, especially in collision sports, during adolescence it is especially important that proper conditioning, proper leadership, proper equipment, and proper medical attention be provided for the adolescent athlete.

Sex and Maturity Matching In Adolescence

Prior to adolescence boys and girls are relatively equal in size and potential ability. As noted in previous chapters, boys and girls may participate and compete together in sports in childhood given adequate maturity and ability matching. However, in adolescence there are many who warn against cross-sex or unisex competition. These people feel that if boys compete with girls and lose, the result will be very damaging to the boy. Michener (1976) for example suggests in his book *Sport in America* that ". . . that the traditional athletic separation of boys and girls during the ages of 12 to 22 conforms to some permanent psychological need of the human race and that to reverse this custom might produce more harm than good (p. 130)." He further suggests that losing to a girl is figurative "castration" and an "ego shattering" experience for the typical American boy.

Martens (1978) in response indicates, "Michener's thoughts are in left field in my opinion. I know of no evidence—none whatsoever—to suggest that male domination and separation of the sexes at this age is biologically based. On the contrary, all evidence indicates that these are learned attitudes— attitudes which incidently are not found universally (p. 168)." Even though Martens rejects entirely Michener's suggestions, he too warns against unisex or cross-sex competition. He recommends that ". . . boys and girls should play all sports demanding speed, strength, and endurance separately beginning at the age of 11 (Martens, 1978, p. 169)." Though he does acknowledge the potential psychological dangers of post-pubescent unisex competition, he bases his recommendation for separating the sexes for competition after 11 are based principally on differences in body size and physical maturation during adolescence.

Based on the research findings and commentary of qualified scholars, the following guidelines for adolescent cross-sex, competition seem warranted.

1. There is little doubt that in America differences in the socialization process have resulted in different sex-role expectations for boys and girls. While time will undoubtedly see significant changes in the socialization process and the sex-role expectations, both boys and girls may experience some problems associated with cross-sex competition in adolescence. Research by Corbin and Nix (1979) suggests that boys may *not* have problems if they and their peers perceive that it is possible that a girl might be "good" in the activity in which they are competing. For example it might be embarrassing to lose to a girl for many boys but it might not be embarrassing to lose in tennis to Chris Evert. Furthermore, girls may exhibit more confidence in activity if they are encouraged to feel that girls can and should be able to achieve in sports. Teachers and adolescent sports leaders would do well to help boys and girls learn that the sex of the opponent is not the important factor. There is a wide range of skill ability for both sexes and in many sports adolescent girls who excel perform better than most boys.

2. Just as girls who excel in activity may perform better than most boys, there are many girls who cannot perform as well as the poorest boy performers. Research results clearly establish this fact. In our society, especially for tasks requiring speed, strength, and power, the performance of the average adolescent girl is considerably poorer than for the average boy. If we are to truely increase the opportunities for young women in sports, it is essential that unisex

sports teams *not* be the only opportunity for participation for females. If this were the case, most teams would be dominated by boys simply because of their experience and strength, power, and speed advantage. Girls would not only fail to receive the opportunity to participate now, but would be deprived of the opportunity to improve for the future.

3. As with youth or children's sports, maturity matching is important. Injuries increase in adolescence and at least part of the reason is the increased size and ability of the participants. When boys and girls compete together on the same teams against each other, the problem of maturity matching becomes a more difficult problem. Because of size, strength, speed, and power differences between the sexes, not to mention the differences in maturation rates, injury potential in contact and collision sports would be great if all adolescents where to compete together on the same teams without regard for these factors. If unisex or cross-sex competition in adolescence is to become a reality, *effective maturation, body size, and ability matching is an absolute must.*

4. When we think of unisex or cross-sex competition we frequently think of a boy wrestling or playing tennis against a girl. To many, girls and boys competing together on the same football or basketball team is the vision conveyed by unisex or cross-sex competition. An alternative to what is generally called unisex or cross-sex competition is mixed-sex competition. In some sports, such as tennis doubles, males and females have competed together against mixed-sex teams of opponents with good results. This type of *mixed-sex* competition is particularly good for certain sports if maturity, body size, and ability matching is considered. Mixed relay teams (an equal number of each sex per

team) seem reasonable for such sports as track and swimming. In cases where a decision is made to have separate teams for each sex group, there appears to be no good reason why the teams cannot compete together at the same time and location against opponents of the same sex. This has worked well with sports such as gymnatics and skating for years.

Guidelines For Adolescent Sports Competition

Adolescence is a time when all people, regardless of ability can refine their skills and benefit from a wide variety of sport and activity. Each person can learn to assess his or her own abilities and pick a form of exercise, sport, or physical activity for a lifetime of use. The less skilled must learn to realistically assess their own abilities and learn to set realistic goals. This will allow these individuals to enjoy activity and will reduce the chance of failure in activity and sports.

For the gifted individual, adolescence is a time for developing high levels of proficiency in a sport. As with any worthwhile pursuit, it is reasonable for the adolescent to strive for excellence in physical activity and sport. For both boys and girls, sport is a legitimate arena for demonstrating achievement. However, it is important that sports achievement not be emphasized to the exclusion of other areas of development. As noted in Chapter 1, total development of the person is of ultimate concern. When any highly specialized area of development is overemphasized it can have detremental effects on total development. Since adolescence is a time of rapid development in many areas, it is especially important that the adolescent attend to many developmental experiences including intellectual, social,

and emotional. Not to be overlooked is total motor development.

For the adolescent excellence in sports is *one* legitimate pursuit. At the same time it is important that the adolescent become involved in social activities including dating, academic activities, and other interest activities such as art and music which have a lifetime of application. As Edwards (1973) has pointed out, sports for most people are only a small part of life after adolescence. Few people will have the opportunity to become college or professional athletes and even these people will have a limited number of years of involvement in sports as a vocation. It is important that adolescents establish a sound academic, prevocational, social, and emotional foundation. Sports involvement should contribute rather than detract from the development of this foundation for effective living.

In addition to the important point discussed above, the same general guidelines for participation in sports for children apply to adolescents. For more details refer to page 263.

References

AAHPER. *AAHPER Youth Fitness Test Manual.* Washington: AAHPER Publications, 1976.

American Amateur Athletic Union. "Effects of Athletic Competition in Girls and Women." New York: AAAU, 1953.

Blyth, C. S. and Mueller, F. O. "Football Injury Survey." *The Physician and Sportsmedicine* 2(1974):45.

Clarke, H. H. "Physical Activity during Menstruation and Pregnancy." *Physical Fitness Research Digest* 8(1978):1.

Chourbagi, Z. Y. "The Age Factor in Competitive Sports." In *Sport in the Modern World,* edited by O. Grupe et al. Heidelberg: Springer-Verlag Berlin, 1973.

Cooper, K. H. "An Aerobic Conditioning Program for the Fort Worth Schools." *Research Quarterly* 46(1975):345.

Corbitt, R. W. et al. "Committee Statement on Exercise and Sports for Girls and Women." *Journal of Physical Education and Recreation* 46(1975):45.

Corbin, C. B. and Nix, C. "Sex Typing of Physical Activities and Success Predictions of Children Before and After Cross-Sex Competition." *Journal of Sport Psychology* 1(1979):43.

Edwards, H. *Sociology of Sport*. Homewood, Ill.: Dorsey Press, 1973.

Ekblom, B. "Effect of Physical Training on Adolescent Boys." *Journal of Applied Physiology* 27(1969):350.

Erdelyi, G. J. "Gynecological Survey of Female Athletes." *Journal of Sports Medicine* 2 (1962):174.

Godshall, R. W. "Junior League Football." *Journal of Sports Medicine* 3(1975):139.

Hirata, K. "The Age of Olympic Champions." In *Sport in the Modern World*, edited by O. Grupe et al. Heidelberg: Springer-Verlag Berlin, 1973.

Landry, F. "Sport for Youth and Sport Medicine." In *Sport in the Modern World*, edited by O. Grupe et al. Heidelberg: Springer-Verlag Berlin, 1973.

Martens, R. *Joy and Sadness in Children's Sports*. Champaign, Ill.: Human Kinetics Publishers, 1978.

Michener, J. A. *Sports in America*. New York: Random House, 1976.

Nash, J. B. *Philosophy of Recreation and Leisure*. Dubuque: Wm. C. Brown Company Publishers, 1960, chapter 13.

Motor Development Throughout Life

31

Joel Rosentswieg
Texas Woman's University

The effects of aging on motor development present what seems to be an obvious result in our youth oriented society: aging after adolescence is deleterious. Yet, what seems to represent a truism is not nearly so clear in reality. Research has shown that aging, other than as a chronological event, is a very complex phenomenon involving multiple relationships many of which are still unknown. The terminology related to aging is in constant flux. For this chapter adolescence refers to the teen years (13-19). A "young adult" is post adolescence (20 yrs.) to 29 years of age. An adult ranges in age from 30 to 65 years. The "aged" will be anyone older than 65 years of age.

During the young adult period of life most of ones' powers are at a zenith. It is fairly well established that speed, strength, power and flexibility activities are the province of the young. The generality frequently heard is speed in the 20's, strength in the 30's and endurance in the 40's. Many exceptions to this concept have been noted so that it may be as much a societal factor as a biological fact. Disuse rather than degeneration of the muscular apparatus is characteristic of a technological society. In activities that are less physically demanding and where experience is also a factor, the age of peak performance occurs later in life but always before old age. Lehman (1953) noted that the peak age of intellectual performance and the peak age of athletic proficiency in many of the less violent neuro-muscular skills are almost identical. Jokl (1964) studied the athletes at the 1952 Olympics in Helsinki, Finland, and found that the younger competitors were involved in the anaerobically demanding activities (i.e. swimming, boxing, running short distances) while the older participants (over 30) competed in events as fencing, marathon running and horsemanship.

It has been suggested that with aging there is an irreversible dystrophy of cells that occurs as a result of the "wear and tear" of living (Bertolini, 1969). Along with this general weakening there is a progressive loss of tissue structure. These physical changes are reflected in the wrinkling of the skin, the increasingly flabby abdominal wall, the loss of elasticity in the arteries, and a reduction in the terminal circulation. The relative amount of body fat increases with aging, especially in the trunk (Skerlj, 1954).

The world can only be known through the sensory organs and the relationship of perceptual ability to aging remains controversial. Kleemeier (1959) indicates that a loss of sensory acuity occurs with aging. Compensation for a sensory loss may sometimes be achieved by increasing the environmental stimuli, such as increasing the lighting or using a hearing aid, or by limiting one's attention to a selected range of stimuli. There appears to be a rise in the visual threshold and a decline in night vision for the aged. The lens loses some of its power to accommodate with aging. Hearing in the high frequency range gradually declines. This is found more often in males than females. Visceral and cutaneous senses seem to decline with the aging process, yet the sense of position as determined by the joint receptors do not seem to vary. The threshold to pain remains constant. The sense of smell and taste decline also. These changes may or may not be a factor in behavior depending upon the specific task; in some situations it may actually be an advantage to not receive certain types of stimulation.

Brain volume and weight have been reported to diminish with age (Himwick, 1959). The number of cells in the higher nervous centers decrease. Some brain areas have been reported to retain only 30 percent of their original number of neurons (Andrew, 1955). The cerebral circulation appears to be significantly reduced in the aged although it should be noted that as long as a person is active intellectually our present tests do not indicate a consistent deterioration in mental abilities.

AGING AND MOTOR BEHAVIOR

Strength

Asmussen (1968) has noted that isometric strength starts to decline for men after age 30. Shephard (1972) states that the North American male maintains his level of strength until age 45 and then the decline is slow. At age 65 only about 15 percent of the peak maximum strength has been lost. After age 65 the loss of strength becomes more rapid. After 25 years of age there is a gradual decrease in muscular endurance until the male of 75-79 equals the performance of the 12-15 year-old boy (Watson, 1971). The studies involving women are far fewer and far less valid. Espenschade and Eckert (1967) report that post-puberty to approximately age 17 is the time of maximum strength for girls. That this is a culturally tainted observation is becoming clear as opportunities for women expand and they become involved with heavy resistance exercises during young adulthood. Strength has been found to continue throughout the college careers of women athletes (Rosentswieg, note). The results of data obtained on the AAHPERD Performance Tests indicate that after age 13 little improvement is noted for women. Women have long been reported to develop only about 2/3 the peak strength of men of the same age, although when muscle mass alone is the criteron little difference is believed to be evident when training is considered.

Flexibility

A loss of flexibility with aging is a common finding. This is not surprising because of the changes that occur to connective tissue over time. Espenschade and Eckert (1967) report that flexibility is greatest during the adolescent years. Flexibility is important for graceful movement as well as directly related to specific performance skills. Each joint is independent of all other joints in terms of flexibility, therefore the general condition of being flexible demands considerable effort. Wright and Johns (1960) believe that the reduction in flexibility that many individuals notice as they grow older may be associated with muscle rather than joint deviation. Chapman (1972) suggests that exercise may have a positive role to play in relieving some of the inflexibility related to aging. The exact point where flexibility changes from acceptable to limiting is not known, nor measurable, as the area of acceptability varies with all types of professions and activities.

Balance

The balance mechanism seems to be relatively stable after childhood. Espenschade (1971) reports that other than an increase in pathological conditions with aging, the reflexes controlling balance remain at a remarkably stable level throughout life. Begbie (1967) found that age did not effect postural sway. Backman (1961) noted that for balance tasks the performance after adolescence does not vary much for young adults. For females, performance in balance tasks tend to decrease during the third decade of life. Slatter-Hammell (1956) found that balance ability discriminated between levels of performance in athletic skills for college age subjects. With the onset of old age any variation noted is probably a result of changes in strength and other related factors rather than in the vestibular organs of the inner ear or the proprioceptors involved in balance.

Coordination

Coordination, the ability to control the muscles involved in a movement so that they work cooperatively to achieve a task efficiently, appears to be age related. Shock and Norris (1970) found that coordination declined steadily after 39 years of age. Body density decreases after age 40 (Behnke and Wilmore, 1974). The loss of muscle tissue, the demineralization of bone and the increased amount of fat, all of which change the body composition, may be related to the loss in coordination. Long term physical activity has a positive effect on body composition. Coordination is a factor that is aided by experience. In activities that are moderately demanding or less, the adult and sometimes the aged, can function very

effectively. When it is physically demanding the older adult shows a decrement in coordination.

Nervous Organization and Other Physiological Variables

Birren (1959) states that one of the most significant implications of aging is that there is a slowing down of all voluntary responses. It is interesting that there is little evidence that the nervous processes change in a qualitive manner with aging. Nerve conduction may slow with time but it is believed to be inconsequental (Weiss, 1956). In fact, the perpheral processes do not appear to be a significant factor in age related motor behavior (Birren and Botwinick, 1955). The literature supports the concept that it is the inability of the central nervous system to integrate the myriad of input that lengthens performing time with age. Welford (1968) states that with increasing age an impairment in short term memory is found and that problems that can be categorized as serial tasks are not performed as well as younger individuals. Skinner (1973) proposes that because of a decrease in strength, flexibility and speed of movement, in addition to the increased reaction time for nervous integration, a reduction in the ability to perform many motor skills with advancing age is logical. It would seem that the greater the stress and the more physiological mechanisms involved the greater the loss of function with age.

At rest the aged maintain many of the basic physiological regulating mechanisms at the same level as young adults. During submaximal, low or moderate level work there is little or no difference in the performance abilities of younger and older persons but the efficiency of the younger person in doing the work is greater. Older individuals may expect positive results from training but the percentage of improvement will be less than it is for the younger participants.

It is under stressful conditions that the relationship of aging to performance becomes clearer (Figure 31.1). With aging there is a loss of active muscle tissue which produces a lower metabolic rate. A number of cardiovascular functions become altered with the change in life style that often occurs with the advancing years. It has been found that less time is needed to reach a given heart rate and that more time is needed to return to homesostasis. For a specific work load older persons have a higher systolic blood pressure, a higher level of blood lactate and a greater pulmonary ventilation per liter of oxygen consumed (Skinner, 1973). The stroke volume of the heart decreases very little with age but with a slower heart rate the cardiac output is reduced. This limits aerobic work. Morehouse (1976) states that after age 25 the ability of men to perform maximum work declines about 1% each year. The amount of decline is believed to be slightly greater for women. Skinner (1973) indicated that after age 30 most tissues show some structural and chemical alteration. Robinson (1938) found that inactive males decline in their cardiovascular ability about 25% from age 17 to age 44. Dill and Consolazio (1962) used themselves as the subjects on a study of work performance under normal conditions and those of excessive heat (50°C.) over a 29 year interval. They found that their work output decreased with aging but their tolerance to a hot environment was relatively constant. In cold environments the aged individual reacts slower to a given task than do younger persons and they cannot main-

tain a uniform skin temperature, probably as a result of inadequate vascular tonus (Bertolini, 1969).

AGING AND PHYSICAL ACTIVITY

Acquired vs. Time-Dependent Aging

Research now indicates that there are two different types of aging. Loss of function which occurs simply with increased age is time-dependent aging. Acquired aging is loss of function resulting from forced inactivity or voluntary sedentary lifestyles. Lamb (1975) indicates that active people do not "acquire" many of the characteristics commonly associated with old age. Elrich (1975) and Radd (1975) support the contention of Lamb citing the fact that individuals over the age of 65 in different cultures who are very active do not show signs commonly associated with aging.

Not only does the research indicate that older adults can participate in physical activity, there is increasing evidence that regular activity (both intellectual and physical) is a must for preventing "acquired" aging and delaying time dependent aging. Butler (1975) suggests that ". . . exercise is the closest thing to an antiaging pill now available (p. 67)." Klumpp (1975) indicates that continued mental and physical activity is ". . . the only antidote for aging that I know (p. 93)."

Appropriate Physical Activity for Adults

Regular physical activity seems to be as important, if not more important, for adults as for children and adolescents. Barring medical problems, the young adults can par-

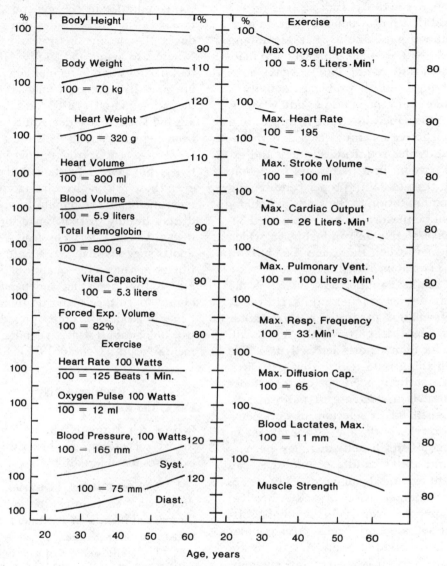

Variation in some static and dynamic functions with age. Data have been collected from various studies, including healthy male individuals. For data on the same function, only one study was consulted. The values for the twenty-five-year-old subjects = 100 percent; for the older ages, the mean values are expressed in percentage of the twenty-five-year-old individuals' values. The mean values cannot be considered as 'normal values,'' but their trends illustrate the effect of aging. Note that the heart rate and oxygen pulse at a given work load (100 watts or 600 kpm·min⁻¹, oxygen uptake about 1.5 liters·min⁻¹) are identical throughout the age covered, but the maximal oxygen uptake, heart rate, cardiac output, etc., decline with age.

Figure 31.1.   Changes in physiological variables with age. (From *Textbook of Work Physiology* by Per-Olaf Astrand and Kaare Rodahl. © 1977 by McGraw-Hill Book Company. Used with permission of McGraw-Hill Book Company.)

ticipate in any activity. Indeed, it is during this period that performance is best. In middle adulthood hypokinetic diseases can and most likely will occur in those who are inactive (Kraus and Raab, 1961). Again however, barring medical problems, activity is appropriate for the middle adult years. While performance in strength, speed, and endurance activities may decrease, performance in activities requiring strategy and experience may be best performed by people in this age group. With proper conditioning there is no limitation to the kinds of activity which can be performed by people aged 30-65. Because of the shift in factors in which the adult can excel, there may be shifts in interests in various activities.

Older adults can perform many of the same activities as younger adults. However, as the information presented in this chapter indicates, absolute performance levels will decrease for many sports and activities. The important thing is to realize that participation in an activity need not cease just because there is a decrease in performance. Some adjustment in selection of opponents in competitive sports and establishment of realistic goals in all activities may be necessary, but older adults of *all* ages can participate in most activities. There are many documented cases of active involvement of people over 70 in handball, softball, racquetball, and tennis. Also popular are golf and bowling. Many Americans are now involved in Masters (over 50) competition in track and swimming. Because they do not require exceptional amounts of skill jogging, walking, swimming, and bicycling are particularly suited for older adults including those who did not participate in activity in their younger years.

For those who exercise regularly the benefits are significant. Shepard (1978) notes that masters athletes are much more fit than contemporaries in the general population. Pollock et al. (1978) notes that exercise reduces the decline in fitness normally attributed to aging and Fardy (1978) notes that participation in regular activity early in life may have benefits long after the participation. Kasch (1976) presents convincing evidence that older adults can benefit from regular training. It is clear that older adults can benefit from regular vigorous activity, but more important is the fact that even those not involved in vigorous activity must maintain a minimum level of activity to stay healthy. A spokesman for the President's Council for Physical Fitness and Sports suggests that ". . . a state of physical fitness enhances the quality of life for the elderly by increasing independence. The ability to 'go places and do things' without being dependent on others provides a strong psychological lift which is conducive to good mental health (Conrad, 1975)."

Benefits of Regular Activity For Older Adults

Research supports the following statements concerning the benefits of regular exercises for older adults.

1. A recent study (DeVries, 1975) indicates that exercise can be more effective than tranquilizers in treatment of nervous tension in older people.

2. The shaky hand syndrome and tottery gait which is responsible for many incidences of dependency in older adults may be remediated through shifting from inactive to active lifestyles (Swartz, 1975).

3. Studies at Duke University at the Center for the Study of Aging indicate that active older adults have fewer illnesses and greater longevity than the inactive (Radd, 1975).

PHYSICAL ACTIVITY
GUIDELINES FOR ADULTS

Unlike children and even adolescents who participate in activity programs which are highly organized, many of the programs for adults are unorganized. For this reason, and because adults are fully capable of making decisions for themselves, leadership is a factor of less significance to adult exercise programs but proper medical attention is paramount. Before beginning regular exercise programs everyone, but especially adults, should have a medical exam. With age, continued medical monitoring is essential for all people including those who are active. There are many other guidelines for adults who are physically active. For more details on these and a discussion of contraindicated exercises for adults, the reader is referred to Corbin et al. (1978, Chapter 18).

References

Andrew, Warren. "Amitotic Division in Senile Tissues as a Probable Means of Self-Preservation of Cells." *J .Gerontology* IV (1955):1.

Asmussen, E. "The Neuromuscular System and Exercise." Chapter 1 in *Exercise Physiology,* edited by H. Falls. New York: Academic Press, 1968.

Bachman, John C. "Motor Learning and Performance as Related to Age and Sex in Two Measures of Balance Coordination." *Research Quarterly* 32(1961):123.

Begbie, G. H. "Some Problems of Postural Sway." In *Myotatic, Kinesthetic and Vestibular Mechanisms,* edited by A. V. S. de Reuck and J. Knight. Boston: Little, Brown and Company, 1967.

Behnke, A. R. and Wilmore, J. H. *Evaluation and Regulation of Body Build and Composition.* Englewood Cliffs, N. J.: Prentice-Hall, 1974.

Bertolini, Alberto M. *Gerontologic Metabolism.* Translated by V. de Sabata. Springfield, Ill.: C. C. Thomas, 1969.

Birren, James E., *Handbook of Aging and the Individual.* Chicago: The University of Chicago Press, 1959.

Birren, J. E. and Botwinick, J. "Age Differences in Finger, Jaw, and Foot Reaction Time to Auditory Stimuli." *J. Gerontology* 10 (1955):429.

Birren, J. E.; Imus, H. A.; and Windle, W. F. *The Process of Aging in the Nervous System.* Springfield, Ill.: C. C. Thomas, 1959.

Butler, R. N. "Psychological Importance of Physical Fitness." *Testimony on Physical Fitness for Older Persons.* Washington, D.C.: National Association for Human Development, 1975.

Chapman, E. A. et al. "Joint Stiffness: Effects of Exercise on Young and Old Men." *J. Gerontology* 27(1972):218.

Conrad, C. C. "Physical Fitness for the Elderly." *Testimony on Physical Fitness for Older Persons.* Washington, D. C.: National Association for Human Development, 1975.

Corbin, C. B. et al. *Concepts in Physical Education.* Dubuque: Wm. C. Brown Co., 1978.

DeVries, H. A. "What Research Tells Us Regarding the Contribution of Exercise to the Health of Older People." *Testimony on Physical Fitness for Older Persons.* Washington, D. C.: National Association for Human Development, 1975.

Dill, D. B. and Consolazio, C. F. "Responses to Exercise as Related to Age and Environmental Temperature." *J. Applied Physiology* 17(1962):645.

Espenschade, Anna S. and Eckert, H. M. *Motor Development.* Columbus, Ohio: Charles Merrill, 1967.

Espenschade, Anna S. "Balance" in "Influence of Activity." V(D)3 in the *Encyclopedia of Sports Sciences and Medicine,* edited by Leonard A. Larson. New York: Macmillan, 1971.

Elrich, H. "Exercise and the Aging Process." *Testimony on Physical Fitness for Older Persons.* Washington, D. C.: National Association for Human Development, 1975.

Fardy, P. S. "Cardiovascular Function in Former Athletes." *The Physician and Sportsmedicine* 6(1978):33.

Himwich, Harold E. "Biochemistry of the Nervous System in Relation to the Process of Aging." In *The Process of Aging in the Ner-*

vous System, edited by J. Birren. Springfield, Ill.: C. C. Thomas, 1959.

Hunsicker, P. A. and Greey, G. "Studies in Human Strength." *Research Quarterly* 22 (1957):109.

Jokl, E. *Medical Sociology and Cultural Anthropology of Sport and Physical Education.* Springfield, Ill. C. C. Thomas, 1964.

Kasch, F. W. "The Effects of Exercise on the Aging Process." *The Physician and Sportsmedicine* 4(1976):64.

Kleemeier, Robert W. "Behavior and the Organization of the Bodily and the External Environment." In *Handbook of Aging and the Individual,* edited by J. Birren. Chicago: The University of Chicago Press, 1959.

Klumpp, T. G. "Physical Activities and Older Persons." *Testimony on Physical Fitness for Older Persons.* Washington, D. C.: National Association for Human Development, 1975.

Kraus, Hans and Raab, Wilhelm. *Hypokinetic Disease.* Springfield, Ill.: C. C. Thomas, 1961.

Lamb, L. E. "Staying Youthful and Fit." *Testimony on Physical Fitness for Older Persons.* Washington, D. C.: National Association for Human Development, 1975.

Lehman, H. C. *Age and Achievement.* Princeton: Princeton University Press for the American Philosophical Society, 1953.

Morehouse, Laurence E. and Miller, A. T. *Physiology of Exercise,* 7th ed. St. Louis: C. V. Mosby, 1976.

Pollock, M. L. et al. "Effects of Fitness on Aging." *The Physician and Sportsmedicine* 6 (1978):45.

Radd, A. "Statement on Physical Fitness and the Elderly." *Testimony on Physical Fitness for Older Persons.* Washington, D. C.: National Association for Human Development, 1975.

Robinson, S. "Experimental Studies of Physical Fitness in Relation to Age." *Arbeitphysiologie* 10(1938-39):251.

Rosentswieg, Joel. Personal Observation at the Texas Woman's University.

Shepard, R. J. "The Effects of Training on the Aging Process." *The Physician and Sportsmedicine* 6(1978):32.

Shepard, R. J. *Alive Man.* Springfield, Ill.: C. C. Thomas, 1972.

Shock, N. W. and Norris, H. H. "Neuromuscular Coordination as a Factor in Age Changes in Muscular Exercise." In *Physical Activity and Aging,* edited by D. Brunner and E. Jokl. Baltimore: University Park Press, 1970.

Skerlj, Bozo. "Further Evidences of Age Changes in Body Form Based upon Material of D.A.W. Edwards." *Human Biology* 26 (1954):330.

Skinner, J. S. "Age and Performance." In *Limiting Factors of Physical Performance,* edited by J. Keul. Stuttgart: Georg Thieme, 1973.

Slatter-Hammel, A. T. "Performance of Selected Groups of Male College Students on the Reynolds Balance Tests." *Research Quarterly* 27(1956):34.

Swartz, F. C. "Statement on Physical Fitness and the Elderly." *Testimony on Physical Fitness for Older Persons.* Washington, D. C.: National Association for Human Development, 1975.

Talland, G. A. "The Effect of Age on Speed of Simple Manual Skills." *J. Gen. Psychology* 100(1962):67.

Watson, Helen B. "Muscular Endurance" in "Influence of Activity," V(D) 9 in the *Encyclopedia of Sports Sciences and Medicine,* edited by Leonard A. Larson. New York: Macmillan, 1971.

Weiss, A. D. "The Motor Component of Auditory Reaction Time as Related to Age." *American Psychologist* 11(1956):374.

Welford, A. T. *Fundamentals of Skill.* London: Methuen, 1968.

Wright, V. and Johns, R. M. "Physical Factors Concerned with the Stiffness of Normal and Diseased Joints." *John Hopkins Hospital Bulletin* 106(1960):215.

Section 11

The Evaluation of Motor Behavior

The Evaluation of Motor Behavior 32

Joel Rosentswieg
Texas Woman's University

Evaluation is central to learning. All theories of learning emphasize the importance of knowing what has occurred in order to make the necessary behavioral adjustments to attain a desired goal. It may appear trite to state that behavior is goal directed and rarely, if ever, random, yet this fact is sometimes ignored when judging motor performance. Peiper (1963) illustrates the primacy of goal directed behavior by noting that in human development the responses of an infant are directed toward the achievement of specific actions that occur in an orderly, phylogenic sequence. As development continues the range of movements and the choice of goals increase but the fundamental truth of moving for a purpose remains. Ultimate reasons directing behavior may never be known but the observable aspect of a performance can and should be evaluated in terms of the achievement of extrinsic, known goals.

Superior physical performances have always been of interest. The Olympic Games represent the kinds of athletic performances most people notice. Robinson (1927) cites many of the feats of Greek athletes that would be remarkable even today. Milo of Crotona, who won six Olympic wreaths in wrestling during the golden days of Greece —and remember the Olympic Games were, even then, held only every four years—is said to have carried a four-year-old bull on his shoulders around the stadium after a win, and then with a single blow to the animal he killed it and ate it all in the same day. The Guinness Book of World Records lists similar unique feats. Too often such performances, both the extremely good and/or the unusually funny, are believed to be within the reach of everyone if they only "work hard," "follow our directions," "or just want to." Unfortunately normal development portends that only a small minority will be able to achieve championship feats while a similar group will fail to meet minimal performance standards. Recognition of either group requires evaluation and frequently demands measurement.

This chapter is designed to provide a broad overview of the evaluation of motor behavior, yet, an attempt will be made to be specific as to why and how physical activities should be evaluated.

SPECIFICITY OF MOTOR EVALUATION

Research has indicated that motor behavior is specific. Factor analytic studies (Cumbee et al. 1957; Fleishman and Ellison 1962; Ismail and Gruber 1967) have divided movement skills into a number of independent factors each of which contributes to a performance but to different degrees in different tasks. This is made obvious by the importance balance has for a gymnast in comparison to the need for balance for a weight lifter.

Some of the analytical studies have further indicated that motor abilities are unique to different body segments as well as to the factors isolated (Guilford 1958; Lotter 1960). Guilford found seven factors of motor ability for four divisions of the body. Table 32.1 presents one possible matrix of psychomotor factors. Other investigators (McCloy, 1937; Fleishman, 1964) have found considerably more than seven ability factors.

Specificity of motor activities implies that to be skilled in one task has little general relationship to performances on another task. The relationship between the two tasks would depend upon their specific similarities. Juggling, a skill demanding considerable coordination, would not be expected to correlate highly with dribbling a soccer ball which also requires great coordination. The factor of coordination, like all skill factors, appears to be task specific. A good floor-exercise gymnast would be expected to be a good diver because of the similarity of the tasks. Some persons are fortunate to be able to perform a wide variety of tasks extremely well and they are recognized as superior in motor abilities. Just as there are few geniuses found in the cognitive domain, so there appear to be few in the psychomotor domain.

Specificity appears to be a concept applicable to much more than just motor skills. Guilford (1959) found that specificity exists for cognitive skills, and Williams (1963) states that the uniqueness of individuality extends to the cellular level on a biochemical basis as well as at the obvious personal level. The exercise physiologist is becoming as aware of this uniqueness at the cellular level as the sports psychologist is at the behavioral level. With an acceptance that each person is different from every other person, it follows that each person must be evaluated on an individual basis. Group comparisons or a comparison of one person with a standard or norm can be considered acceptable only if the results are used to help individuals grow and increase their capabili-

TABLE 32.1
Matrix of the Psychomotor Factors, with Columns for Kinds of Abilities and Rows for Parts of the Body Involved.

Part of Body Involved	Type of Ability						
	Strength	Impulsion	Speed	Static Precision	Dynamic Precision	Coordination	Flexibility
Gross	General strength	General reaction		Static balance	Dynamic balance	Gross bodily coordination	
Trunk	Trunk-strength	Time					Trunk-flexibility
Limbs	Limb-strength	Limb-thrust	Arm-speed	Arm-steadiness	Arm-aiming		Leg-flexibility
Hand		Tapping			Hand-aiming	Hand-dexterity	
Finger			Finger-speed			Finger-dexterity	

From J. P. Guilford. "A System of Psychomotor Abilities." *American Journal of Psychology* 71 (1958):165.

ties. This is extremely difficult to do with large hetergeneous groups. In order to foster optimal growth, guidance must be done on an individual basis.

Tests can be categorized into a number of divisions. One common differentiation of tests is into subjective and objective classifications. Subjective tests depend upon the expertise of the testor in the interpretation of the actions or results of the person taking the test. Subjective testing is only as good as the person giving the test. Variability and validity are inconsistent. In essence this is why a person must become an "expert" in subject matter in order to evaluate any area of endeavor. Objective tests are much easier to give and to use. They are standardized to provide information in an exact and consistent manner. If the instructions for an objective test are faithfully followed the results should be valid and reliable.

Norm referenced and criterion referenced tests describe the types of objective tests. Norm referenced tests are those that have been given to large numbers of subjects and the results tabulated so that the interpretation of a score may be made that is based upon the relative position within this group. Evaluation based upon norm referenced testing is actually a comparison to peer group performance. Criterion referenced tests, as opposed to norm referenced tests, are not necessarily based upon what other people do. Such tests are the product of what someone believes to be appropriate for the situation. This type of testing is only valuable as long as the criterion task is logical. Both types of tests must be frequently reviewed to be sure that they are suitable to the group being tested. "Home-made tests" are used in the same way as standardized objective tests but, unfortunately, they often lack validity and/or reliability.

EVALUATION OF FUNDAMENTAL MOTOR SKILLS

Fundamental motor skills, those skills believed to underlie all movement, probably should be considered extremely well learned developmental tasks which are composed of many specific subskills rather than basic skill factors in or of themselves (Gange and Fleishman 1959). Another way of understanding the complexity of motor behavior is to consider the evolution of a fundamental skill. Kay (1969) notes that walking, a developmental task, is not one simple skill but a combination of carefully controlled motor activities that include posture, balance, and locomotion. Underlying or prerequisite to walking, just as in the case with most gross motor skills, is strength (Espenschade and Eckert 1967). The developmental studies of Bayley (1935) and Gesell and Amatruda (1947) clearly illustrate that achievement of the orderly sequence of skills is dependent upon adequate strength as well as the neurological growth of the infant. Figure 32.1 indicates this relationship during the first year of life. It should be remembered that many changes in motor ability occur as the result of maturation alone. However, as noted in Sections 3 and 4, fundamental skills are not learned and refined exclusively as a result of maturation. Practice, especially practice including emphasis on the proper mechanics, is essential if optimal performance is to be achieved. The reader is referred to the Levels of Performance outlined in Chapters 8 and 9 for information concerning the evaluation of learning of fundamental skills and the Developmental Analysis Checklists in Chapters 10 and 11 for information concerning the evaluation of fundamental skill refinement.

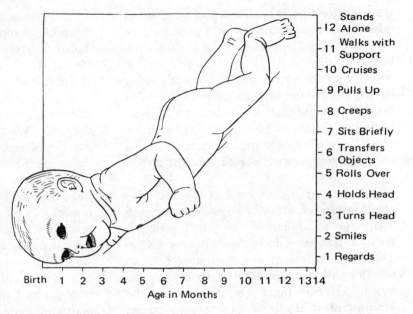

The infant's figure represents a diagonal line on which is plotted the progress of behavior (right of the diagram) against chronological age. The cephalocaudal pattern of behavior is diagrammatically illustrated by position of the figure. (From *Growth and Development of Children* by Watson and Lowrey, 5th ed. Copyright © 1967, Year Book Medical Publishers. Used by permission.)

12 Stands Alone
11 Walks with Support
10 Cruises
9 Pulls Up
8 Creeps
7 Sits Briefly
6 Transfers Objects
5 Rolls Over
4 Holds Head
3 Turns Head
2 Smiles
1 Regards

Birth 1 2 3 4 5 6 7 8 9 10 11 12 13 14

Age in Months

Figure 32.1. Developmental Diagram for the First Year of Life.

TESTS OF GENERAL MOTOR ABILITY

Previous to the work of Henry (1958), researchers of motor activities looked for, and teachers taught on the basis of general factors. The belief that strength, flexibility, agility, and similar general variables were completely inherited or could be developed and transferred to any or all activities, guided the teaching and evaluation of motor skills. Specialists attempted to develop tests of motor ability, motor capacity and motor educability.

Motor ability represents present status as determined by a particular measure or test. Ability is known to fluctuate and is dependent upon many variables. Climate, personal health and the manner in which test directions are provided are among the many factors which affect measurements (Brown 1970). When a test of motor ability is given, the result is a measure of ability in a specific task at a specific time. The interpretation of the data must be somewhat restricted because of the knowledge that variation in performance is normal.

The concept of general motor ability testing implies the ability to predict performance in many different kinds of activities. The earliest measurements of motor ability were strength tests. In 1921, Sargent introduced the famous "Physical Test of a Man," the vertical jump, one of the first measurements other than strength that had been purposed to predict motor ability. Since that time a large number of tests have been designed to measure general motor ability.

The Strength Index (Rogers 1952) has been included in tests and measurement textbooks as a measure of general ability. This index is composed of six strength tests and a measure of lung capacity. The relationship of this test to general motor ability was deduced by a coefficient of correlation which was found to exist with performance in track and field events, basketball free throw ability, and throwing accuracy. A comparison of scores on the strength index between athletes and nonathletes was also used to validate this test. As previously mentioned, strength is believed to be a major factor in most motor performances but it is not by itself a predictor of specific skilled performance.

Strength, in and of itself, is specific. The relationship of static (isometric) strength measures to dynamic (isotonic) strength measures appears to be low (Berger 1962). The value of taking static strength tests to predict ability in any kind of dynamic, gross motor activity must be questioned. The amount of strength needed for any game, sport, or dance is specific and it is even specific to the muscles involved. It has been found that individuals differ in strength as the type of contraction (isometric, isotonic, isokinetic) differs. Also one extremity may produce the greatest tension under one method while another extremity produces the greatest muscular tension using another method (Rosentswieg and Hinson 1972). Therefore, the use of one kind of maximum strength test to suggest abilities in skills demanding another type and/or amount of strength may be meaningless.

The Brace Test (1927), the Johnson Test (1932), the Humiston Motor Ability Test for College Women (1939), the Larson Motor Ability Test for College Men (1941), the Hanson Tests of Achievement for Elementary School Children (1965), and more recently the Texas Physical Fitness-Motor Ability Test (1973) were designed or are used to differentiate between levels of general motor ability. These and similar tests, have sometimes been used to indicate motor

educability or motor capacity. Modern theory does not support the use of these tests because they are contrary to the concept of specificity (Lawther 1968; Sheehan 1971). Unfortunately, there is no valid way to generalize about motor ability; thus we cannot predict ultimate potential to acquire motor skill (motor capacity) or the ease that skills can be learned (motor educability) from a motor performance test, general or specific. Prediction can only be made for the specific tasks measured with any assurance that the results will be valid. It is likely that everyone could do well in at least one motor skill yet do poorly in a number of others. This would not necessarily be reflected in a test of a general nature. Performance in general tests probably indicate an interest in motor activities more than ability for any one game, sport or dance. In situations where only one activity is taught to a group it is considered sound educational practice to organize on the basis of ability or competencies which can facilitate the teaching-learning process (Lockhart and Mott 1951). Wilson (1966), in a study of competencies in selected sports, carefully avoids the error of generalization of motor skill by using standardized tests for each activity considered.

The next chapter discusses tests of physical fitness, perceptual-motor, and motor and motor creativity that have been used in assessing motor development.

References

Bayley, Nancy A. "The Development of Motor Abilities during the First Three Years." *Monographs for the Society for Research in Child Development*, Washington, D.C. 1935.

Berger, Richard. "Comparison of Static and Dynamic Strength Increases." *Research Quarterly* 33:329.

Brace, David K. *Measuring Motor Ability*. New York: A. S. Barnes and Co., 1927.

Brown, Frederick G. *Principles of Educational and Psychological Testing*. Hinsdale, Ill.: The Dryden Press Inc., 1970.

Cumbee, Frances Z.; Meyer, Margaret; and Peterson, Gerald. "Factorial Analysis of Motor Coordination Variables for Third and Fourth Grade Girls." *Research Quarterly* 28 (1957):100.

Espenschade, Anna S. and Eckert, Helen. *Motor Development*. Columbus, Ohio: Charles E. Merrill Books, Inc., 1967.

Fleishman, Edwin A. and Ellison, Gaylord D. "A Factor Analysis of Five Manipulative Tests." *Journal of Applied Psychology* 46 (1962):96.

Fleishman, Edwin A. *The Structure and Measurement of Physical Fitness*. Englewood Cliffs, N.J.: Prentice-Hall, Inc., 1964.

Gagne, Robert M. and Fleishman, Edwin A. *Psychology and Human Performance*. New York: Henry Holt and Co., 1959.

Gesell, Arnold L. and Amatruda, Catherine S. *Development Diagnosis*. New York: P. B. Hoeber, Inc., 1947.

Guilford, J. P. "A System of Psychomotor Abilities." *American Journal of Psychology* 71 (1958):164.

———. "Three Faces of Intellect." *American Psychologists* 14(1959):469.

Hanson, Margie R. "Motor Performances Testing of Elementary School Age Children." An unpublished Ph.D. dissertation, University of Washington, Seattle, Washington, 1965.

Henry, Franklin. "Individual Differences in Motor Learning and Performance." In *Psychology of Motor Learning*, edited by Leon Smith. Chicago: The Athletic Institute, 1969.

Humiston, Dorothy. "A Measurement of Motor Ability in College Women." *Research Quarterly* 8(1937):181.

Ismail, A. H. and Gruber, J. J. *Motor Aptitude and Intellectual Performance*. Columbus, Ohio: Charles E. Merrill Publishers, 1967.

Johnson, Granville B. "Physical Skill Tests for Sectioning Classes in Homogeneous Units." *Research Quarterly* 3(1932):128.

Kay, Harry. "The Development of Motor Skills from Birth to Adolescence." In *Principles of Skill Acquisition*, edited by E. A. Bilodeau. New York: Academic Press, 1969.

Larson, Leonard A. "A Factor Analysis of Motor Ability Variables and Tests, With Tests for College Men." *Research Quarterly* 12 (1941):499.

Lawther, John D. *The Learning of Physical Skills*. Englewood Cliffs, N.J.: Prentice-Hall, Inc., 1968.

Lockhart, Aileen and Mott, Jane A. "An Experiment in Homogeneous Grouping and Its Effect on Achievement in Sports Fundamental." *Research Quarterly* 22(1951):58.

Lotter, Willard S. "Interrelationships among Reaction Times and Speeds of Movement in Different Limbs." *Research Quarterly* 31 (1960):147-55.

McCloy, Charles H. "An Analytical Study of the Stunt Type Test as a Measure of Motor Educability." *Research Quarterly* 8(1937): 46.

Peiper, Albrecht. *Cerebral Function in Infancy and Childhood*. New York: Consultants Bureau, 1963.

Robinson, Rachel Sargent. *Sources for the History of Greek Athletics*. Cincinnati: The Author, 1955.

Rogers, Frederick R. "Physical Capacity Tests in the Administration of Physical Education." *Contributions to Education*, no. 173. New York: Teachers College, Columbia University, 1925.

Rosentswieg, Joel and Hinson, Marilyn. "Comparison of Isometric, Isotonic and Isokinetic Exercises by Electromyography." *Archives of Physical Medicine and Rehabilitation*, in press.

Sargent, Dudley A. "The Physical Test of a Man." *American Physical Education Review* 26(April 1921):188.

Sheehan, Thomas J. *An Introduction to the Evaluation of Measurement Data in Physical Education*. Reading, Mass.: Addison-Wesley Publishing Co., 1971.

Texas Governor's Commission on Physical Fitness. *Physical Fitness-Motor Ability Test*. Austin: The Commission, 1973.

Williams, Roger J. *Biochemical Individuality*. Science Editions. New York: John Wiley and Sons, Inc., 1963.

Wilson, Ruth M. *Assessing Competency in Physical Education Activities*. Springfield, Ill.: Charles C. Thomas, 1966.

Testing Physical Fitness and Perceptual-Motor Development

33

Joel Rosentswieg
Texas Woman's University

Testing is the process of measuring ability at a point in time. Testing is very temporal. Evaluation is a term derived from the word value and is essentially a subjective assessment usually involving a number of tests which may be formal and standardized or informal and possibly even indirect. To evaluate the motor development of an individual requires testing in a wide variety of skills. In this chapter an attempt has been made to provide guidance in the use of tests to measure physical fitness, which underly all motor performances, as well as the perceptual-motor and motor creativity components of behavior. It should be realized that there are other measures that will provide appropriate information for the informed person besides those mentioned here.

TESTS OF PHYSICAL FITNESS

Physical fitness measures have always been based on a "cafeteria" rational. This may be a result of the inability of authorities to agree on a definition of physical fitness.

Many different types of instruments have been developed to measure physical fitness. Exercise physiologists examining one or more physiological parameters have probably come the closest to a valid measure of physical fitness, especially when it is defined as the ability to do work. As is all too often the case, the tests considered most appropriate by research oriented personnel require expensive equipment and/or prolonged training to use (Consolazio et al. 1963). Physical fitness is usually thought to consist of many specific factors. Investigations of physical fitness conclude with a battery of tests, each of which is believed to measure a different fitness factor. Total fitness, an elusive concept that implies maximally effective living, is unmeasurable. Physical fitness may be measured when the terms are defined. Many of the tests of physical fitness suffer from lack of specificity and often from misapplication. The majority of physical fitness tests have been designed for young adults. A number of the tests suggested for younger and older age groups as well as girls and women are suspect because of the limited number of subjects originally involved in the development of the measures. Teachers, psychologists, and most medical doctors must rely on secondary, more easily obtained measures of physical fitness than are available to the exercise physiologist.

The close relationship of cardiovascular fitness to physiological measures of work provides a rationale for the many kinds of step tests used as physical fitness indices (Brouha 1943; Kuruz et al. 1969; Skubic and Hodgkins 1963). The variability inherent in heart rate measurements, especially at submaximal levels, suggests that they are appropriate for screening instruments but that they are not adequate as clinical procedures. The use of cardiovascular measures as the

TABLE 33.1
Physical Fitness Items Included in the Basic Fitness Test
Reliabilities and Factor Loadings of the Tests

Test	Primary Factor Measured	Reliability	Primary Factor Loading	Other Factor Loading
1. Extent Flexibility	Extent Flexibility	.90	.49	-
2. Dynamic Flexibility	Dynamic Flexibility	.92	.50	-
3. Shuttle Run	Explosive Strength	.85	.77	.39 (DS)
4. Softball Throw	Explosive Strength	.93	.66	.32 (SS)
5. Hand Grip	Static Strength	.91	.72	-
6. Pull-Ups	Dynamic Strength	.93	.81	-
7. Leg Lifts	Trunk Strength	.89	.47	.32 (DS)
8. Cable Jump	Gross Body Coordination	.70	.56	-
9. Balance A	Gross Body Equilibrium	.82	.72	-
10. 600 Yd. Run-Walk	Stamina (Cardio-Vascular Endurance)	.80	-	-

Fleishman, E. A. *The Structure and Measurement of Physical Fitness.* 1964.

sole component of physical fitness is irreconcilable with good evaluation techniques because no single factor can provide sufficient information to be considered descriptive of "being fit" without defining the term in the most limited of ways. However, as the American population becomes more sedentary, cardiorespiratory measures become more important.

Fleishman (1964) has proposed a test battery based on a factoral study that minimizes equipment. Analysis of the Fleishman battery in comparison with other tests purporting to measure physical fitness indicates that many popular tests have been empirically derived and are of relatively low validity. The Fleishman Test is an example of a test designed to test many of the specific factors of fitness. While the Fleishman Test can be used with adolescents and young adults, the Kirchner Test (1970) is an example of a multifactor test for elementary school age children (Table 33.2). The Kraus-Weber

Test (1954) reactivated interest in physical fitness measures by indicating that American elementary school age children were not as fit as a similar group of European children. This test is typical of the shortcoming of many of the measures of physical fitness. Some of the tests do not measure what was

TABLE 33.2
Physical Fitness Test for Elementary
School Age Children

1. Standing broad jump
2. Bench pushup (With feet on the floor and hands on a bench 14-17 inches high, the student executes pushups to exhaustion.)
3. Curlups (This is identical to the bent-knee sit-up.)
4. Squat jump (From a crouched position, the student jumps approximately four inches above the mat. One point is awarded for each execution up to 50, when the student is stopped.)
5. 30-yard dash

Kirchner, G. *Physical Education for Elementary School Children.* Dubuque, Iowa: Wm. C. Brown Company Publishers, 1970.

intended and frequently learning and interest rather than ability are the crucial factors. The Cooper 12 minute run-walk test (1968) is also often misunderstood in terms of exactly what it measures. The AAHPERD Youth Fitness Test (1958) may be criticized for all of these reasons, yet because of the wide use of the test, it can be useful. Comparing an individual's score to the national norms of the Youth Fitness Test, or other standardized test, provides a measure that may help direct a person toward the satisfaction of believed and expressed needs. It must be remembered that high success in a physical fitness test only means the ability to do that test well and not that any other test of the same factor may be done equally well.

The relationship of tests of fitness or any other concept, are not always high. This means that although many tests are called physical or motor fitness tests they do not measure the same things (Doolittle and Bigbee 1968; Tharp 1969; Crowley 1972). Progressive participation in any factor of fitness will produce improvement in that factor and it may be assumed that the improvement measured by the test will be carried over to other activities using that same factor, but not necessarily in an amount proportional to the improvement of the fitness test.

TESTS OF PERCEPTUAL MOTOR SKILLS

Considerable energy has recently been put forth in an attempt to measure and evaluate perceptual-motor skills. Perception, or awareness, is requisite to any behavior. The exact neurological processes accompanying perception are discussed in detail in Section 7. The linking of the term perception with motor skills is an attempt to describe the internal and external relationship of movements; however, many so-called authorities use the term "perceptual-motor" as an esoteric flippancy to imply that practice in various kinds of motor skills will produce developmental changes in cortical processes that can aid cognition. The implication is obviously unwarranted. It is interesting to note that Cratty et al. (1970) believe that the relationship of motor ability tests to measures of intelligence, which tends to be very low but positive, probably can be accounted for in the cognitive aspects of the motor ability tests (i.e. comprehension of what or how to do something) that are built into a test rather than upon the motor factors involved.

The Oseretsky Motor-Development Scale (Sloan 1954) is probably the most common perceptual-motor test in use today. The Oseretsky Scale was originally developed to provide a motor ability test that would be comparable to an intelligence test in that maturation as well as individual differences in motor performance would be manifest. The reported validity of this test varies from very good (Rabin 1957) to invalid (Vandenberg 1964). The Oseretsky test and others modeled after it (Stott 1966; Cratty 1966; Roach and Kephart 1966) seem to be of primary value for the very young and/or the retarded individual. It may be hypothesized that the very young and the retarded are not as "culturally contaminated" as are other populations and thus the results of perceptual-motor testing may be a more valid representation of the innate ability of these groups than it is for the others. This possibility may be seen from the following studies. Singer and Brunk (1967) developed a Figure Reproduction Test as a measure of perceptual-motor ability and attempted to determine the relationship of such ability with intelligence of third and forth grade children. The Figure Reproduction Test required subjects to reproduce pictured designs by manipulating rubber bands upon pegs on a small board. The results indicated a low, positive, generally non-significant relationship. Another study by Singer (1968), investigating similar relationships for sixth graders, produced the same results. Herndon (1970) redesigned the figures and used the Figure Reproduction Test technique and a modification of the Oseretsky Motor Development Scale as measures of perceptual-motor ability, and a standardized test of intellectual ability to determine if significant correlations existed for kindergarten age children. The two perceptual tests correlated highly (r=.89) and the relationship of each perceptual-motor test and the intelligence measure was significant (P>.001) but only moderately high (r=.55). This illustrates the fact that these tests may be valid perceptual-motor tests for the young. However, it also suggests the need for all tests to be applied to large groups and longitudinally as well as cross-sectionally in order to verify findings obtained from few subjects at a given level before unquestioningly accepting or rejecting test results. The Pearman modification of the Osertsky test (1968) is suggested for general use because it is relatively simple to give and interpret and most of the other tests purposed to measure perceptual-motor abilities have been validated with some type of Oseretsky test (Table 27.3).

Above the primary level, few if any of the perceptual-motor tests distinguish between important motor abilities except for students with gross deviations. Until further studies are made, perceptual-motor tests should be considered clinical rather than appropriate for group use. It is suggested

TABLE 33.3
Pearman Modification of the
Lincoln-Oseretsky Test

Description of Item
Describing circles in air.
Tap feet and describe circles.
Making a ball.
Placing coins and matchsticks.
Touching fingertips.
Winding thread.
Tapping for 15 seconds.

From "An analysis of the Lincoln-Oseretsky Motor Development Scale with an emphasis on the reduction of total test items" by Roger Pearman. M. A. Thesis, Western Kentucky University, Bowling Green, Kentucky, 1968.

that teachers and clinicians carefully consider the purpose of using motor ability tests, perceptual-motor tests, and physical fitness tests to determine if the potential information that may be obtained can or will be used in a manner that will enhance learning or focus on methods of improving behavior. Motor tests are not tests of total human behavior. Tests that are directed toward school readiness, as are most of the perceptual-motor measures, are only one aspect of the total developmental process and a relatively small part at that.

MOTOR CREATIVITY

Motor creativity has received much emphasis with the renewed interest in the arts and humanities. To what extent the creative abilities of human beings can be fostered is unknown. Some evidence suggests that creativeness can be learned but such a belief is not universal. With the understanding of the concept of specificity it was assumed that cognitive tests of creativity would not measure motor aspects of creativity. Torrance (1962) has been the leader in the study of verbal and written forms of creativ-

.ity and his work has been the basis of much of the research in motor creativity as well.

Wyrick (1968) developed a measure of motor creativity that has been used with some frequency. This test included the factors of motor fluency, the quantity of movement, and motor originality. Most of the reported research does not support the validity of the Wyrick or any other measure of motor creativity. This should not be too surprising because the concept "Creativity" probably cannot be manifested in a structured format. Quantifying movements may be indicative of familiarity with certain objects or even just exuberance rather than creativeness. The testing of dancers has not indicated unusual motor creative abilities. At present it is believed that the concept of motor creativity may be a useful one but any measurement or evaluation of this factor should be used with trepidation.

SYNTHESIS

Motor behavior cannot be directionally changed without evaluation, and evaluation is by definition subjective in nature. The goal of measurement is to provide valid and reliable data in an objective fashion; yet it should be recognized that there are relatively few tests, other than for sport skills, that can provide such data. Thus, the person studying motor behavior must rely on a knowledge of kinesiology to provide a basis for the understanding of efficient movement, and experience and training in the evaluation of performance.

It is important that standard procedures be followed in the collection of data. Such procedures help define and limit the inherent errors of evaluation. A specific test can only indicate what may be achieved at that moment, not what might ultimately be accomplished. Ultimate performance cannot be predicted. Expertise is needed to interpret a measure and make effective evaluations.

It has been emphasized that it is not wise to rely solely on one method of evaluation or on a single instrument. What is believed necessary is a combination of many instruments and procedures that take into account the needs of each individual while motivating everyone to do the very best that they are capable of doing.

AAHPER. *AAHPER Youth Fitness Manual.* Washington, D.C.: The Association, 1965.

Brouha, Lucien. "The Step Test: A Simple Method of Measuring Physical Fitness for Hard Muscular Work in Young Men." *Research Quarterly* 14(1943):31.

Cooper, Kenneth H. *Aerobics.* New York: Bantam Books, 1968.

Consolazio, C. Frank; Johnson, Robert E.; and Pecora, Louis J. *Physiological Measurement of Metabolic Functions in Man.* New York: McGraw-Hill Book Co., 1963.

Cratty, Bryant J. *The Perceptual-Motor Attributes of Mentally Retarded Children and Youth."* Unpublished Monograph, sponsored by the Mental Retardation Services Board, Los Angeles County, 1966.

Cratty, Bryant J.; Ikeda, Namiko; Martin, Sister Margaret M.; Jennet, Clair; and Morrison, Margaret. *Movement Activities, Motor Ability and the Education of Children.* Springfield, Ill.: Charles C. Thomas, 1970.

Crowley, Marian. "A Modification of the Ohio State University Step Test for Junior High School Age Girls." An unpublished Master's Thesis, Texas Woman's University, Denton, Texas, 1972.

Doolittle, T. L. and Bigbee, Rollin. "The Twelve-Minute Run-Walk: A Test of Cardiorespiratory Fitness of Adolescent Boys." *Research Quarterly* 39(1968):491.

Flinchum, Betty. *Motor Development in Early Childhood.* St. Louis: C. V. Mosby, 1965.

Herndon, Daisy E. "The Relationship of Perceptual-Motor Ability and Intellectual Ability in Kindergarten-Age Children." An unpublished Master's Thesis, Texas Woman's University, Denton, Texas, 1970.

Kirchner, Glenn. *Physical Education for Elementary School Children*. Dubuque, Iowa: Wm. C. Brown, 1970.

Kraus, Hans, and Hirshland, Ruth. "Minimum Muscular Fitness Tests in School Children." *Research Quarterly* 25(1954):178.

Kuruz, Robert L.; Fox, Edward L.; and Mathews, Donald K. "Construction of a Submaximal Cardiovascular Step Test." *Research Quarterly* 40(1969):115.

Pearman, Roger. "An Analysis of the Lincoln-Oseretsky Motor Development Scale with an Emphasis on the Reduction of Total Test Items." A Master's Thesis, Western Kentucky University, Bowling Green, 1968.

Rabin, Herbert M. "The Relationship of Age, Intelligence, and Sex to Motor Deficiency." *American Journal of Mental Deficiency* 62 (1957):507.

Roach, Eugene G. and Kephart, Newell C. *The Purdue Perceptual Motor Survey*. Columbus, Ohio: Charles E. Merrill Publishers, 1966.

Singer, Robert N. "Interrelationship of Physical, Perceptual-Motor and Academic Achievement Variables in Elementary School Children." *Perceptual and Motor Skills* 27 (1967):1323.

Singer, Robert N. and Brunk, J. W. "Relation of Perceptual-Motor Ability and Intellectual Ability in Elementary School Children." *Perceptual and Motor Skills* 24(1967):967.

Skubic, Vera and Hodgkins, J. "Cardiovascular Efficiency Test for Girls and Women." *Research Quarterly* 34(1963):191.

Sloan, William. *Manual for the Lincoln-Oseretsky Motor Development Scale*, no. 37018. Chicago: C. H. Stolting Co., 1954.

Stott, D. H. "A General Test of Motor Impairment for Children." *Developmental Medicine and Child Neurology* 8(1966):523.

Tharp, Gerald D. "Cardiac Function Tests as Indexes of Fitness." *Research Quarterly* 40 (1969):818.

Torrance, E. Paul. *Guiding Creative Talent*. Englewood Cliffs, N.J.: Prentice-Hall, Inc., 1962.

Vandenberg, Steven C. "Factor Analytic Studies of the Lincoln-Oseretsky Test of Motor Proficiency." *Perceptual and Motor Skills* 19(1964):2.

Wyrick, Wyneen. "The Development of a Test of Motor Creativity." *Research Quarterly* 39 (October 1968):756.

Section 12

Motor Development: A Synthesis

Motor Development: A Synthesis

34

Charles B. Corbin
Kansas State University

As outlined in chapter 1, the purpose of this text was (1) to describe characteristic motor development patterns; (2) to suggest reasons, whether familial or environmental, regarding why humans develop as they do; and (3) to project ideas regarding the possible "potential" of humans for motor performance when given optimal conditions for development. Now that the reader has had an opportunity to study motor development in this context, some brief comments on each of the three purposes seems appropriate.

CHARACTERISTIC MOTOR DEVELOPMENT PATTERNS

How important is it for a child to be able to walk, skip or to perform other basic motor tasks? In our society, many of these performances are taken for granted. As long as a person performs most of the expected developmental tasks at approximately the same time as others of the same age, there is little concern about motor development. In fact, it is the individual with extremely poor motor function or extremely good skill abilities who receives our attention. While it is appropriate that special attention should be given to the exceptional person, it does not seem reasonable to take motor development of the normal individual for granted.

Motor development is an important part of total development. To take motor development for granted is to ignore the concept of totality of people. Accordingly the study of motor behavior should be concerned with more than, "How can better motor performance help improve academic performance?" or "How much skill do I need to do my job?" Rather the concern should be for helping each person to achieve full motor potential as part of becoming a total individual. Motor performance ability is necessary to normal functioning but to assume that motor development is only important to meeting these functions places motor development as a secondary aspect of one's development. Movement has meaning in itself and characteristic motor development patterns should reflect not what typical people can do but what fully functioning people can do. It is up to the reader to decide to what extent characteristic motor development patterns, as described in this text, reflect optimal performance levels at any given age.

REASONS FOR TYPICAL MOTOR DEVELOPMENT PATTERNS

After reading the preceding chapters of this text, it is no doubt obvious that there are many complex and diverse reasons *why* children develop as they do with regard to motor performance. Some aspects of motor behavior happen quite automatically while others occur only after considerable instruction or task experience. Given normal diet, rest and reasonable environmental conditions, most individuals develop normally with respect to many basic motor functions. However, even these basic motor functions can be refined with experience or instruction. On the other hand many types of motor performances do not just happen, they must be learned and refined. Society to a great extent dictates which types of motor performances are valued and, therefore, which tasks will be learned. Thus, societal values are one of the major reasons *why* humans develop as they do. Society values football skill, so children emphasize the learning of this type of motor response. Boys are supposed to excel in motor performance so they do. Girls are less likely to be encouraged and performances so indicate. These and similar examples illustrate the relationship of societal values to motor development. Those skills valued by society may not be of greatest importance in helping *all* people achieve optimal motor development.

The reader, after carefully reading some of the reasons for "typical motor development", is encouraged to evaluate the importance of different types of motor responses in an effort to establish "new reasons" for promoting specific types of motor responses. These "new reasons" may provide a better blueprint for helping each person to achieve optimal motor development. These "new reasons" may well become the future's reasons for typical motor development patterns for all people.

THE POTENTIAL FOR MOTOR PERFORMANCE

While little concrete research evidence is available to reveal the full potential for motor performance, one thing is clear; we can achieve much more than we have previously assumed. We have, it appears, grossly underestimated the potential of humans for motor performance. It is likely that children can learn earlier, learn more, and learn better than most people think.

Children can learn motor tasks very early in life! Of importance is not that children learn motor tasks very early in life but that they learn important motor tasks during critical learning periods. The reader is encouraged to study the potential of children for learning motor tasks in an effort to more realistically set motor performance expectations for children. Learning of such tasks should, of course, be sequential and adapted to the physical capabilities of children.

Children can learn many motor skills! We tend, however, to value how many chins a child can perform, or how many times a child can hit a ball rather than how many different skills a child can perform. Perhaps the emphasis for *children* should be on broad exposure to many types of motor performance.

Children can achieve quality in performing motor tasks. Emphasis on quantity often overshadows concern for the quality of a child's movement response. Whether it be walking, throwing, or performing any other motor task, quality of motor performance is important. The realization of full motor potential is more than merely being able to perform a skill, it requires efficient and effective motor performance.

And what of the performance of adolescents and adults. It is hard to learn at an older age what could have been learned early in life. But motor skills can be learned at any age. There is evidence that most adolescents, and especially most adults, could perform much more than "typical" adults actually do perform. Humans never stop developing and never stop learning. This is as true for motor development as for any area of development. We cannot be content to allow maximal performance to occur for most people in adolescence rather than in adulthood. Neither can we be content with severely restricted motor function which are characteristic of many older adults.

SUMMARY

Motor development is but one part of a human's total development. Given optimal circumstances motor development can be promoted through a logical progression of experience and learning. The net result, coupled with commensurate development in other areas, is the emergence of a total, yet individual, human being. The challenge to the reader is to clearly define and provide "optimal circumstances," "logical progression of experience and learning," and to "couple motor performance with all other aspects of total human development."

Index

Author Index

136

210
156
———
366